T0323404

Pornography and Public Health

Pornography and Public Health

Emily F. Rothman

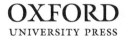

OXFORD
UNIVERSITY PRESS

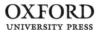

OXFORD
UNIVERSITY PRESS

Oxford University Press is a department of the University of Oxford. It furthers
the University's objective of excellence in research, scholarship, and education
by publishing worldwide. Oxford is a registered trade mark of Oxford University
Press in the UK and certain other countries.

Published in the United States of America by Oxford University Press
198 Madison Avenue, New York, NY 10016, United States of America.

Library of Congress Cataloging-in-Publication Data
Names: Rothman, Emily F., author.
Title: Pornography and public health / by Emily F. Rothman.
Description: New York, NY : Oxford University Press, [2021] |
Includes bibliographical references and index. |
Identifiers: LCCN 2021013438 (print) | LCCN 2021013439 (ebook) |
ISBN 9780190075477 (hardback) | ISBN 9780190075491 (epub) |
ISBN 9780190075507 (online)
Subjects: MESH: Erotica | Public Health | Communications Media |
Sex Offenses—prevention & control | United States
Classification: LCC HQ472.U6 (print) | LCC HQ472.U6 (ebook) |
NLM HQ 472.U6 | DDC 306.77/1—dc23
LC record available at https://lccn.loc.gov/2021013438
LC ebook record available at https://lccn.loc.gov/2021013439

DOI: 10.1093/oso/9780190075477.001.0001

1 3 5 7 9 8 6 4 2

Printed by Integrated Books International, United States of America

Contents

Preface

The purpose of this book is to provide information about pornography to students of public health, public policy, communications, and other fields. My intention is to introduce the reader to some of the intriguing arguments that have been made about pornography, to contextualize those arguments in history, and to encourage further critical thinking about these issues. This book is not exhaustive—there is a lot of ground yet to cover, and I hope that some of what is presented here can serve as a useful base for others who will improve upon my contribution.

Many scholars, and nonscholar activists, have picked a side in the pro-pornography vs. anti-pornography ideological debate. I am not one of them. I've been researching and thinking about pornography and public health every day for nearly a decade and it has become clear to me that pornography is too diverse to either condemn or absolve. My read of the results of the existing peer-reviewed research is that some pornography is harmful to some people in some situations and may have some negative effects on social norms and other societal-level factors. However, not all pornography is inherently dangerous, and it's harmful to the public to suppress access to sexual information and sexually explicit material in general.

The mission of this book is to enrich the discourse about pornography and public health—not to advance an anti-pornography or pro-pornography agenda. I do worry, specifically, about the impact of free, mainstream, internet pornography on youth sexual norms and the risk for sexual aggression perpetration and victimization. But I also worry about the repressive agenda of the anti-pornography movement. When we begin to chip away at sexual freedom, we start down a slippery slope that ends in tyranny. Whether pornography is harmful to public health cannot be turned into a simple question.

While this book covers 14 topics that, in my experience as a teacher, are foundational for understanding how we approach pornography in public health research and practice, there are an almost equal number of topics that I left out but are nevertheless essential for a comprehensive understanding of the issue. In particular, it is a limitation that there is no chapter on racism and pornography, no chapter about porn for, or featuring, people with disabilities, and no chapter on gay or lesbian porn. These are profoundly important topics that have not yet been adequately addressed by empirical studies.

Feminist studies scholars, film scholars, cultural studies scholars, and others have written essential reading on these topics that I have found thought-provoking and worthwhile. I have considered racism, ableism, homophobia, and classism in my digestion of the existing research, and I have commented on these themes to the extent possible in my chapters while focusing on peer-reviewed, published studies. I am hopeful that students of public health and students from related disciplines will be able to pursue research on these topics and that 10 years from now there will be an array of evidence to review. There are other topics that I also found myself underprepared to address from an evidence-based perspective, including whether pornography causes erectile dysfunction or depression, and the extent to which condomless sex is featured in pornography. Information on virtual reality pornography, sex dolls and robots, and other technological advances in pornography would also benefit the field. These are important topics for public health consideration.

I thank the individuals who generously contributed their time to review chapters: Ashley Fires, Lisa Goldblatt-Grace, Sarah Leonard, Michael Meltsner, Carol Queen, Kenneth Rothman, Alice Richmond, Richard Saitz, and Jay Wexler. Thank you to Ryan Cassidy for the research trip. Thank you to David Hemenway, Jonathan Howland, Elizabeth Miller, Deb Bowen, Megan Bair-Merritt, and Greg Stuart for mentorship. Thank you to Kim Nelson, Debra Herbenick, Jess Alder, and Nicole Daley for our collaborations. My gratitude to Sandro Galea for facilitating this opportunity. I am grateful to my parents, parents-in-law, and my siblings. I would also like to thank the three people and one dog that I love most in the world for their unending support and making it possible for me to pursue my career-related dreams. Miluji tě.

Abbreviations

AAML	American Academy of Matrimonial Lawyers
AASECT	American Association for Sexuality Educators, Counselors and Therapists
ACLU	American Civil Liberties Union
AIM	Adult Industry Medical Healthcare Foundation
AMA	American Medical Association
APA	American Psychiatric Association
APAC	Adult Performer Advocacy Committee
APAG	Adult Performers Actors Guild
ASAM	American Society of Addiction Medicine
AVN	Adult Video News
BBW	Big Beautiful Women
BDSM	bondage, discipline/dominance, submission/sadism, and masochism
BIPOC	Black, indigenous, and other people of color
BRFSS	Behavioral Risk Factor Surveillance System
CDA	Communications Decency Act of 1996
CDC	Centers for Disease Control and Prevention
COPA	Child Online Protection Act
CPPA	Child Pornography Prevention Act
CSBD	compulsive sexual behavior disorder
DSM	*Diagnostic and Statistical Manual of Mental Disorders*
ED	erectile dysfunction
EEG	Electroencephalography
ERP	event-related potential
fMRI	functional magnetic resonance imaging
FOSTA	Fight Online Sex Trafficking Act
FSC	Free Speech Coalition
GSS	General Social Survey
IEAU	International Entertainment Adult Union
IITAP	International Institute for Trauma and Addiction Professionals
I-PACE	Interaction of Person-Affect-Cognition-Execution
LPPs	late positive potential
MILF	Moms I'd Like to Fuck
MRI	magnetic resonance imaging
MSM	men who have sex with men
NCMEC	National Center for Missing and Exploited Children
NFSS	National Family Structure Survey
NHIS	National Health Interview Survey
NIH	National Institutes of Health

OSHA	Occupational Safety and Health Administration
OSS Program	"On Set Steward Program"
PALS	Portraits of American Life Study
PASS	Performer Availability Screening Services
POC	Person of Color
POV	Point of View
PPU	problematic pornography use
RCT	randomized controlled trial
RIA	Relationships In America
SESTA	Stop Enabling Sex Traffickers Act
SFW	Safe For Work
SIECUS	Sex Information and Education Council of the United States
SOCE	Sexual Orientation Change Efforts
STIs	sexually transmitted infections
TLDR	"Too long; didn't read"
TVPA	Trafficking Victims Protection Act
VSS	visual sexual stimuli
YISS	Youth Internet Safety Survey
YRBS	Youth Risk Behavior Surveys

1
Pornography as a US Public Health Problem

When I first proposed to teach a class on pornography and public health at the Boston University School of Public Health in 2014, the curriculum committee had a few questions for me. Specifically, they wondered how a class about pornography would complement existing courses on acknowledged public health topics like cancer prevention, maternal mortality, and health care organization and management. I understood why pornography seemed like an unserious topic in comparison. To be honest, it hadn't been my life goal to become a pornography scholar or teacher. I find looking at pornography boring. I've seen some that has held my interest, but on the whole sexually explicit images don't turn me on. That said, I'm also not outraged or disgusted by the concept of legal, consensual, erotic material. I was raised in a sex-positive family, and since an early age have been a fan of nonconformists. And, like many public health and antiviolence activists, I'm a feminist. Objectification of, and cruelty toward, other people are not merely a turn off to me—fighting them is my reason for being. So in 2011, when one of my research analyses uncovered that pornography was an important variable in a study of dating abuse, I was inspired to learn more about it. As I discovered, there was a lot to think about, and there was much that public health tools and training could add to the discourse.

But a decade ago, when I was starting out on my pornography scholarship journey, I understood why we would wrestle with devoting resources, time, or attention to the topic. Public health professionals are tasked with managing threats with high mortality rates, such as pandemics, obesity, substance use disorders, access to healthcare, pollution, climate change, and many more acute health threats. On the other hand, we don't have the choice to continue to ignore the topic of pornography, both because of mounting scientific evidence about the ways in which some of it may influence some people's health and because of politics. In 2016, the Republican Party platform included a section titled "Ensuring Safe Neighborhoods: Criminal Justice and Prison Reform," which included, rather curiously—given that pornography

Pornography and Public Health. Emily F. Rothman, Oxford University Press. © Oxford University Press 2021.
DOI: 10.1093/oso/9780190075477.003.0001

is not neighborhood-based, illegal, or germane to prison reform—the statement that: "pornography, with its harmful effects, especially on children, has become a public health crisis that is destroying the lives of millions. We encourage states to continue to fight this public menace and pledge our commitment to children's safety and well-being"[1] (p. 40).

Has pornography truly become a public health crisis? Whether it has or not, it is being indicted as one, and not just at the federal level. In the United States, the following states have passed resolutions affirming the crisis and condemning pornography: Utah (2016), Virginia, Tennessee, South Dakota, Louisiana, Kansas, and Arkansas (2017), Florida, Idaho, Kentucky, and Pennsylvania (2018), and Arizona, Montana, and Ohio (2019).[2] State resolutions are nonbinding, meaning that there is little that changes about day-to-day life in a state when they are passed, but the 2018 and 2019 versions of the resolutions call upon state district attorneys and the US Department of Justice to enforce federal obscenity laws and call upon Congress to "address the crisis problem of children accessing pornography on the Internet," meaning that the intention is for action to be taken, public dollars to be spent, and public officials' time to be allocated accordingly.[2] A good question is whether these expenditures in the name of public health would be worth it, diverting funds that could have been directed toward the list of other public health priorities that need to be addressed.

The professional public health community is not behind the recent push to declare pornography a public health crisis. One might think that if pornography is a public health menace, "destroying the lives of millions,"[1] public health entities and professional societies must have a viewpoint on the topic, perhaps a clearly outlined health-promotion agenda related to the problem, and a strategic plan. At least one of the National Institutes of Health (NIH) must have named it as a priority, the Centers for Disease Control and Prevention (CDC) must have a branch devoted to putting a stop to it, and the World Health Organization must have at least one infographic on its harms. But none of these things exists or has happened. In fact, there is no public health professional presently in any position of public health leadership or authority who has gone on record to say that pornography is a public health topic of interest—let alone a public health crisis. In 2016, in a written statement to CNN, the CDC said it "does not have an established position on pornography as a public health issue. Pornography can be connected to other public health issues like sexual violence and occupational HIV transmission."[3] But if public health entities are not behind the movement to declare pornography a public health problem, who is? And why are they using the language of public health for their cause?

The Definition of a Public Health Crisis, Problem, and Issue

Before solving the mystery of how pornography became a public health issue without the involvement of any public health professional organizations, it makes sense to define our terms. Pornography has been called a public health crisis, emergency, problem, and issue. The definition of these words matters, because calling something a public health crisis is often used to justify muscular government action. *The Oxford Handbook of Public Health Practice*[4] defines a public health crisis as: "an event(s) that overwhelms the capacity of local systems to maintain a community's health. . . . Crises can range from specific health issues, such as a disease outbreak in an otherwise unaffected community, to a full-scale disaster with property destruction and/or population displacement and multiple public health issues" (pp. 210–211). Similarly, the CDC defines a crisis as an unexpected and threatening event requiring an immediate response.[5]

In short, a crisis is defined as a critical moment in a dangerous situation that can be reasonably expected to lead to death, infectious disease morbidity, property destruction, or population displacement, and that overwhelms the capacity of local systems to do the job of maintaining a community's health. Consistent with this definition, the first time the word "crisis" was used in the *American Journal of Public Health* was in 1914, in an opinion piece about public health in a time of war. The crisis in question was World War I, which ranks among the deadliest conflicts in human history, and in which over 117,000 US lives were lost.[6]

Journalists are under pressure to attract attention to their articles, and it is no secret that some indulge in sensational language. By my count, in the years 2002 to 2015, media reports paired the words "public health crisis" with no fewer than 27 different topics, including AIDS, Ebola, opioids, air pollution, tainted food, energy drinks, school start times, and childhood obesity, among others. Some of these may, in fact, rise to level of true emergencies, while others may be harder to defend as crises. The harm in calling something a "public health crisis" when it is not demonstrably so is that it may motivate lawmakers to consider new policy or shifts in funding that may not be warranted and may activate the public health infrastructure to use all the tools at its disposal to address the problem. For example, government agencies may spend money to convene experts for high-level meetings; authorities may require businesses and individuals to comply with regulations, such as pulling possibly tainted food (or explicit magazines) from shelves;[7] or healthcare professionals may quarantine infected individuals in a hospital. Calling something a public health crisis means invoking a fast and potentially powerful response from federal, state, and municipal government, the press, and members of the public. Another harm is that the public may get burned out on hearing that yet another topic is a public health crisis that requires immediate action and expenditures. If the public health workforce wants to save its power to mobilize people when an acute threat is imminent (for example, when a global pandemic strikes), reserving the phrase "public health crisis" for strategic, select times is advisable.

Pornography is not always portrayed as a public health crisis or emergency. It has also been referred to as a "problem," "issue," and "concern."[8,9] There is no hard and fast definition of what counts as a public health problem, issue, or concern—and perhaps that's for the best. Spending time and energy nailing down a definition of a public health problem seems futile, given that new concerns emerge all the time and warrant consideration. But, if there is no definition, should anything—can anything—count as a public health issue? For example, could any one of us declare that something is a public health issue (e.g., pumpkin spice lattes, TikTok dances), and voilà, make it so? We might be able to do that, but for reasons of avoiding wasted resources and watering down bona fide public health efforts, we shouldn't. And for this reason, it's a good thing that we have at least some guidance from the field about what should be counted as a public health problem, issue, concern, or priority.

In 1999, Dr. Thomas Durant argued in the journal *Sociological Spectrum* that it was time to view violence as a public health problem. In doing so, he laid out what constitutes a public health problem, and he wrote that a public health problem "contributes to both morbidity and mortality, mental and physical injury, and health and medical costs"[10] (p. 274). Consistent with this definition, in 2013, the CDC created a guide to teach people how to prioritize public health problems. The guide uses the following criteria for determining if something should be prioritized: (1) The prevalence of the problem; (2) the potential of the problem to result in severe disability or death, using disability-adjusted life years, for example; (3) monetary and societal costs, such as medical expenses, social services, public services, costs to employers, and loss of productivity; and (4) the availability of effective interventions (where more availability makes it more likely that something should be prioritized).[11] In short, while there is no bright line that helps define which issues are worthy of public health consideration, there are some general principles that help public health professionals decide how to spend limited resources, such as money, energy, the attention of the public, and lawmakers' time. Because pornography does not result in severe disability or death except in the rarest of cases, it is not clear that it should be considered a public health priority. Sexual and dating violence victimization, as well as sexually transmitted infections, are without question public health issues because they demonstrably cause death and disability, and pornography may be a factor contributing to these problems. However, unless it can be established that pornography is responsible for a substantial percentage of violence victimization cases or cases of sexually transmitted infections, the public health focus should remain on these important outcomes of interest and not zero in on pornography. Pornography is one possible causal exposure for the outcomes of interest, so what would be the justification for declaring it a public health crisis when so many other possible causal exposures remain understudied?

Mary Calderone: The First to Ask the Question

The first person to ever pose the question about whether pornography should be considered a public health problem in a scholarly journal was Dr. Mary Calderone, who wrote on this theme in a 1972 issue of the *American Journal of Public Health*.[12] Calderone was an American physician and is famous for being the mother and champion of sex education. She worked as the medical director of Planned Parenthood from 1953 to 1964 and also served as the president and co-founder of the Sex Information and Education Council of the United States (SIECUS) from 1964 until 1982.[13] She is perhaps best known for successfully fighting the American Medical Association (AMA) on their policy that physicians should not disclose information about birth control to patients, which they overturned in 1964. And, in the height of her effectiveness, she was called "witch, mistress of the Devil, prostitute of hell" by Christian opponents to sex education.[14]

In her 1972 discussion of pornography in a public health context, Dr. Calderone made several important points.[12] First, she argued that the erotic is essential to good public health, and therefore public health professionals should recognize that while in some contexts the erotic could be harmful, in other contexts it's not just appropriate but necessary for individuals and societies. Second, she objected to the use of the term "pornography" to lump together all kinds of erotic material, because some sexual material may be, in her words, innocent. Third, she encouraged her readers to acknowledge that what seems objectionable to one person might be entirely normal for another person, and that neither should interfere with the privacy and rights of the other. Fourth, she pointed out that because we are a pluralistic society with diverse values, it was difficult to imagine who would be qualified to arbitrate whether pornography was noxious to society.[12] She also emphasized that a public health response to pornography would be supportive of sex workers, advocate for effective sex education, partner with faith-based groups that are in favor of evidence-based and scientific approaches, and promote positive eroticism for both youth and adults alike. Even though it was 50 years ago, Calderone's response is the same response that we should be embracing today. She answered the question "Is pornography a public health problem?" by suggesting that the context of pornography use matters and that we must be very careful not to substitute morality-based judgments about sexually explicit material for scientific conclusions about the etiology of sexual violence and sexually transmitted infections.

Surgeon General C. Everett Koop

After Calderone, the next official to offer a position on pornography as a public health issue was Surgeon General C. Everett Koop, who served under President Ronald Reagan from 1982 to 1989. Koop was a lifelong Republican and politically conservative, but he was not one-dimensional. He supported sex education in schools during the AIDS epidemic. In 1986, he convened a 3-day workshop in Arlington, Virginia, on pornography and public health. The stated goal of the workshop was to summarize the evidence about the effects of pornography, particularly on children. Twenty experts from the fields of communications, medicine, mental health, and social science were in attendance, including Dolf Zillman, Ann Burgess, Albert Bandura, Jon Conte, Neil Malamuth, Edward Donnerstein, and Murray Straus. A 252-page report was produced.

In the report, the Surgeon General summarized the five papers that were presented at the conference and concluded that "pornography does stimulate attitudes and behavior that lead to gravely negative consequences for individuals and for society."[15] But a close read of the five papers reveals that Koop's synopsis misrepresented what was presented. The experts found insufficient scientific support for the influence of pornography on violence against women (pp. 28–29), stated that the effect of pornography on children less than 12 years old was unknown (p. 37), and that it wasn't possible to say anything definitive about the effects of pornography on children at the time (p. 38). While the experts did express concern that sexual violence may be caused, in part, by people's attitudes about using coercion during sex—and that those attitudes may be influenced by watching pornography depicting coercive sex—they said "it is not clear that exposure to pornography is the most significant factor in the development of these attitudes"

(p. 23). But Koop's summary statement aligned with the views of the Christian anti-pornography movement, who espoused the view that pornography was causing the "moral decline of America" and waged what has been called a "symbolic crusade" against pornography as a way to protest changing gender and sexual norms more generally.[16] Anti-pornography organizations linked pornography to homosexuality and gay rights, abortion, and sex education and mobilized support against all of these issues simultaneously by invoking the idea that pornography was a threat to public health.[16] Public health became a politically useful frame for those with a right-wing social agenda.

State Resolutions on Pornography as a Public Health Crisis

In 2016, Utah became the first US state to declare pornography a public health hazard.[17] As of November 2020, 14 states had passed such resolutions. Here I summarize the text of the 2018 model state resolution on pornography as a public health crisis presented by the National Decency Coalition.[18] The document is of interest to public health professionals because it asserts that pornography has a direct and negative influence on at least 11 measurable outcomes, such as low self-esteem, body image, acceptance of rape, difficulty maintaining intimate relationships, and others.

The resolution text begins with the statement that pornography is creating a public health crisis. It continues with the declaration that pornography "perpetuates a sexually toxic environment," and "efforts to prevent pornography exposure and addiction, to educate individuals and families concerning its harms, and to develop recovery programs must be addressed systemically in ways that hold broader influences accountable." Next, it builds the case against pornography and states that it contributes to the following outcomes [some paraphrased, some quoted directly]:

1. The hypersexualization of teens, and even prepubescent children, in our society
2. Low self-esteem and body image disorders
3. An increase in problematic sexual activity at younger ages
4. Greater likelihood of young adolescents' engaging in risky sexual behavior, such as sending sexually explicit images, hookups, multiple sex partners, group sex, and using substances during sex
5. Bad information reaching children and youth about sex

6. The treatment of women as objects—"It teaches girls they are to be used and boys to be users"
7. The normalization of violence and abuse of women and children
8. The normalization and acceptance of rape and abuse—"It often depicts rape and abuse as if they were harmless"
9. The increase in the demand for sex trafficking, prostitution, and child sexual abuse images (i.e., child pornography).
10. Potential detrimental effects on pornography's users affecting their brain development and contributing to emotional and medical illnesses
11. Influence on deviant sexual arousal
12. Difficulty in forming or maintaining intimate relationships, as well as problematic or harmful sexual behaviors and addiction
13. Biological addiction to pornography, which means the user requires more novelty, often in the form of more shocking material, in order to be satisfied; and this biological addiction leads to increasing use of pornography featuring themes of risky sexual behaviors, extreme degradation, violence, and child sexual abuse images (i.e., child pornography).
14. The lessening of desire of young men to marry, dissatisfaction in marriage, and infidelitya detrimental effect on the family unit.

The text concludes with the statement that: "Overcoming pornography's harms is beyond the capability of the afflicted individual to address alone. . . . NOW, THEREFORE, BE IT RESOLVED, that the Legislature of the State of _____ recognizes that pornography is a public health hazard leading to a broad spectrum of individual and public health impacts and societal harms."

The remaining chapters of this book review the research evidence on several of the assertions made in this model state resolution.

Pornography from a Public Health Perspective

A typical public health strategy is to observe that there is an outcome we wish to change and then to consider the full spectrum of risk and protective factors that may influence it. For example, if the problem is diabetes, we may work on solutions that have to do with diet, exercise, access to care, and racism. One of the problems with declaring pornography a public health problem is that pornography is an exposure—not a disease, condition, or behavior. Sometimes an exposure is solidly linked to numerous health outcomes, in which case we consider the exposure itself a public health problem. Racism and lead, for example, are exposures that are considered public health problems. But pornography is not yet clearly established as a risk factor for multiple health outcomes. Evidence suggests that certain types of pornography may cause aggression and compulsive use in some people and negatively influence youth sexual behavior, and it is implicated in some cases of human trafficking. But there are also drawbacks to, and even possible harms from, eradicating pornography—including harms to those who create it consensually and earn an income from it, harms associated with limiting the availability of information about sex generally, harm related to stigmatizing nondominant sexualities or sexual behaviors, harm in denying that eroticism is important for human health, and harms associated with controlling what adults say, do, or can see, which influence whether they can live safe, fulfilling, and free lives.

For these reasons, it is problematic when advocacy groups appropriate public health language to try to advance their cause without engaging in an authentic public health agenda-building process. However, it would be a mistake to discount what may also be real threats to health posed by pornography just because advocacy groups have framed their message in ways that do not resonate with the standard public health approach. As a field, public health has much to offer if our task is to contemplate whether pornography has relevance for individuals' health and well-being, and excellent tools that we can use if we decide there is some aspect of pornography production, dissemination, or use that we wish to address. Below I provide my own top five ways that public health tools can be applied to questions about the impact of pornography on human health: (1) Using the four steps of a public health approach; (2) The social-ecological model; (3) Harm reduction; (4) Ethics; and (5) Coalition-building.

The Four Steps of a Public Health Approach

There is a best practice, or recommended way, to approach any public health problem.[19] The first step is to define the problem, and typically the problem is a health outcome, such as becoming ill. The problem could also be engaging in a behavior that we know to be a strong risk factor for becoming ill. Once we have identified the problem in as precise terms as possible, the second step is to identify risk factors or protective factors for that problem. In the case of pornography, the outcome of interest might be sexual assault, and pornography may emerge as one of the risk factors that we seek to address. After identifying the outcome and one or more risk or protective factors, the third step is to develop and test prevention strategies. Finally, once we have evidence that our prevention strategies work, we promote adoption of those strategies. This can be useful to us as we consider whether pornography should be part of a public health action agenda because it will guide us to start with an outcome, to consider the full constellation of potential risk and factors that may lead to that outcome, and to weigh pornography's role in relation to the others. It will also guide us in the strategic development of prevention strategies that have a logical connection to the outcome of concern, and then to advocate for adoption of the prevention strategies only if they prove to be effective. In other words, we would not begin the process by advocating for a ban on pornography, then try to determine if pornography had ill effects on sexual assault. A logical flow of steps would be: to agree that sexual assault is an outcome of interest; to look at the array of factors that might influence it; to zero in on pornography due to its connection to sexual assault, if warranted; to develop prevention strategies that are expected to influence the impact of pornography use as it pertains to sexual assault; and to evaluate whether our prevention strategy was effective.

The Social-Ecological Model

The social-ecological model is a way of organizing risk and protective factors that emphasizes the dynamic interplay between what are referred to as levels of the social ecology.[20] For example, according to this model, determinants of health problems or their solutions can be arrayed according to the following levels: intrapersonal (including, for example, personal characteristics, such as gender, sexual orientation, socioeconomic status, and psychological traits), interpersonal (including family and peer factors, such as experiences of child abuse or affiliating with a delinquent peer group), institutional factors (such as school climate or workplace policies), community factors (including neighborhood features, community resources, and the built environment), and societal-level factors (including social norms and public policies).

The social-ecological model can help us think about pornography and its possible influence on public health in different ways. First, if we are investigating sexual assault as an outcome, we can picture pornography in the community factors level, one of perhaps fifty or more factors arrayed across the multiple levels. Other factors will include self-concept and sexual drive at the intrapersonal level, experiences of parent-to-child abuse and childhood sexual abuse at the intrapersonal level, school-bonding and employment support for health and wellness in the institutional factors level, and policies that harm or help people who are convicted of sex offenses to manage their behavior at the public policy level. Visualizing pornography as one of many factors across multiple levels of the social ecology that may relate to sexual assault helps to put into perspective the idea that we should focus all or most of our time, money, and attention on fighting pornography. A second way that we might use the social-ecological model is to think about what causes problematic pornography use. If we take problematic pornography use as the outcome, we might use a social-ecological model approach to map out intrapersonal factors that put people at risk for such problematic use, as well as interpersonal, institutional, community, and societal-level factors. Arraying risk factors for problematic pornography use this way would enable us to see that the right solution to problematic use is not simply to tell people "pornography is bad, stop using it," but would necessitate responses that support people with intrapersonal risk factors, such as a lack of knowledge about sex, interpersonal factors, such as experiences of abuse victimization, and institutional factors, such as lack of access to behavioral healthcare through their workplace. Finally, the social-ecological model can help us to array our proposed solutions to some aspect of pornography production and use so that we ensure we have at least one or two strategies at every level, working conjointly.

This type of rich and fully elaborated consideration of pornography as a risk factor for an outcome of interest has much higher odds of success than the scattershot approach currently being used by those who say that they object to pornography as a public health issue. Their approach is to say pornography is bad for many reasons, let's declare it a problem and limit access to it. A public health-informed multilevel consideration of the potential impact of pornography on human health will yield a wider variety of, and more effective, solutions.

Harm Reduction

Harm reduction is a "pragmatic public health approach encompassing all goals of public health: improving health, social well-being, and quality of life."[21] Harm reduction was initially developed as a way to improve the lives of people who use drugs "in partnership with those served without a narrow focus on abstinence from drugs."[21] The idea is simple. Instead of an abstinence-only perspective, the public health professional embraces the idea that helping a person move one step further along the continuum of behavior change is for the best. For example, even if someone is not ready to quit chronic alcohol use, they might be ready to use less alcohol. A harm-reduction practitioner would be enthusiastic about the change from high use to low use.

When it comes to pornography use, a harm-reduction approach would celebrate small victories in moving people from harmful use toward less harmful use—rather than insist upon an "all or nothing" outcome. The idea that all people should cease and desist from pornography use 100% is an abstinence-only goal. The idea that people could be motivated to use less pornography, or less extreme pornography, and less frequently, is a harm-reduction goal. The harm-reduction approach has been found to be effective at reducing a number of negative health behaviors, most notably substance use.[22]

Ethics: Balancing Benefits over Harms for Most People

People sometimes call the public health system the "nanny state" or "big brother," which is a way of saying that the public health infrastructure has the goal to influence and sometimes limit behavior and freedom. There are always factions of the public that object to public health regulation. For example, during the COVID-19 pandemic, many have had strong objections to wearing masks. Another example from the field of injury prevention is that there are people who do not want to wear motorcycle helmets, despite evidence that helmets can reduce brain injury and death substantially. There have been bitter debates about whether public health and government entities should have the power to impose requirements to wear helmets on people who would rather be free to enjoy riding without a helmet. There have been similar debates about seatbelt laws, lifejacket requirements on water crafts, infant car seats, texting and driving laws, and mandatory HIV testing. As a field, public health has wrestled for nearly two centuries with how to strike balances between protecting the health of the public and imposing on the public's freedom. We agonize over how to ensure that the largest percentage of the public benefits substantially without impinging too drastically on freedoms or safety. As a result, when it comes to policy choices about pornography, trained public health ethicists and policy experts should be able to offer sound guidance. Principled action that carefully weighs the costs and consequences of controlling media against the supposed benefits is needed. Public health professionals have the right preparation and training to undertake this type of difficult determination, in collaboration with experts from other fields, and to make recommendations.

Coalition-Building to Solve Problems

A final strength that public health practice has to offer those who are grappling with whether and how to manage the influence of pornography on the public is its capacity to bring diverse communities and individuals together. "Nothing about us without us" is a slogan that has been used for decades to express the idea that policymakers need to partner with the people affected by the proposed legislation that they craft. It was popularized in the United States in the 1990s by disability rights activists[23] and was adopted by the sex worker rights movement shortly thereafter. What the slogan means in the context of pornography-related policy and intervention development is that it is best practice to be inclusive of people who have performed in pornography and who work in pornography production, retail, or businesses related to pornography sales (e.g., payment processing systems). However, sex workers are not the only stakeholders who may need to be included in policy and intervention development processes. Formerly exploited people (e.g., those who have experienced human trafficking) also deserve to contribute their experiences, as do concerned parents, youth, violence-prevention advocates, artists, first amendment experts, anti-racism activists, Internet technology specialists, and perhaps a lengthy list of others. Is it possible to have a table large enough for everyone to have a seat? And who decides which individuals are truly representative of their stakeholder groups, whether participation will be remunerated and how, and how decisions will be made in cases of disagreement? These questions are not necessarily easily answered, but the field of public health has prior experience establishing participatory processes to benefit communities and members of the public. There are best practices and how-to manuals that describe how to establish fair, inclusionary, balanced groups of collaborators who share equitable access to information and a voice in decision-making processes. With good stewardship, and grounded in the principles of social justice, even diverse groups of stakeholders who may have fundamental disagreements on particular aspects of a problem can be brought together for meaningful collaboration on public health topics. Experienced public health professionals with expertise in community-based participatory research and in policy and intervention development should take leadership to address pornography-related concerns through coalition-building.

Conclusions

Sexual violence, partner violence, anxiety, depression, compulsive pornography use, and commercial sexual exploitation are public health problems, and there is a possibility that pornography exacerbates these problems. Given that possibility, we need to know more about whether, how, and why pornography influences social norms as well as individuals' behavior, and what we can do to address that influence if it is harmful. It is also important to be aware that framing pornography as a public health issue has been used as a rhetorical trick by right- wing groups to promote a conservative social agenda at odds with public health goals. Public health professionals should sponsor rigorous research on the possible negative effects of pornography on society and individuals, counter misinformation, and use evidence to move forward with policy decisions.

References

1. Republican Platform. 2016. https://prod-cdn-static.gop.com/media/documents/DRAFT_12_FINAL%5B1%5D-ben_1468872234.pdf
2. National Decency Coalition. 2019. https://nationaldecencycoalition.org/updates/
3. Howard, J. 2016. "Republicans Are Calling Porn a 'Public Health Crisis,' But Is It Really?" https://www.cnn.com/2016/07/15/health/porn-public-health-crisis/index.html
4. Guest, C., W. Ricciardi, I. Kawachi, and I. Lang. 2013. *Oxford Handbook of Public Health Practice*. OUP Oxford.
5. US Centers for Disease Control and Prevention. 2014. "Crisis and Emergency Risk Communication." https://emergency.cdc.gov/cerc/ppt/cerc_2014edition_Copy.pdf
6. Byerly, C. R. 2017. "War Losses (USA)." in: 1914–1918-online. *International Encyclopedia of the First World War*, ed. by Ute Daniel, Peter Gatrell, Oliver Janz, Heather Jones, Jennifer Keene, AlanKramer, and Bill Nasson, issued by Freie Universität Berlin, Berlin 2014-10-08. doi:10.15463/ie1418.10162. https://encyclopedia.1914-1918-online.net/pdf/1914-1918-Online-war_losses_usa-2014-10-08.pdf
7. Kelly, K. J. 2015. "Stores Urged Not to Openly Display 'Pornographic' Cover." https://nypost.com/2015/02/10/stores-urged-not-to-openly-display-pornographic-cover/
8. Fight the New Drug. 2018. "Why Is Porn Being Considered a Public Health Concern?" https://fightthenewdrug.org/porn-considered-a-public-health-concern/
9. Caplan, A. L. 2019. "Pornography: A Public Health Problem?" http://www.medscape.com/viewarticle/880510
10. Durant, T. J. 1999. "Violence as a Public Health Problem: Toward an Integrated Paradigm." *Sociological Spectrum* 19, no. 3: 267–280.
11. US Centers for Disease Control and Prevention. 2013. "Prioritizing Public Health Problems." https://www.cdc.gov/globalhealth/healthprotection/fetp/training_modules/4/prioritize-problems_fg_final_09262013.pdf
12. Calderone, M. S. 1972. "'Pornography' as a Public Health Problem." *American Journal of Public Health* 62, no. 3: 374–376.
13. Mary S. Calderone, Pioneer in Sex Education, Dies at 94. 2019. https://www.washingtonpost.com/archive/local/1998/10/25/mary-s-calderone-pioneer-in-sex-education-dies-at-94/ec3e0b6e-2b31-4ad8-85b3-e37173e9a4ef/
14. Petrzela, N. 2019. "Witches Get Stuff Done" (Podcast). https://www.caveat.nyc/podcasts/nevertheless-she-existed/witches-get-stuff-done
15. National Criminal Justice Reference Service. 2019. "NCJRS Abstract—National Criminal Justice Reference Service." https://www.ncjrs.gov/App/Publications/abstract.aspx?ID=109837

16. Burke, K. 2019. "Why the Christian Right Opposes Pornography but Still Supports Trump." http://theconversation.com/why-the-christian-right-opposes-pornography-but-still-supports-trump-94156

17. Hamblin, J. 2016. "Inside the Movement to Declare Pornography a 'Health Crisis.'" https://www.theatlantic.com/health/archive/2016/04/a-crisis-of-education/478206/

18. National Decency Coalition. 2019. "Pornography: Public Health Crisis Resolution." https://nationaldecencycoalition.org/updates/

19. US Centers for Disease Control and Prevention. 2019. "The Public Health Approach to Violence Prevention." https://www.cdc.gov/violenceprevention/publichealthissue/publichealthapproach.html

20. Bronfrenbrenner, U. 1979. *The Ecology of Human Development*. Cambridge, MA: Harvard University Press.

21. Stancliff, S., B. W. Phillips, N. Maghsoudi, and H. Joseph. 2015. "Harm Reduction: Front Line Public Health." *Journal of Addictive Diseases* 34, no. 2-3: 206–219.

22. Dick, S., E. Whelan, M. P. Davoren, et al. 2019. "A Systematic Review of the Effectiveness of Digital Interventions for Illicit Substance Misuse Harm Reduction in Third-Level Students." *BMC Public Health* 19, no. 1: 11.

23. Charlton, J. 2006. "Nothing About Us Without Us." In *Encyclopedia of Disability*, edited by G. I. Albrecht. Thousand Oaks, CA: SAGE Publications.

2

Defining Pornography

When I teach graduate students about pornography, I always begin the semester with an introduction to the history of erotic art and a short summary of key obscenity cases. I'm neither a historian nor a legal scholar, so admittedly I am outside my comfort zone. However, I have found that it's essential to ground discussions of pornography and public health in the context of how and why pornography became such a contentious issue. As we grapple with the debates about pornography today—and try to sort out why pornography is considered dangerous, objectionable, and offensive to some stakeholders and not to others—it helps to have a basic, working knowledge of when pornography was first indicted as possibly harmful, by whom, and for what reasons. This chapter presents a condensed version of the history of erotic art and a review of important legal decisions that continue to influence how pornography is perceived and regulated today.

The idea that certain drawings, statues, or written texts should be considered "pornographic" is a relatively recent one. Evidence from ancient Sumeria (4500–1900 BC), and later Babylon (2300 BC–1000 AD) suggests that sex and nudity were accepted as a natural part of life.[1,2] Many cultures around the world incorporated representations of sex into poetry, woodblocks, carvings, paintings, and other forms of art, from India, to Japan, to Turkey, to Bali, to Egypt, to Peru.[3,4] Ancient Greeks and Romans were not shy about sex and celebrated sex through art.[2,5]

In the 2nd- to 4th-century Roman Empire, sex went from being considered a relatively innocuous pleasure to a sin.[6] During the Middle Ages, in the region now known as Europe, the Church started dictating everything from what positions one should use to have sex (i.e., missionary), to whether one should masturbate, use dildos, or have homosexual sex (i.e., No, No, and No).[7,8] It also became more common during the Middle Ages for people or their art to be censored for political or religious reasons, although not on the grounds of sexual lewdness.[2,9] After the moveable printing press was invented in 1428,[2] and people had the means to disseminate information, the first papal mandate to prosecute producers and consumers of politically objectionable materials was issued in 1479.[10]

Pornography and Public Health. Emily F. Rothman, Oxford University Press. © Oxford University Press 2021.
DOI: 10.1093/oso/9780190075477.003.0002

In the late 1500s, the first regulations against sexual images were introduced on the grounds that the images were "ungodly."[2] But the concern wasn't that seeing sexual imagery would impair people's health; it was that it had the potential to give people rebellious political energy. Erotic material was recognized as tremendously powerful, with the potential to motivate people to manifest change and fight oppression. In 1596, the Archbishop of Canterbury explained his concerns about the power of erotic material this way: "The simpler and least advised sorts of her majesty's subjects are either allured to wantonness, corrupted in doctrine or in danger to be seduced from dutiful obedience which they owe unto her highness."[2] In other words, seeing sexually arousing art might encourage people to behave more freely sexually, and that could erode their sense of servitude and obedience to the Queen.

The idea that certain sexually explicit materials should be classified as "pornography" and cordoned off from the public has its roots in a specific event that occurred in the mid-1700s.[11] Explorers from Britain discovered the ancient Roman city of Pompeii, which had been covered in ash during the explosion of the volcano Mount Vesuvius 1,800 years earlier.[4] As they excavated the Roman villas, which had been well preserved by the ash, they were surprised to find detailed frescoes on the walls of many homes showing humans engaged in intercourse—group sex, gay and lesbian sex, oral sex—and not just on walls in the bedrooms, but in dining areas and living rooms. They found sexually explicit statues, too. One artifact that they uncovered in 1752 was a marble statue of the Roman god Pan having sex with a goat, genital details visible.[4] Like everything else that was excavated, the frescoes, statue, and hundreds of sexually explicit vases, figurines, oil lamps, wind chimes, and dishes were stored at the national museum in Naples.[11] This happened during a moment of intense social change in Europe when virtue, restraint, and modesty were becoming fashionable. In this context, in 1819, future King Francis I of Naples visited the collection and took exception to the graphic nature of the artifacts.[4] He ordered everything locked away in a room that became known as The Secret Museum.[11] Meanwhile, in Great Britain, the display of similarly sexually graphic classical artifacts in the British Museum was also causing a stir.[12] The museum director began choosing certain items to take out of public view, and by 1865 the British Museum had secured them in a secret repository where they could be viewed only by those who were specifically approved.[12] The word "pornography," from the Greek words for prostitutes (*porni*) and writing (*graphein*), which had previously been used to describe writing *about* prostitutes, came into common usage to describe sexually explicit materials intended to arouse.[13]

Legal Definitions of Pornography in Britain and the United States

This book is focused on the United States, but US law was derived from English law, so my review of legal cases begins in Britain. As a public health professional, what I find particularly interesting about these legal cases is how difficult it has been for policymakers to clearly define pornography and to lay out rationales for making it illegal to view, possess, create, or distribute. The cases demonstrate that whether pornography is considered a threat to the public rests on something squishy: continuously evolving cultural beliefs about what constitutes healthy sex, sexuality, and mental health.

The first laws pertaining to regulating pornography took aim at obscenity. Pornography is a broad category; a subset of the most objectionable pornography is regulated for being obscene. Historically, writing or art that blasphemed religion or was politically objectionable, even if not sexually explicit, might also be considered obscene. The historic Obscene Publications Act was passed by the British Parliament in 1857 in order to give the state a legal structure for suppressing sexual material and controlling people's access to it.[14] There had never been a law previously that permitted law enforcement to go into private residences or businesses to search for sexually obscene material, to seize it, and to destroy it. The primary justification for the act was that works of obscenity could corrupt the morals of youth, specifically.[14] Medical professionals were among the supporters of the act, because of beliefs that reading sexual novels could cause "desecration" of "pure minds," or mental health problems (p. 614).[14] Many were also of the opinion that masturbation, or "self-pollution," could cause the brain to shrivel, sickness, and death, and that reading erotic texts perverted the imagination dangerously.[15,16] The Obscene Publications Act is important to public health history because it was the first time that the argument was made that legislation was needed to protect people's health because of something that they could see. Many regulations had been passed previously to regulate what people could do, where they could go, and what they could purchase. But no government entity had previously suggested that simply laying eyes upon something was so noxious that people needed government to invade their homes to protect them from it for their own health. Thus, British obscenity laws were established based on the untested (and still unproven) assumptions that (a) the material people view has the power to cause mental health disorders; (b) that masturbation, associated with the use of sexually explicit materials, is harmful to public health; and

(c) government intervention is necessary to rescue youth, in particular, from moral threats.

One British legal case, *R v. Hicklin* (1868 L. R. 3 Q. B. 360), had particularly long-lasting ramifications for obscenity law in England and the United States.[17] The story of *Hicklin* is that in 1868, a Protestant man in Wolverhampton, England, named Henry Scott started disseminating anti-Catholic leaflets titled "The Confessional Unmasked: shewing the depravity of the Romish priesthood, the iniquity of the Confessional, and the questions put to females in confession."[17] The leaflets argued a political point that was relevant at the time, but to win readers, the text went into detail about the sexual nature of confessions that Catholic priests heard from young women. The pamphlets were confiscated by authorities for being too sexually graphic, but the local official in charge of destruction of obscene materials, named Hicklin, felt that they did not meet the definition of obscenity put forth by the Obscene Publications Act and should be returned to their owner. A court disagreed with Hicklin and in deciding the case put a written definition of obscenity on record that remained in place, unamended, until 1959. The judge wrote: "I think the test of obscenity is this, whether the tendency of the matter charged as obscenity is to deprave or corrupt those whose minds are open to such immoral influences, and into whose hands a publication of this sort may fall" (p. 471).[18] Thus, material could be obscene even if it was intended to have, or did have, artistic or literary value.[17,19] Ultimately, this definition, as subjective as it was, was imposed on colonies of the British Empire, including Australia, New Zealand, South Africa, and India, and was used in the United States as well.[20] In the United States, from the *Hicklin* case onward until the mid-1950s, obscenity cases subjected potentially obscene materials to what became known as the Hicklin test (see Table 2.1).

From a public health perspective, one interesting aspect of the *Hicklin* definition of obscenity is that inherent in it was the idea that seeing obscene material has the power to influence mental health (i.e., "deprave"). In 1868 there was no evidence that seeing obscene material caused depravity, but the idea that it did became fundamental to its definition anyway. That the original legal definition of obscene material was predicated upon the idea that it *does* influence mental health negatively means that modern-day questions about the empiric relationship between pornography and mental health problems are part of a historical circular argument. By way of example, imagine that the definition of a cigarette was "material that causes lung cancer." In that case, there would be no need to investigate whether cigarettes caused lung cancer because the definition itself would obviate scientific inquiry.

Table 2.1. Selected US obscenity cases and their impact on the legal definition of pornography

Year	Case	Impact on Definition of Pornography
1896	*Rosen v. United States*	The US Supreme Court explicitly adopted and reified the *Hicklin* case definition of obscenity, which was: all material tending "to deprave and corrupt those whose minds are open to such immoral influences" regardless of its artistic or literary merit.
1957	*Butler v. United States*	A strike against the *Hicklin* definition: The Supreme Court found that the Michigan obscenity statute was not reasonable, overturned it, and wrote that grown men and women should not be shielded from books in order to protect children's innocence.
1957	*Roth v. United States*	New definition of obscenity. Each of three elements must independently be satisfied before a book can be held obscene: (1) the dominant theme of the material taken as a whole appeals to a prurient interest in sex; (2) the material is patently offensive because it affronts contemporary community standards relating to the description or representation of sexual matters, and (3) the material is utterly without redeeming social value. The Court asserted that the constitutional status of an allegedly obscene work must be determined on the basis of a national, not local, standard.
1964	*Jacobellis v. Ohio*	The Supreme Court reaffirmed that "contemporary community standards" refer to community norms at the national, and not local, level. In writing his concurring opinion, Justice Potter wrote, about hard-core pornography: "I shall not today attempt further to define the kinds of material I understand to be embraced within that shorthand description; and perhaps I could never succeed in intelligibly doing so. But I know it when I see it, and the motion picture involved in this case is not that."
1966	*Memoirs v. Massachusetts*	The Supreme Court asserted that to qualify as obscenity, it must be proven that a text is *entirely* (i.e., "utterly") without socially redeeming value, otherwise it is protected by the First Amendment.
1973	*Miller v. California*	The Miller test for determining obscenity was put forth: (1) Whether the average person, applying contemporary community standards, would find that the work, taken as a whole, appeals to the prurient interest; (2) Whether the work depicts or describes, in a patently offensive way, sexual conduct specifically defined by applicable state law; and (3) Whether the work, taken as a whole, lacks serious literary, artistic, political, or scientific value. The *Miller* Court, unlike prior Courts, asserted that "community standards" should be determined at the local, and not national, level. The *Miller* Court also raised the bar for media to be considered protected by the First Amendment by changing the "utterly without socially redeeming value" language to "serious . . . importance."
1997	*Reno v. American Civil Liberties Union*	The US Supreme Court found the Communications Decency Act (CDA), which had been passed into law in 1996, to be unconstitutional. The CDA was crafted in order to protect minors from being exposed to messages or images on the Internet that were either "indecent" or "offensive." However, the Court found that parts of the CDA were too vague and found that the Internet was entitled to the highest protection from government intrusion.

Table 2.1. *Continued*

Year	Case	Impact on Definition of Pornography
2002	*Ashcroft v. American Civil Liberties Union*	The US Supreme Court recommended that the injunction against the Child Online Protection Act (COPA) remain and that it be referred back to the Appeals Court to decide on its constitutionality. COPA was a narrower version of CDA, designed to protect children from harmful material on the Internet, but COPA was more specific about which purveyors of obscenity were of concern and was limited to commercial sellers and only those in the United States. After it passed, COPA was immediately challenged by the ACLU and ultimately was found to be unconstitutional. Of interest, COPA specified that the following should be considered harmful to minors: depictions of simulated sexual acts, sexually explicit drawings, written descriptions of sex, and any depictions of postpubescent female breasts.
2002	*Ashcroft v. Free Speech Coalition*	The US Supreme Court found that the Child Pornography Prevention Act of 1996 (CPPA) was invalid. CPPA prohibited any visual depiction, including computer-generated images or pictures, of a minor or a person appearing to be a minor in a manner that conveys the impression of engaging in sexually explicit conduct. Like CDA and COPA, CPPA was found to be overly broad and to impinge upon the First Amendment.

The History of the Definition of Obscenity in the United States

In the British North American Colonies, which would become the United States, Puritanical censors had been banning materials they considered obscene since 1712, when a Massachusetts law criminalized publication of any "filthy, obscene, or profane song, pamphlet, libel or mock sermon."[21,22] But Massachusetts was particularly prudish. It was the only colony to specifically criminalize obscenity, and the sexual nature of materials wasn't even the core of their concern, it was any material that they felt was blasphemy against the church.[21] That changed over time. In 1821, Massachusetts censors banned a sexually graphic book called *Memoirs of a Woman of Pleasure* (also known as *Fanny Hill*) because of its sexual content.[23] However, the regulation of sexual material wasn't addressed at the federal level until 1842, when the US Tariff Act passed and restricted importation of sexually obscene prints, paintings, and lithographs into the country.[24] Granting the federal government the power to censor access to materials was inconsistent with the values of liberty-loving Americans as outlined, at a minimum, by the First Amendment of the Constitution. At the same time, there was a recognition that it was possible to go too far in the direction of freedom. There was a concern that society wouldn't function if everyone felt free to pursue entirely selfish, criminal, and uncivil behavior, so morality and sexual propriety were promoted, in part, to keep the democracy from sliding into chaos and disorder.[21]

In the late 1800s, the moral crusader Anthony Comstock effected some major legal changes. Anthony Comstock was a devout and theologically conservative Christian from rural Connecticut who moved to New York City after he served in the Union Army in the Civil War.[21] His morality was so strict that when he was a soldier he had poured out his daily military-issued ration of liquor rather than drink it or share it with someone else.[21] After his service, he moved to Brooklyn to sell dry goods, but New York City was not to his liking. He was appalled by the number of prostitutes and the availability of pornography, and he felt that advertisements for birth control promoted lust.[21] Aggrieved, Comstock personally drafted an anti-obscenity bill and took it to Congress in Washington, DC. Hoping to draw a clear connection between printed materials and prostitution, he used the slogan "Books are feeders for brothels!" for this campaign.[19]

Comstock's bill was debated in Congress for less than an hour and was passed into law in 1873.[19] The Comstock Act (18 U.S. Code § 1461) made it illegal to send obscene material through the mail, including medical textbooks or information about abortion or sexually transmitted infections.[19] It also defined contraceptives as obscene and made it a federal crime for anyone to give out birth control either through the mail or across state lines. State-level versions of the act also passed in some states, as well.[25] The Connecticut version made it illegal for married couples to use birth control in the privacy of their own home.[25] Comstock's moral crusading made him popular in Washington, DC. Soon after the Comstock Act passed into law, he became the unpaid US Postal Inspector General, a role that allowed him to make arrests for obscenity violations.[26] During the course of his career, he reportedly destroyed 15 tons of books and 4 million pictures, claimed responsibility for 4,000 arrests, and boasted about driving 15 people to suicide.[27] Two important aspects of Comstock's crusade were: first, that he was motivated by his hatred of lust, of which he said "there is no evil so extensive, none doing more to destroy the institutions of free America,"[21] and second, that he said he was motivated by a desire to protect children, and he called his campaigns against obscenity a fight for the young. Just like Lord Campbell, who presided over the passage of the Obscene Publications Act of 1857 in Britain,[18] Comstock used the idea of safeguarding children to advance a repressive ideology that would affect everyone.

During Comstock's reign as Postal Service Inspector General, US courts used the British *Hicklin* case definition of obscenity to enforce the Comstock

Act. In 1896, a US Supreme Court Case cemented the *Hicklin* definition—*Rosen v. United States* (161 U.S. 29). The case involved a defendant, Rosen, who mailed a 12-page paper depicting naked women titled "Tenderloin, Number, Broadway" through the mail and was caught.[28] The images in Rosen's paper were partially covered with a type of soot called lamp black (also called "smut") that recipients could easily wipe away with bread.[29] Rosen appealed his conviction on the grounds that the material that he mailed was not obscene, but the Supreme Court upheld Rosen's conviction, citing the *Hicklin* test.[28]

US courts continued to use the *Hicklin* test to determine obscenity for more than half a century. Between 1957 and 1997, the US Supreme Court made a series of decisions that redefined obscenity. The first case to chip away at *Hicklin* involved a bookseller in Detroit, named Alfred Butler, who unknowingly sold a copy of an erotic book, *The Devil Rides Outside*, to a police officer.[30] A Michigan court found Butler guilty of selling obscene material and fined him $100. However, Butler appealed to the Supreme Court, on the grounds that his free speech rights were violated. Butler fared well. In 1957, the Supreme Court reversed the Michigan conviction.[30] In the written opinion, the Supreme Court stated that the Michigan law was too broad and curtailed freedom of the press. Specifically, Justice Frankfurter wrote that the Michigan law was so overly broad that it reduced "the adult population of Michigan to reading only what is fit for children."[31] The Justice asserted the idea that the rights of adults to have sexual material needed to be balanced against the protection of children.

In that same year, another case involving a bookseller, *Roth v. United States*, also went to the US Supreme Court and loosened the definition of obscenity.[22] Samuel Roth was a New York City-based bookseller who had sent an erotic book, some circulars, and advertising through the US mail, and was convicted of violating the Comstock Act. He, like Butler, appealed on the basis of free speech. This time, the Supreme Court upheld Roth's conviction and wrote that the First Amendment was not intended to protect materials that were "utterly without redeeming social importance," which it felt applied to Roth's materials. However, whereas the *Hicklin* definition of obscenity stipulated that written material with *any* lines or passages that included obscenity rendered the entire document obscene, the new definition set forth by Justice William J. Brennan, Jr., in the *Roth* case specified that the dominant theme of the material in question had to be obscene for the material to count as pornographic—meaning that a book with a few sexually explicit lines might be acceptable.[22] Moreover, Brennan tried to clarify that each obscenity case would need to be decided on a case-by-case basis, because it was too challenging to lay out an objective definition of pornography. To guide these case-by-case decisions, Brennan wrote that material should be considered pornographic if the "average person applying contemporary community standards" would think was appealing "to the prurient interest." By "community standards," the Court meant the national, not local, community.[22] This broad definition of community was countered by later Court decisions.

The next case to influence legal definitions of pornography was *Jacobellis v. Ohio* (1964).[22] In this case, a movie theater manager (Nico Jacobellis) in Cleveland Heights, Ohio, was fined $2,500 for showing the French film *The Lovers*. The film had been shown in numerous US cities without incident and had only one sexually explicit scene. Jacobellis appealed, and the US Supreme Court found that the film had cultural value, and thus was not obscenity. Further, the Court specified that community standards about what was obscene should be determined by considering the nation as the community, not a local state or city. In writing his concurring opinion, Justice Stewart wrote his now famous line about hard-core pornography: "I know it when I see it." Though often quoted, the statement "I know it when I see it" was not intended to be used, nor was it ever used, by the Court to make determinations about obscenity.

Two years later, in 1966, the Supreme Court made a notable ruling in *Memoirs v. Massachusetts*, also known as the *Fanny Hill* case.[22] The book at the center of the case, as the reader will recall, had a long history of censorship. *Memoirs of a Woman of Pleasure*, also called *Fanny Hill* for short, was written by John Cleland and was published in London in 1748. In 1821, the book had been banned in Massachusetts, but that didn't stop people from circulating it or attempting to publish it again years later. In 1963, the book was once again made available by a US publisher, and it was immediately banned in Massachusetts when a woman complained to the state's Obscene Literature Control Commission. The publisher challenged the ban, and the case went to the US Supreme Court. The 1966 Supreme Court found that *Fanny Hill* was not obscene and therefore was protected by the First Amendment. Furthermore, the 1966 Court took issue with some of the decisions that the 1957 Court had made with regard to *Roth*. Specifically, the *Memoirs* Court argued that "there is no basis in history for the view expressed in *Roth* that 'obscene' speech is 'outside' the protection of the First Amendment" and that "no interest of society justified overriding the guarantees of free speech and press and establishing a regime of censorship."[32] The upshot of this Supreme Court decision was that the new prevailing definition of obscenity was that a text had to be entirely without socially redeeming value to be considered obscene. In other words, even if a work had some small element of social import, it should be considered protected speech.

The most significant US Supreme Court case was *Miller v. California*, a 1973 case that involved a business owner who had mailed advertisements for pornographic materials to a wide, general audience.[22] Marvin Miller was convicted of violating a California state statute related to sending obscene material through the mail. The Court asserted that community standards could not be determined at the national level, only at the local level. What's more, the Court offered new language with regard to the issue of whether material had socially redeeming value. It introduced the idea that material that lacked "serious" social importance could be considered obscene, which was a departure from the language of "utterly" without social value and made it more difficult for material to get protection from the First Amendment. Drawing upon the definition of obscenity created in *Roth*, the Court set forth a three-part test for obscenity that remains in place today: (1) Whether the average person, applying contemporary community standards, would find that the work, taken as a whole, appeals to the prurient interest; (2) Whether the work depicts or describes, in a patently offensive way, sexual conduct specifically defined by applicable state law; and (3) Whether the work, taken as a whole, lacks serious literary, artistic, political, or scientific value.

With the advent of the Internet, a plethora of issues came to the fore regarding access and intent related to pornography online. Three related cases between 1997 and 2002 offer an outline of the constitutionality of laws designed to protect children from being harmed by sexually explicit material on the Internet. The first of these three cases, *Reno v. American Civil Liberties Union*, had to do with the Communications Decency Act of 1996 (CDA).[22] The CDA was broad and criminalized the intentional transmission of any "obscene or indecent" messages over the Internet, as well as depictions or descriptions of "sexual or excretory activities or organs" in a manner offensive as per community standards. The US Attorney General, Janet Reno, appealed to the Supreme Court for a decision about the CDA because a District Court had entered a preliminary injunction against enforcement of the CDA. The American Civil Liberties Union (ACLU) and other litigants objected to the CDA on the basis that it violated both the First and Fifth Amendments because it was overly broad, vague, and criminalized Internet communications meant to convey educational information. The Supreme Court was unanimous in its agreement that the CDA was too vague about what counted as indecent communications, and that the CDA was too broad in its criminalization of Internet messages that could, in fact, have redeeming value. In response to the Supreme Court's problems with the CDA, Congress passed a new version called the Child Online Protection Act (COPA) in 1998 (Public Law 105–277). COPA would have required commercial Web publishers to request proof of age and credit card information from users to prevent children from viewing obscene material, and penalties for failing to do so would include a $50,000 fine and up to 6 months in prison.[33,34] However, COPA never took effect because of litigation against it by the ACLU, which objected that the definition of material that would become criminal to display was too broad, given that it would include anything that "appeals to 'prurient interest' (according to the average person applying contemporary community standards)."[34,35] In 2002, the Supreme Court upheld an injunction against COPA and referred the case back to the Circuit Court to be reviewed for constitutionality.[36] Ultimately, a permanent injunction against COPA was issued in 2007.[37]

The third case was in 2002, when the Supreme Court struck down a federal law that had been passed in 1996, called the Child Pornography Prevention Act (CPPA).[38] CPPA was designed to expand the federal definition of child pornography to include virtual images of children, as well as any image that appears to be of a minor engaging in a sex act. CPPA meant that pornography featuring adults who appeared to be children would be restricted, as well as simulated sexual activity between teenage actors. The Supreme Court found that CPPA was too broad. CPPA did not affirm that sexual depictions would have to be offensive by community standards to be considered obscene, and it would prohibit material that was neither a crime nor create victims in its production (e.g., pornography featuring an adult who looks like a minor). In 2003, Congress passed the PROTECT Act, which contains language similar to CPPA and does outlaw anything, including a drawing or cartoon, if it appears to be of a minor engaging in sexual intercourse and lacks serious social value.[39]

At least one other case shaped current discourse about the definition of pornography, but it is a case that the Supreme Court declined to hear. In December 1983, the city of Minneapolis, Minnesota, passed a city ordinance that defined pornography as a civil rights violation against women and allowed women to sue producers and distributors of pornography in civil court for damages.[40] A key feature of the ordinance was that did not seek to make the production or dissemination of pornography criminal—instead, it was intended to allow women harmed either in the making of pornography or because of its use to sue in civil court for damages and for a future ban on similar material. The ordinance was primarily authored by two feminists, Andrea Dworkin and Catherine MacKinnon, who were an author and a lawyer, respectively. The ordinance held that pornography is the "graphic sexually explicit subordination of women through pictures and/or words," but specified that this was also true for men, children, and "transsexuals" who appeared in pornography. The ordinance set forth the definition of pornography in this way:

> We define pornography as the graphic sexually explicit subordination of women through pictures and words that also includes (i) women are presented dehumanized as sexual objects, things, or commodities; or (ii) women are presented as sexual objects who enjoy humiliation or pain; or (iii) women are presented as sexual objects experiencing sexual pleasure in rape, incest or other sexual assault; or (iv) women are presented as sexual objects tied up, cut up or mutilated or bruised or physically hurt; or (v) women are presented in postures or positions of sexual submission, servility, or display; or (vi) women's body parts—including but not limited to vaginas, breasts, or buttocks—are exhibited such that women are reduced to those parts; or (vii) women are presented being penetrated by objects or animals; or (viii) women are presented in scenarios of degradation, humiliation, injury, torture, shown as filthy or inferior, bleeding, bruised, or hurt in a context that makes these conditions sexual. (p. 205)[40]

An interesting feature of MacKinnon's argument was that she tried to invert the relationship between obscenity and pornography. Whereas, legally, obscenity is typically considered a more harmful subset of pornography, MacKinnon argued "obscenity . . . probably does little harm" but that "pornography causes attitudes and behaviors of violence"(p. 324).[41] While the original ordinance was vetoed by the mayor of Minneapolis,[40] the city of Indianapolis invited Dworkin and MacKinnon to work with them on crafting a similar ordinance that focused on violent pornography, specifically, and it was passed in 1984.[42] The Indianapolis ordinance was then legally challenged by a group of book, magazine, and film distributors and consumers. In 1985, the US Court of Appeals agreed with the group of distributors and consumers that the ordinance was not constitutional. Then the US Supreme Court declined to review the case, and in doing so affirmed the ruling, expressing agreement with the idea that it is not constitutional to define pornography as gender-based discrimination.

Despite the Supreme Court ruling, the Dworkin and MacKinnon case inspired broader nonlegal discussions about pornography in the 1980s and was part of the reason that President Reagan ordered a comprehensive investigation into pornography by Attorney General Edwin Meese, which resulted in the so-called Meese Report on pornography in 1986.[33] The "sex wars," which divided the feminist movement and ended what is called the second wave of feminism (~ 1963–1994), came into full force during this period.[43] In short, in the late 1980s, the idea that women and girls are victimized by pornography began to be accepted as a truism, and anti-pornography feminism became part of a broader critique of the ways in which women were sexualized in all kinds of contexts (e.g., in the workplace, in advertising media). Anti-pornography feminists argued that the fact that women were imagined as sexual objects, or sexual commodities, was a cause of women's economic and social marginalization.[43] However, on the other side of the debate, sex-positive feminist groups argued that anti-pornography feminism was repressive, aligned with conservative political ideals, and threatened free speech and other types of liberty.[43]

Erotica as a Synonym for Pornography

Because in recent decades the word "erotica" has been used to describe certain kinds of written pornography and videos, some people think that there is a clear distinction between erotica and pornography. Technically, there is no difference. Erotica describes art intended to arouse a person sexually, just like pornography. However, attempts to distinguish erotica as a more elevated or high-brow form of sexually explicit art began in the mid-1900s, coinciding with the commercial success of *Playboy* magazine.

In 1959, two US sexologists who studied and wrote about pornography and the law, Eberhard and Phyllis Kronhausen, proposed that "erotic realism" was sexual material that had some artistic merit, whereas pornography made no attempt to be artistic.[44] In 1980, the feminist journalist Gloria Steinem wrote that erotica is "mutually pleasurable, sexual expression between people who have enough power to be there by positive choice,"[45] and in 1983 she contrasted it with pornography. She wrote: "Pornography is about dominance and often pain. Erotica is about mutuality and always pleasure."[46] In 1994, the sexual violence researcher Diana Russell contrasted pornography and erotica and proposed that erotica is: "void of violence, illegal portrayals (e.g., children), sexism, racism, and homophobia, and is respectful of the human beings involved."[47] But whether material is respectful is a subjective judgment, and even sex that appears violent and disrespectful to some onlookers may be consensual and delightful to those having it. In the modern era, some have attempted to distinguish erotica by claiming that it is "an opportunity to experience sensuous delight of a higher order," or the transmission of material that is "ethereal in its beguiling sensuality" that honors "the joys of the flesh," while pornography appeals "exclusively to our senses or carnal appetites," is "inevitably cheapening" and "mechanistic," and is "an exploit almost barbaric in its egoistic lack of caring and concern."[48]

How Social Scientists Define Pornography

The legal definition of a phenomenon does not always sync up with the definition used by scientists. When it comes to pornography, the Miller test definition isn't used by researchers. In fact, one of the challenges to understanding the research evidence about pornography and its impact on human health is that inconsistent definitions of pornography have been used across studies. To summarize and characterize how the definition has varied across articles, public health scholars Ashton, McDonald, and Kirkman (2019) conducted a thematic analysis of definitions of pornography in scholarly articles published in peer-reviewed journals in 2016 to 2017.[49] Two thirds of the 49 papers that they reviewed were found not to include a definition of pornography. Articles that did include a definition based their definitions on everything from the intention of the producer (e.g., the dividing line between pornography and non-pornography is whether someone is trying to make money), to context (e.g., the researcher decides what counts as pornography, while taking into account cultural and historical meaning and public perception), to how a consumer uses the material (e.g., anything that a consumer finds arousing counts as pornography, even if it was not intended to arouse).

Ashton et al. proposed a comprehensive definition of pornography to be used for research in the digital era: "Material deemed sexual, given the context, that has the primary intention of sexually arousing the consumer, and is produced and distributed with the consent of all persons involved."[50] On the face of it, including consent in the definition seems like a useful and public-health-oriented step. On the other hand, there is some material that might otherwise be considered pornographic that could not meet the consent criteria, such as cartoons that do not involve living people or pornography made using computerized digital images that do not resemble any people.

"Pornographies" Instead of Pornography?

When I began teaching a course called "Understanding Pornography" at the Massachusetts Institute of Technology (MIT) in 2015, I had the excellent fortune of being paired with Professor Sarah Leonard, a historian and faculty member at Simmons College. Professor Leonard argued that we should not, in fact, use the word "pornography" to describe sexually explicit media. There are, she argued, so many different types of sexually explicit media to contemplate that sweeping them all up into a sole category is a fundamental mistake. The word "pornographies," signifying the multiplicity of genres, styles, and subtypes of sexually explicit media that have existed throughout history and proliferate today, is an apt and more appropriate term because it reminds us that pornography comprises diverse media.

In my lectures and conversations, as well as in this book, I use the singular form of the word, "pornography," because it is conventional. But in doing so I risk falling prey to the very mistake that bedevils pornography research: treating all sexually explicit media as though it is one and the same thing, when in fact it is so varied that when we employ the term "pornography" we might be discussing 14th-century Javanese poetry or yesterday's top video clips on a free porn Website. To suggest that only mainstream free Internet pornography is real, true pornography is a mistake, and one that disconnects us dangerously from our recent history. The same empirical questions about the potential harms of pornography that we pose today were being asked in the 1960s and 1970s of films like *Deep Throat*, or erotic novels like *Fanny Hill*, and the same charges were used in the 1800s to limit access to reproductive and sexual health information and products. Ignoring the fact that the media has changed while the questions, and criticisms, have remained the same means that we are doomed to repeat ourselves, wasting resources as we do so.

Public health involves a trade-off between what is reasonable and practical and what is ideal for human health. Defining pornography is difficult, and the choices we make have consequences for our research and policy. Thinking of sexually explicit media as a multiplicity is appropriate and correct. Yet, for practical reasons, I refer to it in this book in the singular and vernacular: pornography.

References

1. Leick, G. 2003. *Sex and Eroticism in Mesopotamian Literature*. London and New York: Routledge.
2. Stone, G. 2007. "Origins of Obscenity." *NYU Review of Law & Social Change* 31, no. 711: 711–731.
3. P. F. 2015. "A brief and gloriously naughty history of early erotic in art (NSFW)." https://www.huffpost.com/entry/a-brief-and-gloriously-naughty-history-of-erotica-in-art_n_55b65df9e4b0224d8832ecb9
4. Eko, L. 2016. *The Regulation of Sex-Themed Visual Imagery: From Clay Tablets to Tablet Computers*. New York: Palgrave Macmillan US.
5. Vout, C. 2013. *Sex on Show: Seeing the Erotic in Greece and Rome*. London: British Museum Press.
6. Harper, K. 2013. *From Shame to Sin*. Cambridge, MA: Harvard University Press.
7. Richards, J. 1995. "Sex, Dissidence and Damnation: Minority Groups in the Middle Ages." In *Chapter 2 is Sex in the Middle Ages*, edited by Jeffrey Richards, 34–53. London and New York: Routledge.

8. Berkowitz, E. 2012. *Sex and Punishment: Four Thousand Years of Judging Desire*. Berkeley, CA: Counterpoint.

9. Green, J., and N. J. Karolides. 2014. *Encyclopedia of Censorship*. New York: Facts on File, Inc.

10. Jones, D. 2001. *Censorship: A World Encyclopedia*. London: Fitzroy Dearborn.

11. Kendrick, W., and W. M. Kendrick. 1996. *The Secret Museum: Pornography in Modern Culture*. Berkeley and Los Angeles, California: University of California Press.

12. Gaimster, D. 2000. "Sex and Sensibility at the British Museum." *History Today* 50, no. 9: 10 15.

13. Lane, F. S. 2001. *Obscene Profits: The Entrepreneurs of Pornography in the Cyber Age*. New York, NY and London: Routledge.

14. Roberts, M. J. D. 1985. "Morals, Art, and the Law: The Passing of the Obscene Publications Act, 1857." *Victorian Studies* 28, no. 4: 609–629.

15. Laqueur, T. W. 2003. *Solitary Sex: A Cultural History of Masturbation*. Brooklyn, NY: Zone Books.

16. Tissot, S. A. 1832. *Treatise on the Disease Produced by Onanism*. New York: Collins & Hannay.

17. Fix, M. 2016. "The Evolution of Obscenity Standards in the Common Law World." *Journal of Comparative Law* 11, no. 2: 75–99.

18. Mullin, K. 2018. "Unmasking *The Confessional Unmasked*: The 1868 Hicklin Test and the Toleration of Obscenity." *ELH* 85, no. 2: 471–499.

19. Jones, T. 1967. "Obscenity Standards in Current Perspective." *SMU Law Review* 21, no. 1: 285–305.

20. National Coalition Against Censorship. "English Pamphlet 'The Confessional Unmasked' leads to Hicklin rule." *http://www.thefileroom.org/documents/dyn/DisplayCase.cfm/id/1109*

21. Strub, W. 2013. "Toward Obscenity: Legal Evolution from Colonies to Comstock." In *Obscenity Rules: Roth v. United States and the Long Struggle over Sexual Expression*. Lawrence, Kansas: University of Kansas Press.

22. Harrison, M., and S. Gilbert. 2000. *Obscenity and Pornography Decisions of the United States Supreme Court*. Carlsbad, CA: Excellent Books.

23. Semonche, J. E. 2007. *Censoring Sex: A Historical Journey Through American Media*. Lanham, Maryland: Rowman & Littlefield.

24. James, C. N. P., and M. L. Schwartz. 1957. "Obscenity in the Mails: A Comment on Some Problems of Federal Censorship." *University of Pennsylvania Law Review* 106, no. 2: 214–253.

25. Dennet, M. 1926. *Birth Control Laws: Shall We Keep Them, Change Them or Abolish Them*. New York: Frederick H. Hitchcock.

26. Leonard, D. 2016. *Neither Snow nor Rain: A History of the United States Postal Service*. New York: Grove Atlantic.

27. Faircloth, S., and R. Dawkins. 2014. *Attack of the Theocrats: How the Religious Right Harms Us All—and What We Can Do about It*. Charlottesville, Virginia: Pitchstone Publishing.

28. Fronc, J. 2017. *Monitoring the Movies: The Fight over Film Censorship in Early Twentieth-Century Urban America*. Austin, Texas: University of Texas Press.

29. Rosen v. United States, 161 U.S. 29 (1896).

30. McClure, R. C. 1962. "Obscenity and the Law." *ALA Bulletin* 56, no. 9: 806–810.

31. Butler v. Michigan, 352 U.S. 380 (1957).

32. United States Supreme Court. 1966. *United States Reports: Cases Adjudged in the Supreme Court*. Washington, DC: US Government Printing Office.

33. United States Department of Justice. 1986. *Attorney General's Commission on Pornography: Final Report*. Washington, DC: United States Department of Justice. 1986.

34. Urbina, I. 2007. "Federal Judge Blocks Online Pornography Law." https://www.nytimes.com/2007/03/22/us/22cnd-porn.html
35. American Civil Liberties Union (ACLU). "Speech at Risk Under COPA." https://www.aclu.org/other/speech-risk-under-copa
36. Bates, L. 2002. "*Ashcroft v. ACLU*: Coping with Online Community Standards." *Jurimetrics* 43, no. 1: 29–41.
37. Purdy, E. 2009. "Child Online Protection Act of 1998 (1998)." https://www.mtsu.edu/first-amendment/article/1066/child-online-protection-act-of-1998
38. Sternberg, S. 2000. "The Child Pornography Prevention Act of 1996 and the First Amendment: Virtual Antitheses Note." *Fordham Law Review* 69, no. 6: 2783–2824.
39. Center for the Study of Technology and Society. 2003. "Porn, Privacy, and Kids: Congressional Attempts to Make the Internet Child-Friendly." *The New Atlantis* 2003, no. 2: 100–102.
40. Parent, W. A. 1990. "A Second Look at Pornography and the Subordination of Women." *The Journal of Philosophy* 87, no. 4: 205–211.
41. MacKinnon, C. A. 1984. "Not a Moral Issue." *Yale Law & Policy Review* 2, no. 2: 321–345.
42. Shipp, E. R. 1984. "A Feminist Offensive Against Exploitation." https://timesmachine.nytimes.com/timesmachine/1984/06/10/252077.html?pageNumber=149
43. Bronstein, C. 2011. *Battling Pornography: The American Feminist Anti-Pornography Movement, 1976–1986*. Cambridge University Press.
44. Kronhausen, E., and P. Kronhausen. 1959. *Pornography and the Law: The Psychology of Erotic Realism and Pornography*. New York: Ballantine.
45. Steinem, G. 1980. "Erotica and Pornography: A Clear and Present Difference." In *Take Back the Night: Women on Pornography*, edited by L. Lederer, 34. New York: Morrow.
46. Steinem, G. 1983. *Outrageous Acts and Everyday Rebellions*. New York: Holt, Rinehart, and Winston.
47. Russell, D. E. H. 1994. *Against Pornography: The Evidence of Harm*. Berkeley, California: Russell Publications.
48. Seltzer, L. F. 2019. "What Distinguishes Erotica from Pornography?" http://www.psychologytoday.com/blog/evolution-the-self/201104/what-distinguishes-erotica-pornography
49. Ashton, S., K. McDonald, and M. Kirkman. 2019. "What Does 'Pornography' Mean in the Digital Age? Revisiting a Definition for Social Science Researchers." *Porn Studies* 1–25.

3

Pornography Viewers

In Chapter 1, I argue that pornography may be an exposure of public health interest. However, not every harmful exposure is treated as a public health problem. Typically, the prevalence of the exposure and the severity of the harm it causes are taken into consideration when public health professionals are prioritizing health issues. If only a small percentage of the population experiences the exposure (i.e., pornography), it would have to have the potential to cause severe, acute harms for it to threaten public health. By way of example, a very small percentage of the population is ever infected with the Eastern equine encephalitis virus—in 2019, there were 38 cases in the United States—but because approximately 30% of those exposed die and many survivors have ongoing neurologic problems, we consider it a public health threat.[1] On the other hand, if the exposure does not cause acute harm, but a large percentage of the population has the exposure, we might also consider it a public health threat. A single sunburn, for example, does not elevate risk of mortality substantially, but sunburn is very common, and the Centers for Disease Control and Prevention (CDC) consider sunburn a public health issue.[2–4] The bottom line is that the prevalence of the exposure is relevant to how we decide if something is a public health problem. This is one reason why it is important to estimate the prevalence of pornography use in the general population.

Ninety percent of US adults use the Internet,[5] 80% go online daily, and 28% say that they are "almost constantly" online.[6] In 2018, close to half of US teens 13 to 17 years old said that they were on the Internet almost constantly, and that figure had almost doubled from 2014 to 2015, when 24% said the same.[7] Internet access is common and has been increasing, and of course pornography can be found on the Internet. To many, that is sufficient evidence that pornography is ubiquitous and that a larger and larger percentage of people are watching pornography more and more frequently.[8] Intuitively, it makes sense: the Internet provides anonymity and privacy for pornography viewing that prior generations did not enjoy, it provides a wealth of free content that was also more limited in decades past, and it provides easy, immediate access. This leads to the commonplace assumption that porn is more popular today than ever.

Pornography and Public Health. Emily F. Rothman, Oxford University Press. © Oxford University Press 2021.
DOI: 10.1093/oso/9780190075477.003.0003

Is porn more popular today than ever? The question isn't well specified, so it's difficult to answer. By claiming porn is more popular today than ever in history, and without specifying geographic location, demographic, or operationalizing "popular," it's an unsupportable claim. As explained in Chapter 1, sexually explicit media was so popular in Italy in 79 AD that many homes had pornographic frescoes painted right on the dining room walls. I propose that we consider two more specific, and answerable, questions about the popularity of pornography:

1. Is the percentage of US people under 18 years of age who view pornography at least once per year greater than it was in the 1990s?
2. Do US adults who consume pornography view it more frequently than they did in the 1990s?

You might wonder why we should even bother to be curious about the percentage of people who view pornography. Most people tend to be curious, and worried, about whether pornography has negative effects on the health of viewers.* For sake of argument, let's say that it does. Then, the question of whether there are a lot of pornography viewers or only a few matters—because whether something qualifies as a public health concern depends on the nature and severity of the harm it causes and its prevalence, among other things.[9] The other reason why the percentage of people who are viewing, using, or consuming pornography is important to public health is that increases or decreases in that trend over time may signal other important changes in social norms that have implications for population health. For example, we may be particularly interested in the percentage of elderly adults or young children who are viewing pornography, if viewing pornography is related to depression, well-being, or some other condition in those populations.

Any discussion of the assessment of pornography viewing or pornography using should be prefaced with at least two cautionary notes about the challenges of collecting these data and thus limitations of results. First, asking people, particularly those in sexually repressive or restrictive (also known as "sex-negative") cultures, if they watch pornography may lead to underreports due to social desirability bias. In other words, people may be reluctant to admit that they view pornography. Also, they may be less reluctant to admit to it today than people were 40 years ago, introducing false time trends that have to do with reporting rather than actual viewing. As a result, increases in self-reported porn viewership may reflect either actual increases in viewership or people's feeling more comfortable admitting on surveys that they watch pornography. Second, there are few nationally representative data sources on pornography use. Since pornography use hasn't been considered a public health problem by any public health decision-making entity, no questions about pornography use have been included on our nationally representative surveys, such as the National Health Interview Survey (NHIS), Behavioral Risk Factor Surveillance System (BRFSS), or Youth Risk Behavior Surveys (YRBS). Therefore, our estimates and interpretation of those estimates are limited because we have too few sources of information to triangulate.

A Lot of People Visit the Pornhub Website

Before we dive into the research on the prevalence of pornography use in the United States from best-available population-based samples, it is useful to consider some facts generated by one of the world's largest pornography websites, Pornhub. Pornhub was launched in 2007, and it reached 1 million daily visitors within 7 months, which is only slightly fewer than 20 times the number of people who visit Disney World Orlando every day.[10] Pornhub was the 38th most-visited website on the Internet in 2019, and the 58th in global Internet engagement in the second quarter of 2020, according to Alexa rankings.[11] Every minute, 63,992 new visitors land on the Pornhub webpage and the majority are from the United States.[12] In 2019, there were 42 billion total visits to Pornhub, which is an increase of 9 billion visits over 2018, and an average of 115 million daily average visits.[12] To put it in perspective, Pornhub suggests that the number of daily visits is the equivalent of the population of Canada, Australia, and Poland combined—although it is unlikely that each Pornhub visit is from a unique visitor. Every 5 minutes, Pornhub transmits more data than the entire contents of the New York Public Library's 50 million books.[13] There are 3.6 billion minutes of pornography on the site, which is approximately 7,000 years' worth of pornography.[14] That sounds like a lot, but for comparison: YouTube adds approximately 82.2 years of new video content every day.[15] In any case, the following can be deduced from the information about Pornhub: many humans watch pornography. Whether that has changed over time is less clear.

Are a Larger Percentage of US Adults Watching Pornography Once or More per Year Today Than in the 1990s?

Lifetime experience of pornography use by US adults is almost ubiquitous. A population-based and nationally representative survey of US adults 18 to

60 years old conducted in 2016 found that as many as 94% of adult men and 87% of adult women reported ever having seen pornography.[16] But knowing that virtually everyone in the modern era has seen pornography at least once doesn't get at the question of whether we are more likely than our parents or grandparents to have seen it. There have been multiple claims in mass media outlets that we are experiencing a "sexplosion" of pornography and that pornography use is spiraling ever higher.[17,18] Is this true?

The best source of data for determining how much the percentage of US adults who have watched pornography has changed over time is the General Social Survey (GSS), because the GSS is the only nationally representative survey that has included a question about pornography since the early 1970s. The GSS has been implemented annually since 1972 by National Opinion Research Center (NORC) at the University of Chicago. In 1973, respondents to the GSS were asked if they had seen an X-rated movie in the last year. There are a few peculiarities of that survey question, including the use of the word "X-rated," which may not resonate with today's consumers as much as it used to, and the word "movie," which may not be precisely the term that we would use to describe Internet-based sexually explicit media consumption today. Weaknesses of the survey question wording notwithstanding, in 1973, 43% of 18- to 34-year-olds reported that they had seen an X-rated movie in the past year. In 2018, 49% of 18- to 34-year-olds responded that they had seen an X-rated movie in the past year. In other words, approximately the same percentage of young adults reported having seen porn in the past year in 2018 as in 1973. This does not necessarily square with the idea that substantially more young adults are turning to pornography.

You're probably thinking that these statistics *can't* be right. Given the tremendous popularity of porn sites and the fact so many of us have near continual access to the Internet on personal devices—how can it not be true that a much larger percentage of people today watch porn than people 30 or 40 years ago? First, the GSS question about viewing X-rated movies in the past year does not capture how frequently people watch porn. One possibility is that roughly the same percentage of adults, and young adults, are interested in seeing any pornography (i.e., a little less than half of us) but for those who choose to view pornography, they are choosing to see it more often than they might have in decades past. In other words, maybe the same proportion of people are into seeing porn, but if you are interested in porn today you can see a lot more of it, more often, than your grandparents or great-grandparents did. Second, it appears that pornography viewing has always been popular. Nearly half of 18- to 34-year-olds were viewing X-rated movies in 1973, meaning that we might not have needed the Internet to propel us into high viewership levels. It might be that the Internet didn't change things all that much in terms of pornography viewership, because humans like to think about and look at sex, and that has been a constant reality for much longer than the past few decades. You might never look at your great-grandparents the same way again, but what I'm suggesting is that they may have had roughly the same probability of seeing pornography (or, depending on the era, a saucy lingerie catalog, or pin-up girl calendar, or burlesque performance) as the young adults of today. Prior generations may have been more discreet and better at covering up their trysts, fantasies, kinks, and use of sexual material to fuel their erotic desires, but they were just as human as humans today, and sex has always been popular with humans.

Let's look a bit deeper into the data on the prevalence of use. Several researchers have examined GSS data in order to report on the prevalence of use. One of the first to do so was the media scholar Paul Wright, who examined consumption by US men between the years 1973 and 2010.[19] Wright found generally stable rates of past-year pornography use, although there was a minor increase over the decades from 26% in the 1970s to 34% in the 2000s.[19] The increase was one that occurred gradually over time—there wasn't a sharp uptick in any one year. Admittedly, eight percentage points isn't the same as zero—it's a 31% increase in relative terms. It means that, technically, pornography viewing among men did increase over time. But it increased only 0.5% per year on average, so the idea that "porn is more popular today than ever" is correct but an exaggerated way to describe the trend. Wright didn't look at only men's use. He also studied women, and he found that the percentage reporting past-year porn viewing increased from 14% in the 1970s to 16% in the year 2000. Again, an increase was detected, but it was only a 14% increase in the percentage who reported viewing porn. Among the subset of women 18 to 30 years old, the increase was larger, from 28% in the 1970s to 34% in the year 2000.[20] Still, a six-percentage-point increase, or 21% increase on a relative scale, over three decades doesn't align with the idea there was an acute increase in porn viewership. Wright's findings have been confirmed by subsequent analyses of GSS data that studied cohorts of adults and found that the most recent cohorts (from the 1980s and onward) are using approximately 10% more pornography than the cohorts from the 1970s.[21]

Wright also used the GSS data to determine if factors like age, race, education, and religiosity were associated with increases or decreases in pornography viewing over the decades. He found that, in both men and women, age was inversely correlated with pornography viewing no matter the year—meaning that pornography viewing is less common among older people.[19,20] Wright also found that the more religious a person was (i.e., the more frequently they attended religious services) the less likely they were to report pornography use, and that was true for every year from 1973 to 2010.[19,20] Interestingly, in the 1970s, pornography viewing was more common among those with more education. Things changed during the 1980s and 1990s, though, and the disparity in men's and women's pornography viewing based on years of education disappeared.[19,20] In the 2000s, years of education were inversely associated with pornography viewing. In other words, in more recent times, those with less education are more likely to report pornography viewing, but that wasn't true in the 1970s. In terms of race, Wright found that people who identified as white were more likely to report pornography viewing than those who identified as other races, and that the association between identifying as white and being more likely to report pornography use was particularly strong and steady during 2002 to 2010.[19,20]

Do US Adults Who Consume Pornography View It More Frequently Than They Did in the 1990s?

In the 1970s to 1990s, the GSS had one question about pornography use. It pertained to the past year and viewing one or more X-rated movies. In the years 2000, 2002, and 2004, the GSS also included a question about viewing pornography online in the past month. Using the GSS Data Explorer, a cross-tabulation reveals that for males, in 2000, 2002, and 2004 the percentages reporting past month Internet pornography use were 28%, 40%, and 17%, respectively. For females, the percentages were 3%, 8%, and 4%, respectively. These percentages are for all adults in the data set, which includes those ages 18 and older. Three data points are too few to draw conclusions about increases or decreases over time. What appears to be an uptick in 2002 among males and females might have been more of a random fluctuation than a reflection of an actual trend in an upward direction. Without additional years of data from the GSS or a similar source, it's impossible to know. Doran and Price (2014) generated a similar estimate of past-month online pornography use by examining the responses of all ever-married adults they are 2000, 2002, and 2004 and found that 16% of men reported visiting a pornography site in the last month, and 3% of women did.[22]

There are two other national surveys that have asked US adults about pornography viewing in the past week and past month. A University of Texas researcher, Mark Regnerus, and colleagues investigated the frequency of pornography use in two different nationally representative samples of American adults. The studies were conducted in 2011–2012 and in 2014, respectively, and were the National Family Structure Survey (NFSS) and the Relationships In America (RIA) study.[23,24] According to the RIA, approximately 40% of men 18 to 23 years old as well as 19% of women in that age group reported intentionally seeing pornography within the past week.[24] According to the NFSS, 47% of men ages 18 to 23 and 21% of women in that age group reported seeing pornography more often than once per month in the past year.[24] The studies were one-time-only, so there is no way to know if the percentages have increased or decreased in the intervening years. As Regnerus and co-authors wrote: "An increase in personal pornography use is a plausible hypothesis but one that cannot be confirmed by any data we have evaluated."[24]

While it is disappointing not to be able to assess whether pornography use is becoming more frequent among US adults, Regnerus and colleagues' work is useful because it provides some confirmation of past-year pornography use as estimated by the GSS. Estimates of past-year pornography use from the RIA and NFSS are similar to those found by the GSS: 63%, 68%, and 59% for men 18 to 23 years old, and 42%, 38%, and 27% for women 18 to 23 years old, respectively, meaning that data from multiple surveys converge around the same estimates.[24] So what we can take from these analyses are that they support Wright's findings that pornography use is relatively common among US adults and that there is a disparity between men's and women's use.

The Women Who View Pornography

Analyses of GSS and other nationally representative data sources consistently find disparities between US men's and women's pornography use. Men are more likely to report that they have used pornography during their lifetimes, the past year, and the past month. But there are women, and particularly a substantial percentage of the women born in the 1990s and later, who use pornography. In 2008, 36% of 18- to 26-year-old women reported using pornography at least once in the past year.[21] In the 1980s and 1990s, women in their 20s were already much more likely than women in the previous generation to report using pornography—they were roughly twice as likely.[21] But in the 1999 to 2012 era, the disparity between younger and older women has grown even more. Now young women are three times more likely to report using pornography than the prior generation did at their same age.[21] That said, while the younger generation is more likely to have used pornography in the past year as compared with their elders, it's not by a lot more—younger women are 7% more likely than older women to have used pornography at their same age.[21]

Are Children Seeing More Pornography Than in Decades Past?

In 2016, Utah became the first state to pass a state resolution that declared pornography a public health issue. The text of the Utah state resolution suggested that the rationale for the declaration was at least in part because young children are being exposed to pornography at high rates. The resolution states: "Due to advances in technology and the universal availability of the Internet, young children are exposed to . . . pornography at an alarming rate" and "the average age of exposure to pornography is now 11 to 12 years of age." While it's true that research using convenience samples of youth in the late 1990s and early 2000s found that 42% to 70% of youth < 18 years old had seen pornography at least once,[25] it's not clear if the rates of pornography viewing among young children are truly increasing over time, nor if the average age of first viewing is a strong predictor of health and safety or is decreasing. A third problem is that pornography is diverse, and it might matter if children are seeing something like the statue of David or a free, mainstream, online porn video clip featuring slapping, gagging, and spanking.

In an article summarizing the results of the 1999–2000 wave of the nationally representative Youth Internet Safety Survey (YISS), researchers Michele Ybarra and Kim Mitchell report that 15% of children 10 to 17 years old had viewed pornography (either online or offline) or had called a 1-900 sex chat phone line intentionally in the past year. Those who were older (in the 14- to 17-year-old age bracket), were male, were seriously involved in substance use, had engaged in delinquent behavior, or had poor emotional bonds with their caregiver were more likely to have viewed pornography.[26] Approximately 20% of those in the 14- to 17-year-old age group had intentionally viewed pornography in the past year (either online or offline), but only 8% of those in the 10- to 13-year-old age group had done so.

A different analysis of subsequent waves of YISS data found that in the year 2000, 8% of youth 10 to 17 years old reported intentionally viewing Internet pornography in the past year, and that that figure increased to 13% in the year 2005 and remained at 13% in 2010. Stratifying by gender, this analysis found that in 2010, 21% of boys and 5% of girls 10 to 17 years old had intentionally seen Internet pornography in the past year.[27] The study found that only 2% of 10- to 11-year-olds sought out pornography in 2010, meaning that alarm about high rates of pre-pubescent youth seeking out pornography may be inconsistent with data.[27]

At least one study did find higher rates of youth pornography access. A survey of 13- to 18-year-old US youth conducted in 2005 to 2007 found that

40% of boys and 13% of girls reported seeking sexual content from pornography Internet sites at least once in the past month, and that 18% of boys and 8% of girls sought sexual content from magazines like *Playgirl* and *Playboy*.[28] These rates are almost double what was found using the YISS question, which likely reflects the fact that on this survey "sexual content" was defined broadly as including showing sexy clothes, nudity, sex, or information about homosexuality.

Where does this leave us on the question of the percentage of youth who have seen pornography and if that percentage is increasing? The YISS data are the best available because they are nationally representative, and the YISS asked the same question at three different points in time. The YISS found that only a minority of youth 10 to 17 years old had seen pornography in the years 2000, 2005, and 2010—and these were years when access to the Internet was rapidly expanding, and when parental controls and blocking and filtering software were not yet as sophisticated as they are today. Even the more broadly worded question found that a minority of youth (40% of boys and 13% of girls) 13 to 18 years old had seen pornography in the past year in 2005 to 2007. It is possible that youth substantially underreported their pornography exposure on both surveys. It is also possible that things have changed in the past decade and now a much larger percentage of youth would report that they have seen pornography in the past year. But if we want to go by the numbers, as Ybarra and Mitchell succinctly put it: "Concerns about a large group of young children exposing themselves to pornography on the Internet may be overstated" (p. 473).[26]

Pornography Viewing by Race-Based Subgroup

Some people may be curious about pornography viewership stratified by race, although historically "the concept of race and the subsequent racial groups" have "devalued and degraded those classified as non-European,"[29] so I raise it here with some mixed feelings. Personally, I'm not sure that social justice and thus public health is well served by discussions of race-specific pornography viewing because of the potential that race-specific estimates could be used to stigmatize, blame, or shame Black, indigenous, and other people of color for any amount of pornography viewing. That said, the data exist, and there may be people who have valid and public-health-related reasons for wanting to know more about the topic—for example, wanting to address race-based inequities related to access to sex education—so a brief discussion of the available information is presented.

The first important note about analyses of race and pornography viewing is that too many studies of pornography viewership have used college samples, often because psychology professors who want to conduct this type of research have relatively easy access to these populations and the research is therefore inexpensive. The overuse of college samples means that the quality and type of information that we have about pornography use are limited, and the fact that college samples have lacked racial and ethnic diversity, as well as socioeconomic diversity, is an important weakness of the existing research.[30] But there have been several studies of convenience samples, and some of nationally representative samples, that have included some analysis of pornography viewing by racial subgroup. Generally, these have found that in both adolescent and adult samples, Hispanic and Black individuals have been more likely to report pornography use than white people (for a discussion, see Perry and Schleifer, 2019).[30] But these studies did not control for social class (that is, income, years of education, or wealth), and given that Wright found years of education were related to pornography use, these seem like important potential confounders.

One recent study that analyzed GSS data from more than four decades and did control for respondents' income, education, marital and parental status, frequency of religious service attendance, age, and region of the United States found that Black men were 9% more likely than white men to have viewed pornography in the past year, and that the difference remained even when potential confounders, such as income or education, were controlled for. The study also found that the Black–white viewing difference has increased over time—between 1973 and 2016, white Americans experienced an 8% increase in past-year pornography viewing, while Black Americans experienced an 18% increase. The study authors, Samuel Perry and Cyrus Schleifer, explained in their article that they do not think that there is scientific evidence to support the idea that race (or sex) differences drive differences in pornography viewing patterns.[30] They propose that white Americans, and particularly religious white Americans, are the ones most likely to find pornography morally objectionable, and that although a larger percentage of Black Americans attend religious services than whites, Black Americans "have never targeted pornography use [as] a key moral issue worth opposing, preferring instead to focus on more immediate, structural issues" (p. 6).[30] Separately, a different study by Perry also found that Asian Americans may consume less pornography that white Americans.[31] The bottom line is that it appears that in the United States, on average, there may be more white Americans than Black who never view pornography, and that part of the reason has been ascribed to white conservative Christians' tendency to "connect their religious piety to their sexual norms and behaviors,"[30] which Black Americans are less likely to do.

Religion and Pornography Viewing

There is a fascinating story hidden in the data about religiosity and pornography use in the United States. Readers with an interest the topic are directed to the body of work by Jeremy Thomas (2013), and by Samuel Perry and his colleagues, for in-depth treatment.[32] Here, I relay some basic findings that may help shape thinking about whom pornography harms and why, and why there is such an outcry in the United States about pornography at this time.

Religiosity appears to have a dampening effect on pornography use. The concept of "religiosity" can be operationalized as frequency of religious service attendance, how literally one takes the Bible or other holy book, one's denomination, or how central a role religious beliefs play in one's development of values, identity, and life choices. Perry and colleagues analyzed GSS data from 1973 to 2016 to study religion and pornography viewership.[30] They found that, on average, for decades theologically conservative Christians were less likely to use pornography than other Americans, but that changed in the mid-1990s when affordable Internet-connected home computers became widely available.[30] According to Perry and colleagues, the conservative Christians who attended church regularly and believed the Bible was the literal word of god were *not* more likely to use pornography, but their Evangelical counterparts who were slightly less conservative started to use pornography more often.[30] Specifically, Evangelicals began using pornography at almost the same rates as any other Americans (26% vs. 29% in the past year, respectively),[30] and they used search engines to search for online porn at the same rate as other Americans.[33] As more Evangelical Christians began to use pornography, Church authorities began to use a new frame in their discourse about why pornography use was wrong.[32] According to the sociologist Dr. Jeremy Thomas, Evangelical Christians began to rely less on rhetoric about pornography being sinful (i.e., scripture-based prohibitions against lust, fornication, and adultery), and instead switched over to secular arguments about why pornography is bad for people—including that it harms children and that it harms the user (i.e., has public health effects).[32]

Why would any theologically conservative Christians use pornography, or use it at roughly the same rate as nonreligious people? Whitehead and Perry (2018) outlined three possible explanations.[33] First, religious culture tends to be "sex-negative," condemning sex outside of marriage. Because of this, those who are religious have fewer sexual outlets and tend to get married at younger ages, because if they want to have sex and can't do it outside of marriage, getting married solves that problem. But getting married at a younger age is associated with higher rates of divorce,[34] and uncoupling is associated with pornography use.[22] Living in a sexually unhappy marriage without getting divorced is also associated with porn use.[22] So, getting married at a younger age might be associated with porn use for multiple reasons. Second, the "preoccupation hypothesis" suggests that putting things off-limits can often backfire; religious people may become preoccupied with pornography precisely because it's forbidden and pursue it covertly.[33] Third, children growing up in theologically conservative communities may have fewer sources of information about sex, so they are more likely to search for pornography out of curiosity.[33] So, despite strong cultural forces that might discourage theologically conservative Christians from using pornography, there are other forces related to age, marriage, and sexual outlets that might encourage it.

Conclusions

Research on the prevalence of pornography use in the United States by adults and underage children reveals a few key facts. First, pornography use is not rare and is not restricted to only males, young people, or the nonreligious. A substantial minority of US adults choose to see pornography at least once a month. The most recent nationally representative survey, the NFSS, found that almost half (47%) of 18- to 23-year-old men, and 21% of women in that same age group reported using pornography more than once per month in the past year in 2014.[24] But that isn't a major departure from our past. While pornography use has been increasing over the past four decades, and while there is some evidence of an uptick that corresponds with widespread home Internet access, the increases have not been overwhelming. Young women and older adolescent children, more than any other demographic subgroups, have experienced noteworthy increases. Even so, data suggest that a minority of adolescents and even a minority of young women are choosing to view pornography. On the whole, pornography use has increased, though not tremendously, and so the question for public health practitioners remains: Is there a reason to worry based on the percentages of people who view pornography? I think that the answer to that question is: It depends on the evidence for harm. Statistics about how common pornography use is, alone, should not be enough to propel us into action. But if pornography is harmful *and* widely used, that is a compelling argument for addressing it as a public health concern.

References

1. US Centers for Disease Control and Prevention. 2019. "Eastern Equine Encephalitis." https://www.cdc.gov/easternequineencephalitis/index.html
2. Cancer.gov. 2019. "Melanoma of the Skin—Cancer Stat Facts." https://seer.cancer.gov/statfacts/html/melan.html
3. Dennis, L. K., M. J. Vanbeek, L. E. Beane Freeman, B. J. Smith, D. V. Dawson, and J. A. Coughlin. 2008. "Sunburns and Risk of Cutaneous Melanoma: Does Age Matter? A Comprehensive Meta-analysis." *Annals of Epidemiology* 18, no. 8: 614–627.
4. US Centers for Disease Control and Prevention. 2020. "Sunburns." https://www.cdc.gov/cancer/skin/statistics/behavior/sunburns.htm
5. Anderson, M., A. Perrin, J. Jiang, and M. Kumar. 2019. "10% of Americans Don't Use the Internet. Who Are They?" https://www.pewresearch.org/fact-tank/2019/04/22/some-americans-dont-use-the-internet-who-are-they/
6. Perrin, A., and M. Kumar. 2019. "About Three-in-Ten U.S. Adults Say They Are 'Almost Constantly' Online." https://www.pewresearch.org/fact-tank/2019/07/25/americans-going-online-almost-constantly/
7. Anderson, M., and J. Jiang. 2018. "Teens, Social Media & Technology 2018." https://www.pewinternet.org/2018/05/31/teens-social-media-technology-2018/
8. Paasonen, S. 2011. "Online Pornography: Ubiquitous and Effaced." In *The Handbook of Internet Studies,* edited by Mia Consalvo and Charles Ess, 424–439. Wiley-Blackwell.
9. Prevention USCfDCa. 2012. "Principles of Epidemiology in Public Health Practice, Third Edition." https://www.cdc.gov/csels/dsepd/ss1978/lesson5/section3.html
10. Cox, T. 2017. "10 Interesting Things You Might Not Know About Pornhub." https://finance.yahoo.com/news/10-interesting-things-might-not-141704415.html
11. Alexa Rankings. 2020. https://www.alexa.com/siteinfo/pornhub.com#section_traffic
12. Pornhub Insights. 2020. "2019 Year in Review." https://www.pornhub.com/insights/2019-year-in-review#2019
13. Silver, C. 2019. "Pornhub 2017 Year in Review Insights Report Reveals Statistical Proof We Love Porn." https://www.forbes.com/sites/curtissilver/2018/01/09/pornhub-2017-year-in-review-insights-report-reveals-statistical-proof-we-love-porn/
14. Spitznagel, E. 2019. "Where the Filthy Things Are." *Popular Mechanics* https://www.popularmechanics.com/culture/web/a29623446/pornhub-porn-data-storage/
15. Hale, J. 2019. "More Than 500 Hours of Content Now Being Uploaded to YouTube Every Minute." https://www.tubefilter.com/2019/05/07/number-hours-video-uploaded-to-youtube-per-minute/
16. Herbenick, D, T. C. Fu, P. Wright, et al. 2020. "Diverse Sexual Behaviors and Pornography Use: Findings from a Nationally Representative Probability Survey of Americans Aged 18 to 60 Years." *The Journal of Sexual Medicine* 17, no. 4: 623–633.
17. Brenner, G. 2018. "When Is Porn Use a Problem?" https://www.psychologytoday.com/us/blog/experimentations/201802/when-is-porn-use-problem
18. Friedersdorf, C. 2016. "Is Porn Culture to Be Feared?" https://www.theatlantic.com/politics/archive/2016/04/porn-culture/477099/
19. Wright, P. J. 2013. "U.S. Males and Pornography, 1973–2010: Consumption, Predictors, Correlates." *The Journal of Sex Research* 50, no. 1: 60–71.

20. Wright, P. J., S. Bae, and M. Funk. 2013. "United States Women and Pornography Through Four Decades: Exposure, Attitudes, Behaviors, Individual Differences." *Archives of Sexual Behavior* 42, no. 7: 1131–1144.

21. Price, J., R. Patterson, M. Regnerus, and J. Walley. 2016. "How Much More XXX Is Generation X Consuming? Evidence of Changing Attitudes and Behaviors Related to Pornography Since 1973." *The Journal of Sex Research* 53, no. 1: 12–20.

22. Doran, K., and J. Price. 2014. "Pornography and Marriage." *Journal of Family and Economic Issues* 35, no. 4: 489–498.

23. Regnerus, M. 2012. "How Different Are the Adult Children of Parents Who Have Same-Sex Relationships? Findings from the New Family Structures Study." *Social Science Research* 41, no. 4: 752–770.

24. Regnerus, M., D. Gordon, and J. Price. 2016. "Documenting Pornography Use in America: A Comparative Analysis of Methodological Approaches." *The Journal of Sex Research* 53, no. 7: 873–881.

25. Wolak, J., K. Mitchell, and D. Finkelhor. 2007. "Unwanted and Wanted Exposure to Online Pornography in a National Sample of Youth Internet Users." *Pediatrics* 119, no. 2: 247–257.

26. Ybarra, M. L., and K. J. Mitchell. 2005. "Exposure to Internet Pornography Among Children and Adolescents: A National Survey." *Cyberpsychology & Behavior: The Impact of the Internet, Multimedia and Virtual Reality on Behavior and Society* 8, no. 5: 473–486.

27. Rothman, E., and K. J. Mitchell. 2019. "A Trend Analysis of U.S. Adolescents' Intentional Pornography Exposure on the Internet, 2000–2010." http://sites.bu.edu/rothmanlab/porn-literacy/

28. Bleakley, A., M. Hennessy, and M. Fishbein. 2011. "A Model of Adolescents' Seeking of Sexual Content in Their Media Choices." *The Journal of Sex Research* 48, no. 4: 309–315.

29. Ford, C. L., and C. O. Airhihenbuwa. 2010. "Critical Race Theory, Race Equity, and Public Health: Toward Antiracism Praxis." *American Journal of Public Health* 100 (Suppl. 1): S30–S35.

30. Perry, S. L., and C. Schleifer. 2019. "Race and Trends in Pornography Viewership, 1973–2016: Examining the Moderating Roles of Gender and Religion." *The Journal of Sex Research* 56, no. 1: 62–73.

31. Perry, S. L. 2016. "From Bad to Worse? Pornography Consumption, Spousal Religiosity, Gender, and Marital Quality." *Sociological Forum* 31, no. 2: 441–464.

32. Thomas, J. N. 2013. "Outsourcing Moral Authority: The Internal Secularization of Evangelicals' Anti-Pornography Narratives." *Journal for the Scientific Study of Religion* 52, no. 3: 457–475.

33. Whitehead, A. L., and S. L. Perry. 2018. "Unbuckling the Bible Belt: A State-Level Analysis of Religious Factors and Google Searches for Porn." *The Journal of Sex Research* 55, no. 3: 273–283.

34. Wolfinger, N. H. 2003. "Family Structure Homogamy: The Effects of Parental Divorce on Partner Selection and Marital Stability." *Social Science Research* 32, no. 1: 80–97.

4

Pornography Content

Contemporary Sources of Pornography

As media and technology evolve, so does pornography. At one moment in history, the only sources of sexually explicit material were bawdy poetry, paintings, and statues. When the camera was invented, people began to take sexually explicit photos and to publish them in magazines and books.[1,2] Soon thereafter, when moving pictures were invented, people began to make sexually explicit films.[3]

Today, pornography is easily accessible on the Internet, but there are differences between free, mainstream websites and subscription or pay-per-use pornography sites. The content can vary widely. Not all Internet porn is in video format. In addition to sites where professional pornography production companies post free clips and previews of longer films, there are fan fiction sites where Internet users can upload their own creative writing about sexual encounters between characters in books or movies, there are social media sites where people are permitted to post photos of themselves or others topless, bottomless, or engaged in some sexual acts, and there are websites where users can pay to interact with "cam girls" or women (and nonbinary gender people and men) who will strip, dance, or perform sex acts on camera for them. There are websites where people who are not professional pornography performers can upload their own videos of themselves having sex (i.e., "user-generated content"), which are sometimes called "amateur" sites. There is a website called "Beautiful Agony" that shows faces—and only faces—of people while they are having orgasms. There is even a website where users can listen to audio clips of people having sex, without seeing any visual content to accompany it.[4] In short, the Internet offers a cornucopia of porn styles and genres.

In 2012, when I was first trying to understand the landscape of contemporary pornography, I created the graphics shown in Figures 4.1 and 4.2 to help myself navigate. Figure 4.1 is a simple illustration depicting the different forms of media that could be sexually explicit and therefore describe

Pornography and Public Health. Emily F. Rothman, Oxford University Press. © Oxford University Press 2021.
DOI: 10.1093/oso/9780190075477.003.0004

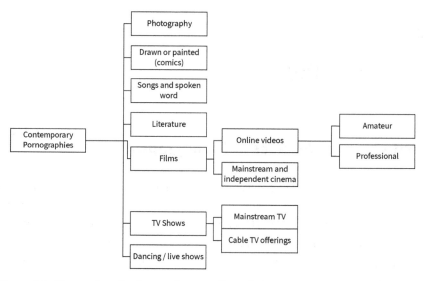

Figure 4.1. Types of media that can be sexually explicit.

categories of pornography. Figure 4.2 is a graphic that describes some genres and subgenres of online pornography, specifically.

Figure 4.2 is not intended to be comprehensive of every type of pornography that is available. There are more than 90 categories of porn available on Pornhub alone. To me, what is useful about the graphic is that it divides pornography into the two primary categories: pornography that is legal to produce and pornography that is illegal. The harms of illegally produced

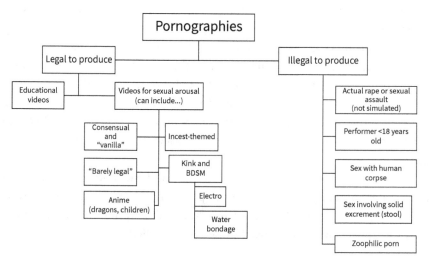

Figure 4.2. A selection of pornography video types that are legal vs. illegal to produce.

pornography are not up for debate. The thornier questions today are about whether legally produced pornography is harmful to public health.

Under legally produced pornography, I propose that there are two main categories. There are educational videos, such as *Bend Over Boyfriend* starring Carol Queen and Robert Morgan, or *Fetish Coaching* and *An Explicit Guide to Squirting*, produced by Erika Lust. These videos are sexually explicit in that they show close-ups of genitals and nonsimulated sex, but they may not be intended to arouse the viewer so much as educate the viewer about sex and sexual techniques. Then there is the very wide variety of content that is specifically designed to sexually arouse viewers that may be mainstream, kink, fetish, or animated and may depict anything from three-person sexual encounters, to BDSM-themed slapping, spanking, gagging, and choking, to humiliation and degradation porn (which might feature someone forcing someone else to lick their foot, or a toilet, or calling them "slut" or "whore"), to videos of actors pretending to be stepmother and stepson, or Dad and the babysitter, and even comic videos of people fully dressed and making jokes about wanting to kiss you on the forehead (i.e., the art of Ryan Creamer) buried among the rest of the explicit content. Of note, in Figure 4.2 I list "electro" and "water bondage" as examples under kink, but I have not listed any other type of kink. The reason is that some people have made the claim that using electric shocks on porno performers, or engaging in water bondage (in which performers may have their head held down under water), is tantamount to torture under the Geneva Convention.[5] It's therefore useful to have these forms of kink included in the space between the legal and illegal forms of pornography, visually, and including them on the graphic reminds me to mention that criticism of these forms of pornography.

Several years after I started using these illustrations in my graduate classes on pornography, scholars Hald and Štulhofer published their 2016 article that presented a taxonomy of pornography subtypes based on a principal factor analysis of the types of pornography that a large sample of Croatian adults reported to have preferred.[6] Although they did not present a visual graphic to accompany their taxonomy, if they had, it would be rather different from mine. Hald and Štulhofer found that there were four main types of pornography, including paraphilic, nonheterosexual, group sex, and female-specific (that is, the made-for-women category). This, too, is an interesting way to organize and group subgenres of pornography. Also useful was Hald and Štulhofer's analysis of the most popular types of pornography that adults in their sample preferred. Another approach, taken by the authors of the book *A Billion Wicked Thoughts*, was to analyze Internet search terms.[7] Ogas and Gaddam used a search engine to analyze searches for porn from July 2009 to

July 2010. They found that 13% of all Internet searches are sexual in nature, and that among the most frequently used sexual search terms were "youth," "breasts," "cheating wives," "gay," and "penises."[8] Hald and Štulhofer, who conducted their survey in 2014, found that the most popular type of porn was "amateur," followed by "oral sex," "big breasts," "threesomes," "anal sex," "MILF/mature," "vaginal sex," "lesbian," and "cumshot." Lolita/teen pornography (i.e., pornography meant to satisfy those seeking pornography featuring underage girls or very young adult women) came in 11th, bondage and dominance came in 19th, and violent sex came in 22nd. In a probability-based sample of US adults, Herbenick and colleagues found that, in their lifetime, 45% of men and 33% of women have seen BDSM (bondage, discipline/dominance, sadism/submission, masochism) porn and 35% of men and 22% of women have seen porn where someone pressures another person to do something that they did not want to do.[9]

The sheer number of categories can be confusing and overwhelming. A now classic 2003 web comic even pokes fun at the width and breadth of modern pornography subgenres. It depicts a young man at a computer feeling overwhelmed by seeing that pornography has been made featuring beloved cartoon characters from his childhood. The caption reads "Rule #34. There is Porn Of it. No Exceptions."[10] Some people wonder if the availability of a wide array of genres of pornography is reason, in and of itself, for concern.

There is little question that there is now a much wider variety of pornography on offer than there was in the prior century. As of February 2021, there were 97 categories of pornography on Pornhub, which is the largest international purveyor of online pornography videos. Pornhub boasts having enough pornography footage that it could play video clips continuously for 68 years without ever repeating one,[11] although the company has also stated it hosts 11 petabytes of content, which works out as close to 7,000 years' worth.[12] In any case, to say that there is a wealth of content available is an understatement. It makes sense, then, that porn websites tag and label the clips and group them into categories for viewers. However, one result of the labeling is that people who have not been keeping up with pornography trends, or newcomers to pornography, might have a difficult time navigating through them. Things were simpler in the 1980s and 1990s. In that era, typically pornography was classified into one of two basic categories: hard core or soft core. Hard-core pornography showed genitals or vaginal, oral, or anal intercourse taking place, whereas soft-core pornography may have featured performers simulating sex or may have alluded to sex acts without depicting them graphically. Within the categories of hard-core and soft-core pornography, one might have found gay or BDSM pornography, but there were few other categories of pornography until the late 1990s. In contrast, today, visitors to the Pornhub site are presented with some categories that they might understand intuitively, such as "Czech," "Ebony," "Feet," "Orgy," "Pissing," and "Vintage," but many others that could have them scrambling for urbandictinoary.com. Some of these newer and more difficult to intuit categories include, for example, verified amateurs, babe, bukkake, cartoon, casting, cosplay, creampie, described video, double penetration, fetish, fisting, gangbang, hentai, interactive, MILF (Moms I'd Like to Fuck), POV (Point of View), scissoring, SFW (Safe For Work), and squirt. These aren't the only new genres. On Kink.com, one will find categories including device bondage, water bondage, ultimate surrender, naked kombat, electrosluts, and wired pussy. The indie site Pinklabel.tv offers eco-sexual porn, edu-porn, feminist porn, trans and nonbinary porn, and POC (Person of Color) porn, among others.

From the standpoint of a researcher trying to understand the impact of pornography on public health, why might it matter that there is now an almost endless variety of pornography on offer, and that consumers can select with such specificity exactly what they want to see? The first point of interest is that pornography is not monolithic. There is such a wide variety of pornography categories and subcategories that virtually any statement that begins "pornography is . . ." is bound to be wrong. Lumping all sexually explicit media together, even all of it that can be found on the mainstream Pornhub website, masks potentially important differences between categories. It's a bit like saying "Food is bad for you," or "Food is good for you." Neither statement can be correct because food is too broad a category.

Second, whether it is inherently harmful that pornography now comes in many categories is an open question. It is not clear that an endless variety of something, even if that something is bad for us, worsens the impact on human health. Consider potato chips, the most popular snack food in the United States. According to the US Department of Agriculture, US consumption of potato chips has remained relatively steady for five decades.[13] In 1970, Americans ate 17.4 pounds of potato chips per person per year, and in 2014 that rate was 17.0 pounds per person per year.[13] In other words, there was no increase in per-person potato-chip consumption during that period, and this is true despite the fact that potato chip flavors expanded dramatically from a handful of varieties in the early 1970s (e.g., barbeque, cheese and onion, and salt and vinegar) to the 2000s, when seasonings included, among others, dill pickle, jalapeno, ketchup, wasabi, paprika, salt and pepper, ranch, bacon, lime, crab, fried green tomato, and many others. It is a marketing strategy to invent new flavors—but it does not appear to be because the variety in flavors nets a substantial number of new customers who are now drawn to the product. In other words, not many of us think: "I've never been interested in potato chips, but now that they have fried green tomato chips, I'm going to be a regular buyer!" The business strategy behind variety is about grabbing attention and free publicity by introducing "stunt" or over-the-top flavors that will generate buzz,[14] which in turn will keep consumer attention focused on the product and brand. In terms of pornography, the seemingly endless expansion of categories and genres may be a strategy to hook new viewers or a strategy to maintain the interest of existing customers by keeping their attention on pornography in general—although not necessarily, as anti-pornography activists have claimed,[15] by converting them to consumers of new, more extreme types of pornography. The one longitudinal study that has tested the hypothesis that pornography viewers tend to become more interested in extreme content over time, also known as the "content progression thesis," found that interest in more violent pornography actually *decreased* over time in a sample of 248 Croatian teenage boys.[16] There has been one cross-sectional study of US adults that found that people who first started using pornography at a younger age were more likely subsequently to have intentionally searched for illegal pornography, such as zoophilic and child sexual abuse pornography, which could mean that their interests broadened over time—in support of the content progression thesis—or it could mean that those with deviant sexual interests develop an interest in pornography at a younger age.[17]

And to be fair, there is at least one counterexample that might give us reason to suspect that the high degree of specialization of pornography clips could be drawing in new consumers as well as securing the loyalty of existing ones. Consider the example of flavored nicotine products. Until 2009, cigarettes came in flavors like berry, vanilla, margarita, and others, when federal legislation banned these flavors because of overwhelming evidence that such flavors were causing minors to start smoking.[18] Working around this legislation, tobacco companies began marketing electronic cigarette products in a wide variety of flavors, and there are now more than 15,500 unique flavors of electronic cigarette e-liquids, which is a substantial increase from 2014 when there were only 7,700.[19] Evidence suggests that while most consumers stick with one e-liquid flavor, there are some adults and youth who continue e-cigarette use longer than they might otherwise because of the array of flavors available to try.[20] In other words, people may remain loyal consumers out of a sense of adventure—whether they are consumers of pornography, e-cigarettes, or other products—if there are always new categories or new flavors still to sample.

Whether the array of pornography categories entices people to initiate pornography use, influences the frequency of pornography consumption, or extends the length of time of pornography viewing sessions, are potentially important questions. But just as the quantities of nonsexualized media on popular viewing platforms like Netflix, Hulu, or Amazon may influence the frequency and length of consumers' media viewing sessions, the amount of time spent viewing is not in and of itself a public health outcome of consequence. If time spent viewing causes depression, anxiety, sexual assault, self-harm, or substance use, or reduces motivation to work, to parent, to exercise, to socialize with friends, or otherwise to participate in a healthful lifestyle—then there would be a clear impetus to attempt to shorten viewing sessions and to reduce viewing frequency. But there is little to suggest that the sheer number of genres is a problem in and of itself.

Categories of Pornography of Public Health Interest

Manga and Anime

While it is not clear that the sheer number of categories of pornography is inherently problematic, the content or plot of some categories of pornography may influence people's health. While this review is far from exhaustive, here I focus on several categories that have come under legal or political fire in the past decade: manga/anime, barely legal, incest porn, and kink. Research findings on whether these types of pornography negatively influence health are reported in later chapters.

Manga are Japanese comics and anime is Japanese animation. Manga and anime aren't exclusively sexual and are available in many nonsexual genres, such as comedy, horror, mystery, romance, and science fiction. Sexual genres of manga include ecchi, same sex, "adult themes" (e.g., failing marriages, problems at work), and hentai.[21] Hentai refers to "extreme, bizarre or inappropriate sexual situations" and may depict gang rape, interspecies sexual encounters, incest, and pedophilia.[21] While hentai is drawn, and thus no humans are harmed in the creating of hentai, some argue that cartoon images that depict children as sex objects, for example, may worsen the risk of child sexual abuse by priming people to view children a sex objects, conditioning them to feel sexual excitement when looking at images of children in general, or giving viewers a sense that the desire to have sexual contact with children is widespread, shared by many, and perhaps acceptable. The legal status of hentai varies by country. Presently in the United States, according to provisions of the PROTECT Act (Public Law 108-21), it is not legal to possess obscene visual representations of minors engaged in sexual conduct. In Japan, it is legal to possess and produce visual representations of minors engaged in sexual conduct, as long as the representations are drawn or are created using computer graphics.[22]

There have been at least four prosecutions and criminal convictions for manga possession in the United States. In one case, a manga collector in Iowa was sentenced to 6 months in prison for possessing and mailing manga depicting children engaged in sexual acts.[23] In 2009, the executive director of the Comic Book Legal Defense Fund said of that case that the drawings were, essentially, lines on a paper. This may sound like a serious case of minimization, given the prevalence of child sexual abuse and the abject harm it can cause. But, public health professionals should also contemplate the implications of the government's having the power to arrest, prosecute, and incarcerate people for sketches.

Incest Porn

Incest is nearly universally taboo across cultures. Incest between consenting adults is illegal in every US state, although it is not a criminal offense in New Jersey and Rhode Island.[24] Most producers of pornography in the United States who want to depict incest typically go out of their way to demonstrate that the actors they are filming are not actually related, and they typically film pornography that features fictional step-relationships rather than fictional biological relationships. Searches for incest porn featuring step-siblings, or step-parents and step-children, began appearing in Pornhub's lists of most popular searches in 2014.[25] In 2015, the Adult Video News (AVN) awards, which is the pornography industry's version of the Oscars, created a new category: "Best Taboo Relations."[25] And in 2016, "step mom" was the most searched term on Pornhub in the United States. Between 2015 and 2017, many of the most widely read Internet pop journalism outlets, including *Esquire, Vice, Maxim, Daily Beast,* and *Cosmopolitan,* ran articles about the surge in popularity of incest pornography. In several of these articles, it was pointed out that non-sexually explicit entertainment like *Game of Thrones, Pretty Little Liars,* and *Arrested Development,* as well as the films *Star Wars, Cruel Intentions,* and *Clueless,* featured storylines that normalized incest even before incest-themed pornography became popular.

Questions of public health relevance related to the availability of incest-themed porn include: (1) Does the proliferation of incest-themed porn influence rates of sexual contact between underage step- or biological sibling who view it? (2) Does it influence rates of consensual or nonconsensual sexual contact between adult step- or biologically related people who view it? (3) Does it influence rates of consensual and nonconsensual sexual contact between step- or biologically related people who are *not viewers* of incest pornography?

Barely Legal

Barely legal is a genre of pornography that uses adult performers made to look like underage teenagers. For example, an 18-year-old woman with small breasts who puts her hair in pigtails may appear to the viewer to be a girl. Technically, according to Section 1466A of Title 18 USC, it is illegal to produce, distribute, receive, or possess with intent to transfer or distribute any image that appears to depict a minor engaged in sexual intercourse, so creators who make content for the barely legal category—if they are worrying about the law—have to ensure that the video does not appear to depict a minor. The term "barely legal" is a direct reference to the fact that the pornography in this category is designed to depict people who are just over the threshold and 18 years old but still technically teenagers.

Viewers of barely legal pornography can find hundreds of thousands of videos of young adult performers dressed as babysitters, step-daughters, sisters, and schoolgirls, and performing the roles of virgins, first-time pornography performers, or teenagers. To my knowledge, the category rarely depicts boys or non-binary people as the barely legal performers. Importantly and unacceptably, some publicly accessible porn websites that host user-uploaded content have hosted pornography featuring actual children.[26] Thus, some viewers who have sought barely legal or "teen" category pornography have watched illegal child sexual abuse material, perhaps without knowing they were doing so.[26] But putting aside the disturbing fact that some "barely legal" porn is in fact illegal porn, and focusing on the idea that there is some legal pornography that depicts very young performers, it is reasonable to wonder if even this legitimate "barely legal" pornography is harmful to the viewers or causes harm to the social environment.

It has been established that legal pornography featuring older teenagers tends to be qualitatively different in content than pornography featuring mature adult performers. A recent study that compared the content of pornography featuring performers who are referred to as "teen" in the title or description of the clip, or otherwise indicated to be between 18 and 20 years old, vs. pornography featuring more mature women who appeared to be 20 to 40 years old (or "adult"), found that teen pornography performers are more likely to experience degrading treatment and risky sex acts.[27] Teen performers were more than twice as likely to be in anal penetration scenes and five times more likely to be in forceful anal penetration scenes.[27] They were also approximately 40% more likely to be in scenes in which the male performer ejaculated in their mouth or on their face.[27] In addition, 90% of the teenage women in videos containing visible aggression displayed pleasure, compared with 54% of the videos in which there was no visible aggression. The author of this study commented that the videos: "celebrate aggression and degradation by portraying these acts as both consensual—showing the dominance and aggression of men over willing women—and sensual—producing pleasure and satisfaction for both men and women."[27]

The concern is that underage viewers may be more likely to develop sexual scripts—that is, beliefs about what should happen during sex, and what they want to have happen during sexual encounters—that are nonconsensual and violent if they are more likely to view barely legal or teen pornography, in part because the performers are supposed to be depicting teenagers and may seem like age-appropriate exemplars for sexual behavior. As of 2021, we lack evidence that underage viewers gravitate toward the barely legal category. It may be that this category is primarily popular with middle-aged or older men, for example, and not underage or very young adult viewers.

Kinky and BDSM porn

"Kink" is the word used to describe sexual behavior that falls outside of the norm or mainstream.[28] Kink is an umbrella term, and there are a variety of sexual behaviors that might fall under kink, including consensual bondage, discipline/dominance, sadism/submission, masochism (BDSM), "age play" (where partners pretend to be older or younger than they are), cuckolding (being aroused by one's partner having sex with someone other than yourself), giving or receiving enemas, role-playing, urophilia (i.e., golden showers, water sports, or peeing on someone during sex), watching other people have sex (with their consent), and others. A fetish is a fixation on an object or body part and deriving sexual pleasure from it, even if it is not usually considered erotic—such as a foot, a bedside lamp, a yoga mat, or gloves. Sex that is not kinky and does not involve a fetish is often referred to as "vanilla."

There may be multiple reasons why some people develop kinks or fetishes. Too little is known about how they develop and change or not over time, and whether kink should be considered a sexual orientation, because some people say that their interest in kink transcends the gender of their partner(s).

An unfortunately common belief is that the reason that people are drawn to BDSM is that they were abused as children or that something is wrong with them psychologically.[29] For example, when a *New Yorker* magazine writer confessed to an interest in BDSM in a written article on the issue in 1996, her mental health was publicly questioned.[30] But multiple studies have found that, compared to nonpractitioners, BDSM practitioners are *less* likely to have experienced sexual coercion[31] and exhibit lower levels of depression, anxiety, PTSD, psychological sadism, psychological masochism, borderline pathology, psychological distress, sexual problems, and paranoia (although they exhibit similar levels of obsessive-compulsive disorder to nonpractitioners and greater levels of dissociation and narcissism).[29,31,32] And a systematic review of the peer-reviewed literature published in *Sexual Medicine* reveals that an interest in BDSM is explained by a number of factors, both biological and psychological.[33] One proposed explanation for BDSM, dating back almost a century, is that it helps to rev up the libido of people with a lower sex drive (i.e., hyposexuality). The idea is that the BDSM acts evoke strong feelings—for example, feelings of shame or disgust—and that physical sensations of pain make neurons fire in the brain. The more powerful the feelings of shame, disgust, or even pain, the easier it is for the libido to borrow that energy and get a kick-start.[34,35] What's more, and perhaps counterintuitively to some, recent research suggests that BDSM can actually increase closeness in relationships. BDSM partners may permit themselves to feel vulnerable with one another, to communicate about intimate thoughts and feelings, and to let their emotional guards down after the sexual encounter (e.g., "aftercare") in ways that non-BDSM practitioners do not.[36,37]

While BDSM and kink may have its benefits for those who enjoy it, the problem with kink pornography that looks like violence to the casual observer is that it *looks like violence.* Alan McKee (2015) has argued that pornography "viewers see consensual sadomasochism as being a different kind of sex act from nonconsensual sexual violence" (p. 85), and that content analyses of pornography tend to mischaracterize pornography as more violent than it actually is because it is impossible to tell from observing the pornography if consent was genuinely given by performers.[38] Indeed, studies of pornography from the past decade reveal that approximately 40% of mainstream website pornography clips contain aggression,[27,39,40] and the percentage of viewers who see those clips and understand that what they are seeing is consensual is unknown. In other words, we do not know, for example, the percentage of sexually inexperienced 18-year-olds who find free porn videos that depict strangulation and slapping and understand that what they are seeing is a type of play-acting and is consensual. Anti-pornography activists seemingly presume that no viewers are capable of seeing BDSM pornography without becoming aroused by thoughts of actual sexual violence, while some pornography defenders seemingly presume that all viewers understand, as they themselves do, that BDSM can be practiced safely and is not necessarily a depiction of abuse. The truth is that we don't know much about how familiar underage children who view pornography, or even adult viewers, may be with BDSM and how susceptible they are to acquiring new schemas about sex and sexuality from seeing BDSM pornography online. A particular problem is that some BDSM practitioners are part of a "BDSM community" that promulgates safer sex guidelines, offers checklists, and offers classes and workshops in safe BDSM—but too many casual observers of BDSM pornography may have no idea that such a community exists, no access to the safety information, and no motivation or capacity to seek out and join an alternative sex community. So, there is still an urgent need for social science to answer the question: Is seeing BDSM pornography bad for viewers if they don't understand what they are looking at? And, if so, how is that best addressed?

Content Analyses

Content analyses of pornography have been published in peer-reviewed publications since at least 1979. Beginning with the unpublished Kinsey Institute Harsanyi analysis,[41] as of July 2020, by my count there have been at least 43 content analyses (see, for example, Malamuth and Spinner 1980; Cowan and Campbell 1994; Monk-Turner and Purcell 1999; Vannier, Currie, and O'Sullivan 2013; and Carrotte et al. 2020).[42-46] Most content analyses are driven by a desire to understand the percentage of pornography that depicts BDSM or aggressive sex. The earliest content analyses found that the percentage of pornography that depicted either violence or bondage and dominance was approximately 5% to 17%.[42,47-49] The most recent studies, those by Fritz (2020), Shor and Seida (2018), Shor (2019), Shor and Golriz (2019), and Willis et al. (2019), also found that 40% to 46% of adult videos feature visible physical aggression, and 17% feature physical aggression with nonconsent.[27,39,40,50,51] Shor and Seida specifically took on the question of whether pornography is becoming "harder and harder," meaning more and more likely to depict nonconsensual aggression or visible aggression, and they demonstrated that over the period 2008 to 2016 there was no increase in aggression in mainstream pornography.[39] While pornography may have become harder and harder over the past 40 years, it is possible that in the past 10 years it plateaued.

Of the list of more than 40 content analyses that have been conducted, there is one that tends to be cited by anti-pornography activist groups or websites. That is the 2010 analysis by Ana Bridges that found that 88% of pornography videos featured an act of physical violence.[52-55] The estimate is notable because it is the only content analysis to have yielded such a high percentage rate of violence for mainstream pornography content. Bridges' methods have been critiqued by other researchers who have used alternative methods for characterizing aggression in pornography.[38] Bridges counted 14 types of physically aggressive behaviors as aggression, whether the target expressed pleasure, displeasure, or responded neutrally. McKee conducted an analysis of aggression in pornography, using a stricter definition of aggression, and found that only 2% of pornography contained aggression. In McKee's study, an act was only counted as aggression if a character stated that they didn't want to partake and were then forced, if the actions were "outside of obviously consensual sadomasochistic role playing," or if the characters appear to be unhappy performing (p. 283).[38] On the other hand, Bridges' list of physically aggressive acts, which were counted no matter how the respondent reacted to them, included: pushing or shoving; biting; pinching; hair-pulling; spanking; open-hand slapping; gagging (defined as when an object or body part, e.g., penis, hand, or sex toy, is inserted into a character's mouth, visibly obstructing breathing); choking (when one character visibly places his or her hands around another character's throat with applied pressure); threatening with a weapon (which 0% of videos depicted); kicking; closed fist punching (which 0% of videos depicted); bondage or confining; using weapons; and torturing, mutilating, or attempting murder (which 0% of the videos depicted). Bridges found that 88.2% of the videos she analyzed contained one or more scenes depicting an act of physical aggression in this list. Of note, 75% of the physical aggression was spanking. Spanking is a relatively common sex act—as many as 30% of US adult men and 34% of women report having been spanked or spanking someone during sex in their lifetimes.[56] The next largest category that Bridges' team uncovered was gagging, which was depicted in 54% of the scenes that they analyzed. The 54% figure is much closer to that found by Shor and Seida, who analyzed top-rated videos uploaded to Pornhub between 2008 and 2016 and found that 40% depicted physical aggression.[39] In summary, Bridges used a more expansive definition of physical aggression and as a result found that 88% of mainstream pornography depicts violence, and that statistic has now been used widely to characterize present-day Internet pornography.

Eran Shor's analysis of 172 Pornhub videos uploaded between 2000 and 2016 found that 36% to 46% depicted aggression.[27] Interestingly, the study revealed that there were differences in how videos were titled, and what they depicted, based on whether the video was in the "teen" category (featuring performers described as being 18 to 20 years old) or in an "adult" category (featuring performers 20 to 40 years old). For example, 18% of video clip titles in the teen category referred to aggression (i.e., "Gigantic Cock Rips Skinny Bitch"), whereas only 7% of pornography featuring someone 20 to 40 years old (i.e., "adult" pornography) did so. However, even though teen videos were more likely to be titled in a way suggesting aggression, pornography featuring adults was more likely to depict aggression: Shor found that 36% of teen and 46% of adult pornography depicted aggression, 15% of teen pornography and 23% of adult pornography showed forceful vaginal penetration, 13% of teen and 3% of adult pornography showed forceful anal penetration, and 22% of teen and 26% of adult porn showed forced gagging.[27] There were also differences in terms of gender equity; only 9% of teen videos showed a woman initiating a sex act instead of a male partner, while 18% of adult porn depicted women as initiators.[27] Worrisomely, in both teen and adult porn, women were unlikely to indicate verbal consent for sex; in 16% of teen porn, and 15% of adult porn, women clearly indicated verbal consent for sex.

Shor's results are consistent with the analysis of 4,009 pornography scenes from Pornhub and Xvideos conducted by Fritz and colleagues (2020) using clips from 2013–2014.[40] The Fritz study found that 35% to 45% of scenes included at least one act of physical aggression, and that spanking, gagging, slapping, hair-pulling, and choking were the five most common forms. Fritz and colleagues also found that women were the target of aggression in 97% of the pornography scenes, men were the aggressors in 76% of scenes, and that women's response to aggression was either neutral or positive and rarely negative.[40] In summary, the results of the most recent and most rigorous content analyses suggest that the content of mainstream Internet pornography often depicts aggression and gender inequity.

Feminist Pornography Is No Less Likely to Show Violence

Because mainstream pornography tends to depict aggression and gender inequity, people often wonder if there is an alternative source of pornography for sex-positive people who want to enjoy eroticism minus the misogyny. I am often asked where one can find feminist pornography. While I do have a list of websites and directors that I think might appeal to those seeking ethically produced pornography, it's a bit tricky to discern what qualifies as "feminist pornography." That often comes as a surprise to my students. Given that there was such a thing as the feminist pornography awards (in Canada, 2013–2014),[57] and there is a book called *The Feminist Porn Book*,[58] there are pornography directors who have described themselves as, or have been described as, feminists (e.g., Nina Hartley, Carol Queen, Candida Royale, Annie Sprinkle, Betty Dodson, Erika Lust, and others), and there are women's studies professors who write about "why feminist pornography matters,"[59] there must *be* feminist pornography—right? This is actually a deceptively difficult question. There certainly is pornography that is directed by women, pornography that centers women's pleasure, and pornography that markets itself as feminist. The Feminist Porn Awards, which bestowed awards upon videos each year from 2005 to 2017, used three criteria for determining if pornography was feminist: (1) Women and/or historically marginalized people were involved in the direction production and/or conception of the work. (2) The work depicted genuine pleasure, agency, and desire for all performers, especially women and historically marginalized people. (3) The work expanded the boundaries of sexual representation on film, challenged stereotypes, and presented a vision that set the content apart from most mainstream pornography.[58,60] In other words, and as summarized by Rebecca Whisnat, the difference between feminist porn and mainstream porn according to The Feminist Porn Awards is "not so much that different things [i.e., sex acts] are being done . . . but rather that more different kinds of people are shown doing them." And, as Whisnat argued, just because pornography shows different kinds of performers, or is made by women—it may nevertheless depict acts of aggression directed at women, celebrate women being sexually dominated, and glorify the sexual humiliation of women.[61] Does that count as feminist pornography? Perhaps.

That there is no way to arbitrate what qualifies as feminist media is not unique to pornography. For example, Amanda Hess recently wrote in the *New York Times* that "there is a growing sense that there is no bright line between feminist material and mainstream material."[62] In my experience, popular conceptions about what feminist pornography might be varies. Some imagine that what is meant by the term "feminist pornography" is pornography that depicts two women engaged in consensual, mutually pleasurable, gentle, and non-kinky sex, in a comfortable or beautiful natural setting— or, as self-described feminist pornography producer Tristan Taormino has written: "romance and flowers and pretty lighting and nothing too hard."[63] Others imagine women in command of a sexual encounter with one or more people. Still others believe that what they see under the "popular with women" category on Pornhub is what is meant by feminist pornography. Importantly, the pornography posted to the "popular with women" category on mainstream sites tends to feature conventionally attractive, heteronormative-looking women.

Research suggests that Pornhub pornography in the "popular with women" category depicts fewer acts of physical aggression than mainstream pornography but is as likely to objectify women as mainstream pornography.[60] A content analysis of 300 pornographic scenes from the For Women category on Pornhub in 2014 compared feminist pornography from the queer feminist CrashPad series, the website of feminist pornographer Erika Lust, the For Women category of Pornhub, and mainstream pornography from Pornhub and found the following: mainstream pornography was four times more likely than queer feminist pornography to show women stripping, but 1.7 times less likely to show physical aggression against women.[60] That finding may surprise readers who would have guessed that feminist porn would be less likely to depict violence against women. Interestingly, some self-described feminist pornographers defend "eroticized depictions of female pain, abject submission, and even violence against women" and insist that these "need not disqualify something as feminist pornography."[61] One line of feminist argument is that women have a right to produce, profit from, consume, and enjoy depictions of female submission.

Public health professionals need to know that classifying pornography as either feminist or mainstream is not a straightforward, and perhaps not a possible, task. It would make things easier if there were certain pornography that could be stamped "feminist" or "organic" or "ethically produced" or "safe to watch" and we could celebrate and protect that pornography while attempting to limit access to more harmful forms. But when producers and directors promote their work as feminist, it may be because there is a commercial market for so-called feminist pornography. The word "feminist" can be used for marketing purposes and does not necessarily indicate anything about the content of the pornography.

Race and Racism in Contemporary Pornography

Given that racism and race-based inequity are two of the largest drivers of public health problems, public health professionals will be curious about pornography content analyses that have examined race. Unfortunately, these are too rare. Exceptions include two content reviews from the 1990s,[43] and one recent content analysis by Zhou and Paul (2016) on videos taken from the

"Asian women" category of Xvideos.com.[64] In addition, some basic information about the race of performers is available. In their analysis of 172 Pornhub videos uploaded between 2000 and 2016, Shor and Golriz found that approximately 55% of pornography featured a white man, 30% featured a Black man, 10% featured an Asian man, and only 5% featured a Latino man. Asian women were comparatively overrepresented. Approximately 37% of pornography videos that they analyzed featured white women, 28% Black women, 16% Latina women, 1% Middle Eastern women, and 17% Asian women.[51] For comparison purposes, according to the 2018 American Community Survey, the population of the United States is 72% white, 18% Hispanic or Latino, 13% Black or African American, and 5% Asian—so Black and Asian men and women appear to be overrepresented as pornography performers.

Cowan and Campbell (1994) analyzed the content of 54 videos and found that Black pornography performers were given lower status in the scenes that they analyzed, that Black women were the targets of more acts of aggression than white women in the pornography scenes, and that Black men engaged in fewer intimate behaviors than white men. Cowan and Campbell also found that interracial pornography was more aggressive than same-race pornography. They concluded that "pornography is racist as well as sexist" (p. 323).[43] Monk-Turner and Purcell (1999) analyzed 40 videos and found that that Black women experienced more violence from both white and Black men than did white women.[44] They also found that white women were more likely to experience violence during sex with a white male partner than a Black man. Zhou and Paul randomly sampled 3,053 pornography videos from Xvideos.com and employed 27 undergraduate students in the coding of the videos in 2013. They found that Asian women were depicted differently than women of other races in pornography, were treated less aggressively, were less objectified, but also had lower agency in sexual activities.[64]

Because so few content analyses have been conducted to answer questions about how depictions of people by race may be evolving over time, and about racism and pornography, this could be a fruitful area for emerging public health and pornography scholars to contribute. Those with an interest in studying race, racism, and pornography will find that guiding theoretical arguments have been made by gender studies scholars, most notably in books by Mireille Miller-Young and Jennifer Nash. Miller-Young and Nash focus on Blackness and pornography.[65,66] Both complicate "the one-dimensional view of race in pornography, in part derived from anti-pornography feminism, which argues that pornography and its aesthetics reduce Black women to the hypersexualized objects of a racist representational discourse."[67] Like

Cowan and Campbell, anti-pornography activists and scholars have proposed that pornography concentrates and amplifies racist stereotypes in its content and perpetuates racism through its labor practices. Both Miller-Young and Nash agree with the idea that Black people have been depicted as hypersexual and particularly objectified in pornography, but both also suggest that a more complicated analysis of Black pornography performance is necessary—that pornography has, for example, helpfully "played with . . . tropes of Black female sexuality."[67] These are important arguments that push back against overly simplistic views on the issue of racism in pornography. Meanwhile, empirical questions remain about the impact of pornography on viewers' racism, and on industry labor practices and policy on the occupational health, safety, and well-being of Black, indigenous, and other people of color (BIPOC) who choose to make pornography.

Conclusions

The primary takeaway from this consideration of the content of pornography is that there is an extraordinarily wide variety. This makes it difficult to generalize any particular statement to all pornography, so public health professionals should specify the precise media type and subgenre they mean to indicate when they are discussing or writing about pornography.

The fact that there is a wide, and perhaps ever-widening, variety is not necessarily in and of itself a threat. The diversity of the content of pornography *may* be a concern. Mainly, though, concerns about the content of pornography tend to focus on two possibilities: that pornography is depicting violence and aggression, and that pornography is objectifying women. Content analyses that have been conducted over the past four decades have generally revealed that a substantial minority of contemporary free online pornography depicts acts of aggression, including strangulation. Multiple content analyses have found that aggression in pornography is overwhelming directed at women by male aggressors, and that women typically react with neutrality or pleasure to the aggression—which is at odds with the fact that only 14.2% of US adult women report that they find the idea of experiencing pain as part of sex very or somewhat appealing.[56] Research also suggests that mainstream, free, online pornography rarely centers female pleasure. Public health professionals should know that it is possible to study the content of pornography and to track changes in the content over time in order to characterize it.

References

1. Pappas, S. 2010. "The History of Pornography No More Prudish Than the Present." https://www.livescience.com/8748-history-pornography-prudish-present.html
2. Marcus, S. 2009. *The Other Victorians: A Study of Sexuality and Pornography in Mid-Nineteenth Century England*. London, UK: Transaction Publishers.
3. Slade, J. W. 2006. "Eroticism and Technological Regression: The Stag Film." *History and Technology* 22, no. 1: 27–52.
4. Meltzer, M. "What If Porn Had No Pictures?" *The New York Times,* November 20, 2019. Fast Forward Series.
5. Dickson, E. J. 2019. "Waterboarding for Pleasure: When Kink Violates the Geneva Convention." https://www.rollingstone.com/culture/culture-features/waterboarding-kink-sex-bdsm-torture-779066/
6. Hald, G. M., and A. Štulhofer. 2016. "What Types of Pornography Do People Find Arousing and Do They Cluster? Assessing Types and Categories of Pornography in a Large-Scale Online Sample." *The Journal of Sex Research* 53, no. 7: 849–859.
7. Ogas, O., and S. Gaddam. 2011. *A Billion Wicked Thoughts: What the World's Largest Experiment Reveals about Human Desire*. Dutton.
8. Yang, W. 2011. "*A Billion Wicked Thoughts,* by Ogi Ogas and Sai Gaddam: Book Review." https://www.nytimes.com/2011/07/31/books/review/a-billion-wicked-thoughts-by-ogi-ogas-and-sai-gaddam-book-review.html
9. Herbenick, D., T. C. Fu, P. Wright, et al. 2020. "Diverse Sexual Behaviors and Pornography Use: Findings from a Nationally Representative Probability Survey of Americans Aged 18 to 60 Years." *The Journal of Sexual Medicine* 17, no. 4: 623–633.
10. Dewey, C. 2019. "Is Rule 34 Actually True? An Investigation into the Internet's Most Risqué Law." https://www.washingtonpost.com/news/the-intersect/wp/2016/04/06/is-rule-34-actually-true-an-investigation-into-the-internets-most-risque-law/
11. Pornhub Insights. 2019. "2017 Year in Review—Pornhub Insights." https://www.pornhub.com/insights/2017-year-in-review
12. Spitznagel, E. 2019. "Where the Filthy Things Are." *Popular Mechanics* https://www.popularmechanics.com/culture/web/a29623446/pornhub-porn-data-storage/
13. PotatoPro.com. n.d. "Potato Statistics." https://www.potatopro.com/united-states/potato-statistics
14. Sedacca, M. 2017. "The Craven Reason for All Those Weird-Ass Oreo Flavors." https://www.gq.com/story/the-business-strategy-behind-oreos-constant-weird-new-flavors
15. Tuohy, W. 2015. "How Porn Is Warping the Male Mind." https://www.dailytelegraph.com.au/rendezview/rougher-harder-violent-how-porn-is-warping-the-male-mind/news-story/504698ce318f551052847f13ac678fd1
16. Landripet, I., V. Busko, and A. Stulhofer. 2019. "Testing the Content Progression Thesis: A Longitudinal Assessment of Pornography Use and Preference for Coercive and Violent Content Among Male Adolescents." *Social Science Research* 81: 32–41.
17. Seigfried-Spellar, K. C., and M. K. Rogers. 2013. "Does Deviant Pornography Use Follow a Guttman-like Progression?" *Computers in Human Behavior* 29, no. 5: 1997–2003.
18. Initiative Truth. 2018. "JUUL e-Cigarette Craze Highlights Why Flavored Tobacco Products Are So Dangerous|Truth Initiative." https://truthinitiative.org/research-resources/emerging-tobacco-products/juul-e-cigarette-craze-highlights-why-flavored-tobacco
19. Hsu, G., J. Y. Sun, and S-H. Zhu. 2018. "Evolution of Electronic Cigarette Brands From 2013–2014 to 2016–2017: Analysis of Brand Websites." *Journal of Medical Internet Research* .20, no. 3: e80.

20. Schneller, L. M., M. Bansal-Travers, M. L. Goniewicz, S. McIntosh, D. Ossip, and R. J. O'Connor. 2018. "Use of Flavored Electronic Cigarette Refill Liquids Among Adults and Youth in the US-Results from Wave 2 of the Population Assessment of Tobacco and Health Study (2014–2015)." *PLOS One* .13, no. 8: e0202744.

21. Joy, A. 2016. "An In-Depth Guide to Erotic Manga." https://theculturetrip.com/asia/japan/articles/an-in-depth-guide-to-erotic-manga/

22. McCurry, J. 2014. "Japan Bans Real-Life Child Sexual Abuse Material but Cartoons Remain Legal." The Guardian, https://www.theguardian.com/world/2014/jun/05/japan-bans-real-life-child-sexual-abuse-material-but-cartoons-remain-legal

23. United States v. Handley, 564 F. Supp. 2d 996 (S.D. Iowa 2008).

24. The Harvard Law Review Association. 2006. "Inbred Obscurity: Improving Incest Laws in the Shadow of the 'Sexual Family.'" *Harvard Law Review* 119, no. 8: 2464–2485.

25. O'Neil, L. 2018. "Incest Is the Fastest Growing Trend in Porn. Wait, What?" @Esquire.

26. Juzwiak, R. 2020. "How Likely Is It That I'm Seeing Actual Kids When I Watch "Barely Legal" Videos Online?" https://slate.com/human-interest/2020/02/barely-legal-videos-online-child-exploitation-explainer.html

27. Shor, E. 2019. "Age, Aggression, and Pleasure in Popular Online Pornographic Videos." *Violence Against Women* 25, no. 8: 1018–1036.

28. Shahbaz, C., and P. Chirinos. 2016. *Becoming a Kink Aware Therapist*. New York: Routledge.

29. Lee, E. M., K. R. Klement, and B. J. Sagarin. 2015. "Double Hanging During Consensual Sexual Asphyxia: A Response to Roma, Pazzelli, Pompili, Girardi, and Ferracuti (2013)." *Archives of Sexual Behavior* 44, no. 7: 1751–1753.

30. Keenan, J. "A Spanking Fetish Is Not Revealed Easily." *The New York Times,* 20121109, 2012.

31. Richters, J., R. O. De Visser, C. E. Rissel, A. E. Grulich, and A. M. A. Smith. 2008. "Demographic and Psychosocial Features of Participants in Bondage and Discipline, 'Sadomasochism' or Dominance and Submission (BDSM): Data from a National Survey." *The Journal of Sexual Medicine* 5, no. 7: 1660–1668.

32. Connolly, P. H. 2006. "Psychological Functioning of Bondage/Domination/Sado-Masochism (BDSM) Practitioners." *Journal of Psychology & Human Sexuality* 18, no. 1: 79–120.

33. De Neef, N., V. Coppens, W. Huys, and M. Morrens. 2019. "Bondage-Discipline, Dominance-Submission and Sadomasochism (BDSM) From an Integrative Biopsychosocial Perspective: A Systematic Review." *Sexual Medicine* 7, no. 2: 129–144.

34. Khan, U. 2014. *Vicarious Kinks: S/M in the Socio-Legal Imaginary*. Toronto: University of Toronto Press.

35. Smid, W. J., and E. C. Wever. 2019. "Mixed Emotions: An Incentive Motivational Model of Sexual Deviance." *Sexual Abuse: A Journal of Research and Treatment* 31, no. 7: 731–764.

36. Sagarin, B. J., B. Cutler, N. Cutler, K. A. Lawler-Sagarin, and L. Matuszewich. 2009. "Hormonal Changes and Couple Bonding in Consensual Sadomasochistic Activity." *Archives of Sexual Behavior* 38, no. 2: 186–200.

37. Cohut, M. 2019. "Why Do Some People Enjoy Experiencing Pain During Sex?" https://www.medicalnewstoday.com/articles/325419.php

38. McKee, A. 2015. "Methodological Issues in Defining Aggression for Content Analyses of Sexually Explicit Material." *Archives of Sexual Behavior* 44, no. 1: 81–87.

39. Shor, E., and K. Seida. 2019. "'Harder and Harder'? Is Mainstream Pornography Becoming Increasingly Violent and Do Viewers Prefer Violent Content?" *The Journal of Sex Research* 56, no. 1: 16–28.

40. Fritz, N., V. Malic, B. Paul, and Y. Zhou. 2020. "A Descriptive Analysis of the Types, Targets, and Relative Frequency of Aggression in Mainstream Pornography." *Archives of Sexual Behavior* 49: 3041–3053. https://doi.org/10.1007/s10508-020-01773-0

41. Harsanyi, M. 1979. *Statistical Survey of Sexual Behavior in Erotic Films, 1910–75.* Bloomington: University of Indiana.
42. Malamuth, N. M., and B. Spinner. 1980. "A Longitudinal Content Analysis of Sexual Violence in the Best-Selling Erotic Magazines." *The Journal of Sex Research* 16, no. 3: 226–237.
43. Cowan, G., and R. Campbell. 1994. "Racism and Sexism in Interracial Pornography: A Content Analysis." *Psychology of Women Quarterly* 18: 323–338.
44. Monk Turner, E., and H. C. Purcell. 1999. "Sexual Violence in Pornography: How Prevalent Is It?" *Gender Issues* 17, no. 2: 58–67.
45. Vannier, S. A., A. B. Currie, and L. F. O'Sullivan. 2014. "Schoolgirls and Soccer Moms: A Content Analysis of Free 'Teen' and 'MILF' Online Pornography." *The Journal of Sex Research* 51, no. 3: 253–264.
46. Carrotte, E. R., A. C. Davis, and M. S. Lim. 2020. "Sexual Behaviors and Violence in Pornography: Systematic Review and Narrative Synthesis of Video Content Analyses." *Journal of Medical Internet Research* 22, no. 5: e16702.
47. Scott, J. E., and S. J. Cuvelier. 1993. "Violence and Sexual Violence in Pornography—Is It Really Increasing." *Archives of Sexual Behavior* 22, no. 4: 357–371.
48. Palmer, C. E. 1979. "Pornographic Comics: A Content Analysis." *The Journal of Sex Research* 15, no. 4: 285–298.
49. Slade, J. W. 1984. "Violence in the Hard-core Pornographic Film: A Historical Survey." *Journal of Communication* 34, no. 3: 148–163.
50. Willis, M., S. N. Canan, K. N. Jozkowski, and A. J. Bridges. 2020. "Sexual Consent Communication in Best-Selling Pornography Films: A Content Analysis." *The Journal of Sex Research* 57, no. 1: 52–63.
51. Shor, E., and G. Golriz. 2019. "Gender, Race, and Aggression in Mainstream Pornography." *Archives of Sexual Behavior* 48, no. 3: 739–751.
52. Bridges, A. J., R. Wosnitzer, E. Scharrer, C. Sun, and R. Liberman. 2010. "Aggression and Sexual Behavior in Best-Selling Pornography Videos: A Content Analysis Update." *Violence Against Women* 16, no. 10: 1065–1085.
53. Hamblin, J. 2016. "How One State Declared Pornography a 'Public-Health Crisis.'" https://www.theatlantic.com/health/archive/2016/04/a-crisis-of-education/478206/
54. Fight the New Drug. 2017. "Study Shows 88% Of Popular Porn Videos Contain Violence." https://fightthenewdrug.org/popular-videos-violence/
55. Parker, K. 2019. "Think Rape Porn Is Just a Kink? Tell That to Victims of Sexual Violence." https://10daily.com.au/views/a190903eswkf/think-rape-porn-is-just-a-kink-tell-that-to-victims-of-sexual-violence-20190904
56. Herbenick, D., J. Bowling, T-C. J. Fu, B. Dodge, L. Guerra-Reyes, and S. Sanders. 2017. "Sexual Diversity in the United States: Results from a Nationally Representative Probability Sample of Adult Women and Men." *PLOS One* 12, no. 7: e0181198–e0181198.
57. Feminist Porn Awards. 2019. http://www.feministpornawards.com/blog/the-feminist-porn-awards-how-did-it-all-start/
58. Taormino, T., Constance Penley, Celine Parrenas Shimizu, and Mireille Miller-Young, eds. 2013. *The Feminist Porn Book: The Politics of Producing Pleasure.* New York: Feminist Press.
59. Potter, C. 2016. "Not Safe for Work: Why Feminist Pornography Matters." *Dissent* 63, no. 2: 104–114.
60. Fritz, N., and B. Paul. 2017. "From Orgasms to Spanking: A Content Analysis of the Agentic and Objectifying Sexual Scripts in Feminist, for Women, and Mainstream Pornography." *Sex Roles* 77, no. 9-10: 639–652.
61. Whisnat, R. 2016. "'But What About Feminist Porn?' Examining the Work of Tristan Taormino." *Sexualization, Media, & Society* 2, no. 2: 2374623816631727.
62. Hess, A. "Women in Pornography: Who Gets to Be Sexy." *New York Times,* May 6, 2018.

63. Taormino, T. 2013. "Calling the Shots: Feminist Porn in Theory and Practice." In *The Feminist Porn Book: The Politics of Producing Pleasure*, edited by T. Taormino, C. Parrenas-Shimuzu, C. Penley, and M. Miller-Young, 79–93. New York: Feminist Press.

64. Zhou, Y. Y., and B. Paul. 2016. "Lotus Blossom or Dragon Lady: A Content Analysis of 'Asian Women' Online Pornography." *Sexuality and Culture* 20, no. 4: 1083–1100.

65. Miller-young, M. 2014. A Taste for Brown Sugar: Black Women in Pornography. Durham and London: Duke University Press.

66. Nash, J. C. 2014. *The Black Body in Ecstasy: Reading Race, Reading Pornography*. Durham and London: Duke University Press.

67. Shah, S. 2015. "Pleasure and Performance." https://www.wcwonline.org/Women-s-Review-Of-Books-Sept/Oct-2015/pleasure-and-performance

5

Pornography and Aggression

Sexual assault is prevalent and often is devastatingly consequential for survivors, their families, and others. In the United States, 43.6% of adult women and 24.8% of men have experienced some form of contact sexual violence in their lifetimes.[1] As many as 16% (1 in 6) US adult women and 9.6% of men have experienced sexual coercion in their lifetimes, meaning that they have been worn down by someone who repeatedly asked for sex or have been otherwise pressured into sex.[1] And the consequences of sexual assault can be long-lasting and debilitating.[2,3] Sexual assault isn't the only problem, though. A recent nationally representative survey found that 23.9% of adult women and 10.3% of adult men in the United States report that at least once during sex someone did something that made them feel "scared," such as holding them down, choking them without consent, engaging in rough sex, or introducing sex toys or bondage play without permission.[4]

As many as 21% of US adult men and 11% of women report having seen pornography depicting simulated rape.[5] Naturally, many people who are concerned about pornography, or wonder if they should be concerned about pornography, want an answer to the question: Does watching pornography cause people to perpetrate sexual assault? This is the billion-dollar question at the heart of much of the controversy about pornography in contemporary society, and which has been the subject of at least three US government commission inquiries (the 1970 US Commission on Obscenity and Pornography, the 1986 US Attorney General's Committee on Pornography, and 1986 Surgeon General's Workshop on Pornography and Public Health).[6] If pornography demonstrably causes harm in the form of interpersonal aggression, many people would be motivated to curtail it. If, on the other hand, it's simply a matter of taste—that is, pornography depicts sexual acts that many people find uninspiring, disgusting, or even horrible, but there was certainty that these depictions do not translate into harms caused by viewers, the "live and let live" or "to each their own" attitude would likely prevail.

In this chapter, I offer a basic overview of the research findings on aggression perpetration and pornography. However, for those who can't wait to know the answer to the billion-dollar question, a "too long; didn't read" (TLDR): as

Pornography and Public Health. Emily F. Rothman, Oxford University Press. © Oxford University Press 2021.
DOI: 10.1093/oso/9780190075477.003.0005

Dr. Neil Malamuth persuasively argued in a 2018 paper in *Aggression and Violent Behavior*, it matters what kind of pornography is being used and the person who is using it.[7] In other words, it depends.

Operationalizing Aggression

In order to study whether pornography influences aggression, researchers must choose how to operationalize "pornography" and "aggression." Studies to date have generally investigated two different types of pornography for effect on viewers: "violent" and "nonviolent" pornography. But the word "violent" isn't really a good fit for the type of pornography that researchers often want to study in this category. A better name for it may be "nonconsensual" pornography because some of the sexual acts are not physically violent. For example, all child sexual abuse imagery (i.e., child pornography) and zoophilic pornography is nonconsensual, as underage minors and animals cannot consent to sex. Other types of pornography can be more difficult to classify. Historically, bondage, discipline/dominance, submission/sadism, and masochism (BDSM) pornography did not always show or depict participants giving consent, which made it straightforward for researchers to classify it as "violent" and "nonconsensual," even if the performers had consented to film it. Today some pornographers precede or conclude BSDM scenes with clips of participants stating that they are eager to participate.[*] This trend has made it more difficult to classify BDSM pornography videos for research purposes. On the one hand, the videos depict what looks like aggression (e.g., one partner receiving physical violence or being humiliated), and some viewers may not see the filmed consent portion of the video, leaving them with the impression it is not consensual. On the other hand, since the performer has given a statement of consent, categorizing it as violent or nonconsensual may misrepresent what is depicted.

Even before BDSM videos began to show consent statements, there was controversy about whether the category violent/nonconsensual pornography should include all pornography that appears violent to the viewer, or whether it should be limited to pornography that is truly nonconsensual. Here is the dilemma: some pornography looks violent to some viewers because what they see are actions that in everyday life, or with a nonconsenting partner, would be violence: slaps, spanks, hair-pulling, pinching, etc. But if what looks like violence isn't intended to harm, damage, or hurt someone, and the participants are enjoying it—should it count as "violence" for pornography research purposes? One the one hand, according to US state laws, if one person harms another physically during BDSM or any other activity, it may indeed count as a criminal offense, even if the act was consensual.[8] But for the people who enjoy BDSM (or getting tattoos or piercings or engaging in other consensual activities that cause scars), this is a problem because it criminalizes what might be harmless pleasure. In brief, for many who choose to engage in BDSM, hard and pain-producing physical contact feels pleasant; they like to experience stinging, pinching, and pressure sensations in sexual contexts.[8] Some also like the theatrical aspect of BDSM that makes them feel like they are in a dangerous or violent scene. Feeling scared-but-safe, whether on a roller coaster, during a horror film, or during sex, can thrill some people in a positive way. In fact, research suggests that those who are hyposexual (that is, with a very low libido) may be particularly likely to benefit from the additional sensational boost that they might get from feeling such a thrill—it jump starts their sexual arousal response.[9] For these reasons, some pornography researchers object to classifying all pornography that appears to depict violence as "violent pornography," because the performers may have consented and may be experiencing it as enjoyable, no matter how it looks from the outside.[10]

But there is a counterargument that favors classifying even consensual BDSM pornography as violent for research purposes. The argument is twofold. First, there is a possibility that some BDSM-themed pornography is coerced or hasn't been safely performed. For example, the performers may not be using a safe word that would stop the sexual activity and may not have had a thorough discussion of what sex acts are alright with them in advance. In other words, what looks like violence may actually be violence, even if it's marketed as BDSM. Second, viewers, and particularly younger viewers, may take what they see at face value. What looks to them like violence may be interpreted by them as violence. This should help the reader to understand one anti-pornography viewpoint. In general, anti-pornography activists are primarily concerned about what the viewer sees, and what pornography looks like—even if the performers are having a good time acting it out. By way of example, anti-violence activists may be concerned that children who watch movies depicting gun battles are affected by that viewing experience regardless of whether the actors enjoyed acting out the gun battle scene. Considering that some viewers may take pornography at face value, some researchers have made the choice to classify pornography according to what the pornography looks like to the viewer, even if performers are in control of the scene and experiencing authentic pleasure.

Returning to the idea that it matters what kind of pornography is being used and which person is using it, let's now consider the viewer. Research suggests that if the viewer is someone who has antisocial personality characteristics or underlying hostility toward women, or other factors that place them at increased risk of sexual aggression perpetration, they are more likely than other pornography viewers to engage in sexually aggressive behavior subsequent to the pornography exposure.[7] But for people who are not at high risk for sexual aggression in general, even viewing violent/nonconsensual pornography does not appear to affect sexually aggressive behavior.[7] In other words, as Malamuth put it, pornography may add fuel to the fire if a person is already at risk of perpetrating sexual aggression, but for the average person, available evidence does not suggest that viewing pornography inspires sexual violence perpetration.

Some people find the idea that pornography may not be a primary driver of sexual assault hard to believe because of their *a priori* beliefs about pornography (i.e., that it is immoral or sinful), misunderstanding about causes of sexual violence (i.e., that it is primarily perpetrated by strangers with psychopathy), and about sexuality (i.e., that it is easily influenced by exposure to short video clips). In general, people have a difficult time accepting science findings that counter their own deeply held beliefs (i.e., confirmation bias). However, I suspect that there are people who may be relieved to find out that the causal relationship between pornography viewing and sexual aggression perpetration may be weak and not clearly established. For example, people who find themselves aroused by kinky pornography and were concerned that seeing it would turn them into sexual aggressors may feel less anxious, and parents who are worried that their children are going to be irrevocably damaged by one exposure to BDSM pornography may be able to avoid panicking.

Caveats about the Evidence about Pornography and Aggression

Before we dive into the research base on pornography and aggression, a few preliminary concerns must be addressed. First, there is evidence that pornography viewing may influence attitudes, and in particular, negative attitudes about women. Here I want to flag a basic concern about this evidence: we don't know how well attitudes predict behavior. In other words, attitudes are one thing, but whether you behave in ways consistent with your attitude is a whole other question. Here's an example: I have a great attitude about exercise, and even intentions to exercise, but this turns out to be a relatively weak predictor of whether I will actually go exercise. When it comes to violence perpetration, social science hasn't yet pinpointed the strength of the association between attitudes and behavior. It's *possible* that attitudes matter a lot, and that watching pornography makes people hold women in lower esteem, which translates into worse treatment of women. It is *also* possible that watching pornography may cause people to hold women in lower esteem, but that attitude does *not* influence actual aggressive behavior against women very much. The problem is that until the link between attitudes and behavior is more firmly established, simply proving that pornography use leads to bad attitudes about women may not be a sufficiently meaningful endpoint.

Another basic consideration is that when we ponder a potential causal link between pornography and aggression, we need to think about how aggression has been defined. Historically, researchers and politicians have been interested in a possible link between pornography and rape, or child sexual abuse perpetration, but not other forms of aggression, such as peer bullying, elder abuse, or self-directed aggression, such as suicide. Moreover, the interest has been primarily in physical forms of aggression as the outcome, but not verbal or psychological abuse, and almost exclusively about a possible link between pornography and men's perpetration of sexual violence against women or children, not about women's sexual violence perpetration. More recently, some researchers have posited that pornography may influence other forms of violence, such as dating violence or partner abuse,[11] and one US representative once even suggested that pornography may influence the propensity for people to perpetrate mass homicide.[12] (NB: No evidence suggests that pornography influences mass homicide.) So as we review the evidence on pornography and aggression, it is important to bear in mind that most researchers have defined aggression as "sexual violence perpetrated by men against women or children." If the definition of aggression was broadened to include psychological abuse, perhaps the measures of association between pornography exposure and aggression-related outcomes would be stronger.

Can People's Sexual Interests Really Be Changed Because of Watching Videos?

Another fundamental question to answer as a prelude to a review of this literature is: In theory, how is it possible that human sexual attraction or sexual behavior can be modified by watching videos, sexually explicit or otherwise? In other words, to what extent are people born with their sexual attractions and desires, to what extent do they also develop over time in response to the environment or culture, and how malleable are our attractions? The answer is debated, but most sexologists agree that sexuality is a complex construct that reflects the interplay of biological, cognitive, and social factors and includes components like romantic attraction, sexual behavior, and sexual identity.[13] While sexual orientation typically remains fixed over the life course for most people, some do experience changes in gender attraction, and most experience changes in other dimensions of attraction, such as feeling less attracted to adolescents as one becomes a mature adult themselves.[14] The strength of humans' sexual response to particular stimuli can change over time, too. For example, sexual desire for one's partner may wane over time due to familiarity, and sexual arousal may be facilitated by the introduction of novel stimuli, such as a new fantasy, new toy, or new partner.

The idea that human sexuality can be manipulated, either by oneself or an external force, is controversial. For example, conversion therapy, which is a type of Sexual Orientation Change Effort (SOCE), seeks to change people's sexual orientation from homosexual to heterosexual and has been opposed by numerous professional medical organizations and has been banned for minors in multiple states due to the documented harms of subjecting people to it.[15] There is no evidence to support the effectiveness of conversion therapy. However, the idea that sexuality is immutable—that one is born with a permanent and inflexible sexual orientation—has been problematized by recent studies suggesting that sexuality and attraction may be more fluid than previously understood, and that the relatively limited categories of gay, straight, and bisexual are not a good fit for how human sexuality actually works.[16] Even if some people may experience sexuality as fluid over the life course, though, there is little evidence to suggest that attraction can be changed by watching pornography videos.

The claim that watching pornography, even BDSM or violent pornography, will transform nonkinky and non-sexually aggressive people into those who want to engage in nonconsensual sadistic sex has been the subject of investigation for decades. One thing that we know currently, but did not know in decades past, was that fantasies about inflicting or receiving pain during sex are uncommon but not exceedingly rare. A nationally representative study of 18- to 60-year-old US adults found that only 9% of men and 14% of women find the thought of actually experiencing pain during sex very or somewhat appealing.[5] However, 21% of US adult women report having been choked (i.e., strangled) by a sexual partner in their lifetimes, 20% report having ever engaged in BDSM, and 66% report having ever been spanked.[5] One reason that some people fantasize about pain and about rape is that things that are off-limits, taboo, or wildly outside our realities typically cause more excitement than things solidly within our realities. (Try fantasizing about winning a billion dollars and about finding a quarter on the sidewalk and see which one gets you more engaged.) Fantasies can serve as an escape, an outlet, a method of self-regulation, a way or reorganizing memories or thoughts to cope or to regulate emotion, and can be used, helpfully, for arousal.[17]

One of the theories about the way that pornography could influence human aggression is through the route of fantasies. Sexual scripting theory suggests that people might observe aggressive sexual behavior in pornography, that it may influence their fantasies, and they may begin to rehearse sexual aggression in their mind, which may facilitate taking action on that fantasy.[18] Other theories that have been used to explain a possible pathway from pornography use to aggression include classical conditioning, or the idea that masturbating to violent pornography could create a positive reinforcement for having violent sexual fantasies, which could lead to sexual violence perpetration.[19] Excitation transfer theory proposes that if people become angry or, essentially, feel pumped up in an aggressive way because of watching pornography, they will unleash that aggression on any convenient target.[20–22] Some feminist and cultural theories posit what I think of as the "it's in the water" theory, meaning that they propose that the existence of nonconsensual pornography contributes in a general way to a social climate that encourages the treatment of women and girls as sexual objects, and that these social norms in turn promote sexual violence.[23] So, even if pornography doesn't directly influence an individual to leap out of his seat and go perpetrate rape after watching pornography, the idea is that steady exposure to sexually violent images as entertainment may enhance cultural norms that encourage sexual aggression. This is entirely possible, just as it is possible that pornography simply reflects our existing cultural norms instead of creating them. Or, it could be both (i.e., recursive): pornography shapes cultural norms, and pornography reflects the norms of the cultures in which it is created.

Pornography and Impersonal Sex

Whether pornography influences people to have sex that can be characterized as less personal, or more casual (also called "recreational"), has been a commonly investigated question in pornography research.[24] Impersonal sex is sex that is believed to lack emotional intimacy and commitment. The concern is that impersonal sex is potentially associated with increased risk of sexual assault perpetration, lower sexual satisfaction, and diminished mental health.[24] Before relaying the findings on pornography use and impersonal sex, I think it's important to consider a few assumptions underlying the research question. First, there is a good chance that the majority of sexual assault is carried out by people who actually feel emotionally or otherwise connected to the victim. Yes, you read that correctly! The idea that sexual assault is primarily perpetrated by people who are strangers to their victims is incorrect. The majority of sexual assault is perpetrated by people who are acquainted with their victims as intimate partners, spouses, friends, coworkers, family members, and other acquaintances.[25] There is no guarantee that being emotionally or otherwise committed to a partner results in noncoercive, nonforced, or pleasurable sex. Though people who don't have an emotional connection to their partner may be at increased risk for using coercive strategies to have sex and may be more likely to ignore nonverbal cues that their partner is feeling hesitant or reluctant to have sex,[24] it is not clear if this is true or how likely this hypothesis may be. What's more, some people have more pleasurable sex with casual partners, perhaps because they feel less inhibited; for those who choose to engage in casual sex, casual sex encounters appear to boost well-being,[26] though some studies find that more personal sex is associated with better sexual satisfaction for women.[27] In other words, impersonal sex isn't inherently bad for people, and sex with emotionally committed partners isn't inherently good for people, but there may be an assumption in some pornography research or advocacy that impersonal sex represents risk.

Most pornography depicts sex between uncommitted partners, and perhaps relatedly, pornography consumption is associated with more positive attitudes toward impersonal sex.[24] Tokunaga and colleagues (2019) conducted a meta-analysis of 70 research studies involving more than 60,000 individuals and found that viewing pornography was associated with more impersonal sexual attitudes, which were in turn associated with increased likelihood of engaging in impersonal sexual behavior. The authors conducted a regression analysis in which impersonal sexual behavior (the dependent variable) was regressed on pornography use (the independent variable) and the model controlled for attitudes about impersonal sex (the potential confounder). Pornography use was associated with impersonal sexual behavior, even when attitudes about impersonal sex were controlled for. However, there could still be confounding at play. It could be that a different confounding factor other than "attitudes toward impersonal sex" drove the relationship between pornography viewing and impersonal sexual behavior. And, because the analysis was cross-sectional, it could have been that people who engaged in impersonal sex were more likely to seek out pornography, meaning that there could be a reciprocal relationship between the behaviors. Nonetheless, the Tokunaga meta-analysis may be taken as one piece of preliminary evidence that pornography viewing could be causally related to viewers' impersonal sexual behavior.

Does Pornography Influence Viewers' Aggression?

There are four research study designs that have been used to investigate whether pornography causes sexual aggression. These are: (1) ecological time-series studies, also called population-level correlational studies; (2) experimental studies, also called laboratory studies; (3) case-control studies; and (4) meta-analyses.

Ecological time-series studies involve assessing the prevalence of an outcome in a place both before and after some kind of policy change or other environmental change. For example, assessing the prevalence of tooth caries both before and after a town began fluoridating its water, and comparing any changes in the tooth caries trends over time for that town and a comparison town that did not begin fluoridating water, might provide some evidence about whether fluoridation protected teeth. The problem with ecological time-series studies is that there is always a possibility that there is some other factor responsible for whatever changes one might observe in the intervention location, other than the suspected causal variable. For example, what if several new dentists moved their practices into town and started offering discounts right at the same time the town began fluoridating their water? This would confound results.

There have been at least 14 ecological studies at the country, state, and city level that examined pornography availability and sexual crimes. The first study was by Kupperstein and Wilson (1970), who studied uniform crime reports for the United States for the 1960 to 1969 period, when there was a surge in pornography availability.[28] The study found an overall decrease in sex crimes during that period, leading some to propose that pornography was providing a good outlet for would-be sexual criminals and decreasing crime, like a steam valve, while others took it more simply as evidence that pornography consumption was not likely to be *increasing* sexual violence. Next, Kutchinsky (1971) studied sex crimes in Copenhagen, Denmark, between the late 1950s and 1970s, because hard-core pornography became legal and widely available there in 1969.[29] He concluded that the increased availability of pornography caused no increase in reported rape and coincided with decreases in reports of exhibitionism and voyeurism. Ben-Veniste (1971) conducted a similar study, also in Copenhagen,[30] and found nearly identical results, though Bachy (1976) and Giglio (1985) used different methods and detected increases in rape rates in Denmark in 1970 to 1982.[31,32] Court (1984) studied data from the United States, England, New Zealand, Singapore, Denmark, Sweden, and states of Australia and argued that his study found that loosening restrictions on pornography was associated with increases in sex crimes, but his claims were challenged by other teams of researchers who argued that he did not interpret his own data correctly and had misunderstood Hawaiian laws.[33] Jaffee and Straus (1987) found that US state-level sex magazine circulation was associated with the rate of reported rape in that state, but they suggested that the correlation was likely attributable to variation in hypermasculinity by state, and not causal.[34] Baron and Straus (1987, 1989) and Baron (1990)[35] studied sex magazine circulation and rape and found that rape was associated with sex magazine circulation, but also negatively associated with gender equality, which they concluded was reason to doubt the relationship between pornography and rape rates was causal.[33,36,37] Scott and Schwalm (1988) found that there was no relationship between the number of adult movie theaters in a state and the state rape rate.[38] Gentry (1991) analyzed sex magazine circulation by metropolitan statistical areas and found that sex magazines were associated with the rape rate, but that the relationship disappeared when the percent of youth in the population was controlled.[39] Kutchinsky (1991) studied the prevalence of sex offenses in Denmark, West Germany, Sweden, and the United States between 1964 and 1984, because pornography restrictions were loosened during this 20-year period.[40] He found that although pornography became easier to find and purchase during that time, sex crimes did not increase any more than crime in general. Winick and Evans (1996) and Kimmel and Linders (1996) found minor increases in rape in specific US cities and states corresponding with increased availability of pornography, but neither team concluded that banning pornography would lead to a reduction in rape.[41,42] In short, as Robert Bauserman summarized in his thorough review of this literature (1996): "Overall, the nonexperimental evidence for a causal role of exposure to sexually explicit material in sex crimes is ambiguous and often contradictory" (p. 422).[33]

Experimental studies on pornography enjoyed their heyday in the 1980s. A series of laboratory-based experiments exposed adults to pornographic materials and then assessed their attitudes and aggressive behaviors, typically by inviting research participants to administer a shock to a female laboratory confederate, and their sexual response to the pornography (by assessing penile response). While the laboratory studies tended to show a small effect on antisocial and misogynistic attitudes, the extent to which attitudes influence sexual aggression is not clear. Models of sexual aggression consistently suggest that while attitudes are relevant to etiology, they are neither a necessary nor sufficient cause.[6] What's more, laboratory studies that have found an association of pornography viewing and subsequent nonsexual aggression in the laboratory setting have been found to have been influenced by the fact that a laboratory confederate typically provoked the respondent in some way.[6]

College students who volunteer to be part of laboratory experiments on pornography have also been found to differ in important ways from students who would not choose to participate in them, including being more willing to use aggression in general.[43] There are other problems with laboratory experiments involving pornography. A brief exposure to pornography in the laboratory may not be a good proxy for at-home viewership, and the effects could be different. For example, people at home may watch pornography for a longer period of time and have a tension-reducing orgasm, whereas in the lab they watch a brief clip, have no orgasm, and then are provoked by a lab confederate—causing them to behave aggressively, but under conditions that may not mirror those of the real world. All told, the experimental evidence is not considered persuasive with regard to a causal relationship between pornography viewing and subsequent sexual violence perpetration. A critical evaluation of the research literature on the association between pornography and sexual aggression published in 2001 found that there was overall "little support for a direct causal link between pornography use and sexual aggression" (p. 46), although the authors urged continued research on the role of pornography in sexual offending because of the seriousness of sexual assault.[6]

Case-control studies involving perpetrators of sexual violence and other criminals have assessed whether pornography is more commonly used by people who have committed sexual offenses than others. A 2019 systematic review of these studies by Mellor and Duff (2019) yielded mixed results.[44] The review identified 21 individual studies published between 1971 and 2014. Of these, five studies found that sexual offenders had less exposure to pornography than controls prior to offending during both preadolescence/adolescence and immediately prior to offending. Only one study found that exposure to pornography prior to offending was greater for those who perpetrated sexual violence as compared to another type of crime.[45] In other words, five studies found that the sexual violence perpetrators had seen *less* pornography than other criminals. The authors therefore concluded: "The consensus is that there is no relationship between early exposure to pornography prior to offending and a person then becoming an offender, therefore suggesting that early exposure to pornography is not a risk factor for sexually offending" (p. 124).[44] In other words, this systematic review found that children who see pornography are not more likely to grow up and perpetrate sexual assault than other people.[44]

The same systematic review did find that, compared to people who perpetrate sexual violence against adults, people who perpetrate violence against children *are* more likely to have used pornography prior to offending.[44] It also found that according to several studies, pornography use immediately prior to committing a crime was linked with less severe offenses—in other words, the individuals who viewed pornography and then perpetrated a crime were *less* likely to use coercive behavior[46] or force[47] and were less likely to commit coital acts, and their crimes involved fewer victims than those of perpetrators who had not been viewing pornography immediately before the crime.[47] However, contradictory results from other studies complicate this finding. Two studies found that pornography use was associated with the use of violence during offending, increased the odds of penetrative sexual acts, and with increased use of physical violence and humiliation during the perpetration of the crime.[48,49] In short, it's difficult to discern from studies of pornography use by sex offenders and other criminals whether, and under what conditions, pornography use exacerbates criminal offending.

A *meta-analysis* by Wright and colleagues (2016) combined effect sizes from 22 studies, comprising 13,234 men and 7,586 women.[50] The studies were published between 1994 and 2014 and used disparate definitions of pornography use and of aggressive behavior. All were studies of people in the general population (i.e., not sex offenders), none were clinical or laboratory studies where people were shown pornography by a researcher, and all of them assessed sexual aggression as a behavior, not attitudes or beliefs. Across the 22 studies, there was a small association between pornography use and sexual aggression ($r = 0.28$, 95% CI 0.24–0.32).[50] The individual estimates of effect size from each of the individual studies ranged from $r = 0.090$ to $r = 0.480$, meaning that none could be characterized as large or very strong. Wright and colleagues looked at the estimates from several different angles, trying to home in on a subgroup for which there was a particularly strong, or no, effect. Re-analyzing stratified by sex (male vs. female), age (adolescent vs. adult), and nation where the study was conducted (United States vs. other nations) found no substantial differences in subgroups. In other words, the effect was similar for men and women, youth and adults, and for people in the United States and other countries. To address the question of whether things have gotten worse since the advent of the Internet, the researchers also looked at the association between pornography use and aggression in or before 1995 or later and found that there was no difference (the r was identical based on year). When Wright and colleagues looked at the results by the content of the pornography that was studied, they found that qualitatively there was a small difference in the strength of the association based on whether the pornography viewed was violent pornography or nonviolent ($r = 0.37$ vs. $r = 0.27$, respectively), but the difference was not statistically significant. They also looked at study design, to see if the association was any different for cross-sectional and longitudinal studies. There was no difference. Wright and colleagues conclude that "the accumulated data leave little doubt that, on the average, individuals who consume pornography more frequently are more likely to hold attitudes conducive to sexual aggression and engage in actual acts of sexual aggression than individuals who do not consume pornography or who consume pornography less frequently" (p. 201). The results are consistent with the results of three prior meta-analyses (Allen et al., 1995; Hald et al., 2010).[51,52] In sum, the weight of the evidence derived from these meta-analyses supports the contention that pornography viewers may be more likely to be sexually aggressive—although whether it is the pornography that causes that aggression remains unclear. Moreover, if pornography influences aggressive behavior, the influence is small. The majority of pornography consumers are not violent, and the prevailing conclusion of research experts is that the simple act of watching pornography is not likely to be enough to activate someone into sexual aggression without other predisposing factors in place. However, whether pornography that features aggressive sexual behavior primarily directed by men at women may influence cultural norms that encourage tolerance for sexual violence in society remains an open question.

Criticisms of the Criticisms of Pornography and Aggression Research

If you are a public health advocate and you are presenting the mixed results of the research on pornography and aggression to an audience, you should be prepared to hear a few critiques—particularly from those who believe that pornography is dangerous. First, even if you acknowledge the possibility that pornography may influence social norms, you may also point out that a major weakness in this body of research is that some of the studies are correlational and causality cannot be determined from them. Those who are wedded to the idea that pornography causes violence may argue that a multitude of cross-sectional or correlational studies are sufficient evidence of a causal relationship between pornography and aggression. This is not true. Whether there are 30 or 30,000 correlational studies that suggest factor X is associated with factor Y, the sheer number of them does not make it more likely that the relationship is causal one. Unmeasured and uncontrolled confounding could be at the root of all 30,000 correlational studies. You may also hear the comment that no study is perfect, meaning that we should overlook flaws in pornography research. However, just because all studies have limitations does not mean that critiques of pornography research studies should be ignored. Importantly, the limitations could be valid, and the truth of the matter could be that the pornography is not causing the harm of which it is accused, and that other factors are responsible. Finally, you may hear that there is no feasible, ethical way to conduct large-scale randomized controlled trials of pornography exposure with longitudinal follow-up, and because it would be too difficult (or impossible) to carry out such a study, we will never solve the puzzle of whether pornography influences aggression and should give up on looking for evidence because public policy decisions can't wait for the far-off day when we have resolved this question. It may indeed be challenging to design research studies that answer questions about pornography and violence. But we should not give up on precision and accuracy and capitulate to advocacy efforts because the research is difficult. There are also costs of implementing public policies based on a lack of evidence. In this case, the costs of presuming that pornography causes violence if it does not should be delineated and weighed prior to taking action.

What Should Be Done

Working with the best available evidence, it would appear that pornography may exacerbate the propensity to perpetrate violence in some predisposed people and may contribute to social norms that encourage some frightening or criminal sexual behaviors,[4] although the strength of association between pornography use and the aggressive behaviors may be small and other factors may be more salient for preventing sexual violence more generally. This creates a bit of a conundrum for public health action. Practically speaking, what should be done about an exposure that appears to be very bad for a small percentage of people, but neutral for others? By way of example, we might consider the problem of Type 2 diabetes. For most people, consuming a few teaspoons of sugar each day is unlikely to cause substantial harm. But for people who have trouble metabolizing glucose, sugar can cause more serious problems. In other words, the very same exposure can cause substantially different outcomes depending upon the characteristics of the consumer. The US Centers for Disease Control and Prevention (CDC) recognizes that sugar consumption is a public health threat for those with diabetes in particular, and in response it urges those with diabetes to participate in a lifestyle change program that helps participants modify diet and exercise with the help of a lifestyle coach and a support group.[53] In other words, the primary public health response to an exposure that can have acute negative effects for approximately 12% of the population is to recommend lifestyle changes for the 12%. In addition, the CDC approach involves attempting to reach the one-third of American adults who are pre-diabetic for healthful lifestyle changes as well.

The analog for pornography would be to focus violence prevention efforts on those who are antisocial and hostile toward women, including limits on pornography use, and to try to reach the rest of the population who have pre-antisocial behavior problems or pre-misogynistic attitudes as well. The problem is that, in practical terms, opportunities to reach only those with antisocial behavioral tendencies and hostility toward women for lifestyle change promotion may be limited. Is it worth reducing everyone's access to BDSM pornography, because those who are antisocial and misogynist should be restricted? This is a question that has yet to be resolved.

Public health professionals have had to make decisions about how we should regulate other issues where only a small subset of the population may be at risk for harm. For example, collectively as a field, we advocate for restricting access to firearms for all people in order to reduce the population-level threats of suicide, homicide, and nonfatal injuries, even though it's only a minority of individuals who use firearms for these purposes and the majority engage in safe storage and handling practices. We advocate for all people to be required to wear seatbelts, life preservers, and ski helmets, even though a relatively small fraction of those who abide by the regulations will ever personally derive a direct benefit from these requirements, and in the meantime, all are denied the pleasure of feeling the wind in their hair or moving unhampered by safety belts and jackets. In 2020, we advocated for all people to stay at home to reduce the spread of COVID-19, even though only a small percentage of the population were expected to experience severe cases of the disease. In other words, in public health, sometimes we advocate to curtail certain products or behaviors even if most people get pleasure out of them because of concern for the small percentage of people who experience adverse effects. There are exceptions, though. For example, we haven't banned cars, or alcohol use, even though a small percentage of people drive cars while intoxicated.

In the case of pornography, perhaps only a minority of individuals will ever be activated by nonconsensual or child pornography to commit crimes, and even in those cases pornography is merely a catalyst for antisocial behavior to which they were predisposed. Should these few "bad apples" spoil the pleasure of the potentially much larger subset of people who enjoy violent-looking pornography with no ill effects? Perhaps, in line with some other public health policy decisions, we should pursue restricting access to violent-looking pornography for all individuals, even if it deprives them of pleasure, if that is what it takes to reduce sexual violence against even a small number of children, teenagers, college students, or adults. But there is a lot at stake: freedom of expression and the potential marginalization, if not demonization, of entire classes of people based on their sexual interests and attractions. And there are other models for regulation besides flat-out banning violent-looking pornography—perhaps we should be considering policies and laws that make it more difficult to put aggressive-looking content in front of certain viewers, but eschewing policies that attempt to eliminate its production entirely. Perhaps there will be ways to encourage pornography content producers to generate content that is less problematic—much in the same way that in the 1980s public health advocates persuaded television program producers to engineer the content of sitcoms to promote designated driving instead of driving under the influence.[54] The bottom line is that public health professionals have an obligation to take seriously the idea that even if it is only a small percentage of viewers who are activated by violent-looking pornography, people's rights to enjoy all types of pornography unfettered must be balanced against our obligation to protect the public from sexual harm.

References

1. Smith, S., X. Zhang, K. C. Basile, et al. 2018. "The National Intimate Partner and Sexual Violence Survey (NISVS): 2015 Data Brief: Updated Release." https://www.cdc.gov/violenceprevention/pdf/2015data-brief508.pdf

2. Rodgers, C., and D. Gruener. 1997. "Sequelae of Sexual Assault." *Primary Care Update for OB/GYNS* 4, no. 4: 143–146.

3. Arditte Hall, K. A., E. T. Healy, and T. E. Galovski. 2019. "The Sequelae of Sexual Assault." In *Handbook of Sexual Assault and Sexual Assault Prevention*, edited by W. T. O'Donohue, and P. A. Schewe, 277–292. Cham: Springer International Publishing.

4. Herbenick, D., E. Bartelt, T-C. Fu, et al. 2019. "Feeling Scared During Sex: Findings From a U.S. Probability Sample of Women and Men Ages 14 to 60." *Journal of Sex & Marital Therapy* 45, no. 5: 424–439.

5. Herbenick, D., T. C. Fu, P. Wright, et al. 2020. "Diverse Sexual Behaviors and Pornography Use: Findings from a Nationally Representative Probability Survey of Americans Aged 18 to 60 Years." *The Journal of Sexual Medicine* 17, no. 4: 623–633.

6. Seto, M. C., A. Maric, and H. E. Barbaree.2001. "The Role of Pornography in the Etiology of Sexual Aggression." *Aggression and Violent Behavior* 6, no. 1: 35–53.

7. Malamuth, N. M. 2018. "'Adding Fuel to the Fire'? Does Exposure to Non-consenting Adult or to Child Pornography Increase Risk of Sexual Aggression?" *Aggression and Violent Behavior* 41:74–89.

8. Safronova, V., and K. VanSyckle. "The Boundary Between Abuse and B.D.S.M." *New York Times*, May 23, 2018.

9. Smid, W. J., and E. C. Wever. 2019. "Mixed Emotions: An Incentive Motivational Model of Sexual Deviance." *Sexual Abuse: A Journal of Research and Treatment* 31, no. 7: 731–764.

10. McKee, A. 2015. "Methodological Issues in Defining Aggression for Content Analyses of Sexually Explicit Material." *Archives of Sexual Behavior* 44, no. 1: 81–87.

11. Rostad, W. L., D. Gittins-Stone, C. Huntington, C. J. Rizzo, D. Pearlman, and L. Orchowski. 2019. "The Association Between Exposure to Violent Pornography and Teen

Dating Violence in Grade 10 High School Students." *Archives of Sexual Behavior* 48, no. 7: 2137–2147.

12. Rosenberg, E. "Pornography Is a 'Root Cause' of School Shootings, Republican Congresswoman Says." *Washington Post,* May 29, 2018.

13. Savin-Williams, R. C., and G. L. Ream. 2007. "Prevalence and Stability of Sexual Orientation Components During Adolescence and Young Adulthood." *Archives of Sexual Behavior* 36, no. 3: 385–394.

14. Frankowski, B. L. 2019. "Sexual Orientation and Adolescents." *Pediatrics* 113, no. 6: 1827–1832.

15. Streed, C. G., J. S. Anderson, C. Babits, and M. A. Ferguson. 2019. "Changing Medical Practice, Not Patients—Putting an End to Conversion Therapy." *New England Journal of Medicine* 381, no. 6: 500–502.

16. Diamond, L. 2008. *Sexual Fluidity: Understanding Women's Love and Desire.* United States: Harvard University Press.

17. Gilbert, F., and M. Daffern. 2017. "Aggressive Scripts, Violent Fantasy and Violent Behavior: A Conceptual Clarification and Review." *Aggression and Violent Behavior* 36: 98–107.

18. Simon, W., and J. H. Gagnon. 1986. "Sexual Scripts: Permanence and Change." *Archives of Sexual Behavior* 15, no. 2: 97–120.

19. O'Donohue, W., and J. J. Plaud. 1994. "The Conditioning of Human Sexual Arousal." *Archives of Sexual Behavior* 23, no. 3: 321–344.

20. Schachter, S., and J. E. Singer. 1962. "Cognitive, Social, and Physiological Determinants of Emotional State." *Psychological Review* 69: 379–399.

21. Dong-ouk, Y., and Y. Gahyun. 2012. "Effects of Exposure to Pornography on Male Aggressive Behavioral Tendencies." *The Open Psychology Journal* 5, no. 1–10.

22. Zillman, D. 1971. "Excitation Transfer in Communication-Mediated Aggressive Behavior." *Journal of Experimental Social Psychology* 7: 419–434.

23. Flood, M. "Young Men, Pornography, and Sexual Socialization." 2020. https://voicemalemagazine.org/young-men-pornography-and-sexual-socialization/

24. Tokunaga, R. S., P. J. Wright, and J. E. Roskos. 2019. "Pornography and Impersonal Sex." *Human Communication Research* 45, no. 1: 78–118.

25. Breiding, M. J., S. G. Smith, K. C. Basile, M. L. Walter, J. Chen, and M. T. Merrick. 2014. "Prevalence and Characteristics of Sexual Violence, Stalking, and Intimate Partner Violence Victimization—National Intimate Partner and Sexual Violence Survey, United States, 2011." *MMWR* 63, no. 8: 1–24.

26. Vrangalova, Z., and A. D. Ong. 2014. "Who Benefits from Casual Sex? The Moderating Role of Sociosexuality." *Social Psychological and Personality Science* 5, no. 8: 883–891.

27. Armstrong, E. A., P. England, and A. C. K. Fogarty. 2012. "Accounting for Women's Orgasm and Sexual Enjoyment in College Hookups and Relationships." *American Sociological Review* 77, no. 3: 435–462.

28. Kupperstein, L., and W. C. Wilson. 1970. *Erotica and Anti-social Behavior: An Analysis of Social Indicator Statistics.* Washington, DC: US Government Printing Office.

29. Kutchinsky, B. 1971. *Towards an Explanation of the Decrease in Registered Sex Crimes in Copenhagen,* vol. 8. Washington, DC: US Government Printing Office.

30. Ben-Veniste, R. 1971. *Pornography and Sex Crime: The Danish Experience,* vol. 8. Washington, DC: US Government Printing Office.

31. Bachy, V. 1976. "Explicit Sex—Liberation or Exploitation: Danish 'Permissiveness' Revisited." *Journal of Communication* 26, no. 1: 40–43.

32. Giglio, E. 1985. "Pornography in Denmark: A Public Policy Model for the United States." *Comparative Social Research* 8: 520–528.

33. Bauserman, R. 1996. "Sexual Aggression and Pornography: A Review of Correlational Research." *Basic and Applied Social Psychology* 18, no. 4: 405–427.

34. Jaffee, D., and M. A. Straus. 1987. "Sexual Climate and Reported Rape: A State-Level Analysis." *Archives of Sexual Behavior* 16, no. 2: 107–123.

35. Baron, L. 1990. "Pornography and Gender Equality An Empincal Analysis." *The Journal of Sex Research* 27: 363–380.

36. Baron, L., and M. A. Straus. 1987. "Four Theories of Rape: A Macrosociological Analysis." *Social Problems* 34, no. 5: 467–489.

37. Baron, L., and M. A. Straus. 1989. "Rape and Its Relation to Social Disorganization, Pornography and Inequality in the USA." *Medicine and Law* 8, no. 3: 209–232.

38. Scott, J. E., and L. A. Schwalm. 1988. "Rape Rates and the Circulation Rates of Adult Magazines." *Journal of Sex Research* 24: 241–250.

39. Gentry, C. S. 1991. "Pornography and Rape: An Empirical Analysis." *Deviant Behavior* 12, no. 3: 277–288.

40. Kutchinsky, B. 1991. "Pornography and Rape: Theory and Practice? Evidence from Crime Data in Four Countries Where Pornography Is Easily Available." *International Journal of Law and Psychiatry* 14, no. 1: 47–64.

41. Winick, C., and J. T. Evans. 1996. "The Relationship Between Nonenforcement of State Pornography Laws and Rates of Sex Crime Arrests." *Archives of Sexual Behavior* 25, no. 5: 439–453.

42. Kimmel, M. S., and A. Linders. 1996. "Does Censorship Make a Difference?" *Journal of Psychology & Human Sexuality* 8, no. 3: 1–20.

43. Wiederman, M. W. 1999. "Volunteer Bias in Sexuality Research Using College Student Participants." *The Journal of Sex Research* 36, no. 1: 59–66.

44. Mellor, E., and S. Duff. 2019. "The Use of Pornography and the Relationship Between Pornography Exposure and Sexual Offending in Males: A Systematic Review." *Aggression and Violent Behavior* 46: 116–126.

45. Carter, D. L., R. A. Prentky, R. A. Knight, P. L. Vanderveer, and R. J. Boucher. 1987. "Use of Pornography in the Criminal and Developmental Histories of Sexual Offenders." *Journal of Interpersonal Violence* 2, no. 2: 196–211.

46. Proulx, J., C. Perreault, and M. Ouimet. 1999. "Pathways in the Offending Process of Extrafamilial Sexual Child Molesters." *Sexual Abuse: A Journal of Research and Treatment* 11, no. 2: 117–129.

47. Beauregard, E., P. Lussier, and J. Proulx. 2005. "The Role of Sexual Interests and Situational Factors on Rapists' Modus Operandi: Implications for Offender Profiling." *Legal and Criminological Psychology* 10, no. 2: 265–278.

48. Mieczkowski, T., and E. Beauregard. 2012. "Interactions Between Disinhibitors in Sexual Crimes: Additive or Counteracting Effects?" *Journal of Crime and Justice* 35, no. 3: 395–411.

49. Mancini, C., A. Reckdenwald, E. Beauregard, and J. S. Levenson. 2014. "Sex Industry Exposure over the Life Course on the Onset and Frequency of Sex Offending." *Journal of Criminal Justice* 42, no. 6: 507–516.

50. Wright, P. J., R. S. Tokunaga, and A. Kraus. 2016. "A Meta-Analysis of Pornography Consumption and Actual Acts of Sexual Aggression in General Population Studies." *Journal of Communication* 66, no. 1: 183–205.

51. Allen, M., T. Emmers, L. Gebhardt, and M. A. Giery. 1995. "Exposure to Pornography and Acceptance of Rape Myths." *Journal of Communication* 45: 5–26.

52. Hald, G. M., N. M. Malamuth, and C. Yuen. 2010. "Pornography and Attitudes Supporting Violence Against Women: Revisiting the Relationship in Nonexperimental Studies." *Aggressive Behavior* 36: 14–20.

53. Prevention USCfDCa. 2020. "National Diabetes Prevention Program." https://www.cdc. gov/diabetes/prevention/index.html

54. Kunkle, F. 2017. "This Harvard Professor Used TV Sitcoms to Fight Drunk Driving. Can He Do the Same for Distracted Driving?" *Washington Post* https://www.washingtonpost. com/news/tripping/wp/2017/04/26/this-harvard-professor-used-tv-sitcoms-to-fight- drunk-driving-can-he-do-the-same-for-distracted-driving/

6

Problematic Pornography Use

On November 5, 2019, the porn star Stoya tweeted to her 258,000 followers: "Porn addiction is not a thing. Not. A. Thing. [Obsessive compulsive disorder] is a thing, compulsive behaviors are a thing, and misuse of sexuality to fill a void are all things. But, porn addiction is not a thing."

Commenters quickly pointed out that Stoya has a financial conflict of interest and that her comment was akin to a tobacco company claiming that nicotine addiction was not real. But putting aside questions about Stoya's fitness as a spokesperson on the topic of porn addiction: What did Stoya mean by her comment? And was she correct? This chapter seeks to answer these questions.

First, some context. During the so-called sex wars of the 1970s and 1980s, questions about whether pornography caused rape and other sexually aggressive behavior were central to debates about pornography and public policy.[1] Porn addiction, or compulsive use of pornography, was not a focal point of concern during that era. In fact, there is little mention of the possibility of porn addiction in the otherwise seemingly exhaustive 546-page Final Report of the Attorney General's Commission on Pornography (1986), which instead focused on a number of possible harms of pornography use, including rape, thoughts of suicide as a result of watching pornography, and child abuse.[1] Things are different today. Whether pornography is addictive, and whether there is an epidemic of pornography addiction in the population, is now a key issue in pornography and public policy debates. In fact, the idea that people can become biologically addicted to pornography is one of the main pillars of the argument that pornography is a public health problem.[2] The model language for state resolutions to declare pornography a public health crisis includes this language: "Recent research indicates that pornography is potentially biologically addictive, which means the user requires more novelty, often in the form of more shocking material, in order to be satisfied."[2] While scientists agree that there are people who cannot control their use of pornography, there is debate about the idea that pornography use is "biologically addictive" rather than compulsive. The debates can get quite intense. Out of all the hotly contested topics pertaining

Pornography and Public Health. Emily F. Rothman, Oxford University Press. © Oxford University Press 2021. DOI: 10.1093/oso/9780190075477.003.0006

to pornography and public health, fights about whether pornography is addictive may be the most fierce.

Public health professionals can play a helpful, bridge-building role between the factions, of which there are at least three: (1) Pro-pornography stakeholders, who argue that pornography is not addictive, but acknowledge that it can be used compulsively or problematically. (2) Anti-pornography activists who want pornography banned or curtailed, and find it politically expedient to leverage the idea that pornography is addictive to make their case. (3) Behavioral health specialists and others who treat and support people experiencing problematic pornography use, and who may develop negative opinions about pornography because of the challenges that their clients experience. There is an important difference between factions 2 and 3: the former promote the idea that pornography is addictive because they have moral objections to all pornography, while the latter are motivated by concern for clients (or partners, family members, parishioners) and are not necessarily judgmental about diverse sexual behavior. I would argue that public health professionals can occupy the spaces in between these factions. On the one hand, we can insist on rigor and precision when it comes to developing the evidence base that will allow us to define, track, prevent, and treat problematic pornography use—and we can point out when ideologues are exaggerating what is known because their real agenda is to eradicate sexually explicit media altogether. On the other hand, we can reject attempts to minimize the evidence that problematic pornography use is too prevalent and bring attention to the need for it to be controlled effectively in individuals and at the societal level.

History of Pornography Addiction as a Concept

Some present-day anti-pornography rhetoric is rooted in the centuries-old beliefs that masturbation is sinful and therefore dangerous. Condemnation of masturbation proliferated in Europe in the 1600s.[3] In 1633, an English physician, religious Puritan, and university fellow named Richard Capel published a book in which he wrote that masturbation was a foul sin that caused bodies to rot and weaken.[4] In 1698, a Dutchman and humanist scholar named Hadriaan Beverland authored a treatise against masturbation in which he wrote that masturbators are "covered in pustules and the like."[5] The problem with masturbation, in the minds of Puritans, Lutherans, and other moralists from that era, was that it "threatened to 'enslave' the victim by constantly stimulating his imagination," that it wasted semen and female sexual secretions, which contained the human soul, and that it was contradictory to marriage and family, and marriage and family were viewed as fundamental bedrock for a functional society.[3] Moralists even used the language of public health to try to promote a sex-negative agenda in the 17th century: Beverland wrote that masturbation "seemed contagious, a veritable 'epidemic disease'" (p. 705).[3]

In the early 1700s, concern about masturbation became increasingly medicalized.[3] Physicians began to write about what they presumed were the dangers of masturbation, and medical specialists in sexually transmitted infections (called venereal disease at the time) wrote that masturbation caused wasting, watery semen, infirm testicles, gonorrhea, constant leakage of semen from the penis, meager jaws, pale looks, scabs, scrawny calf muscles, vertigo, loss of hearing, headache, loss of memory, irregular heartbeat, epilepsy, conjunctivitis, nymphomania, thinning of the penis, and congestion of the labia and caused people to be "fit for nothing in the prime of their years to but to be lodged in a hospital"(p. 711).[3,5] Drug sellers began to market medications to masturbators who had purportedly damaged their genitals through masturbation.[3] Over time, theories about the physiological harms of masturbation gave way to a new set of theories— that masturbating harmed mental health.[6] The first American psychiatric textbook, published in 1812 by Dr. Benjamin Rush, described four cases of patients whose mental health disorder was attributed to masturbation,[6] and in 1839 Dr. Leopold Deslandes wrote that the "last annual report of the State Lunatic Asylum of Massachusetts . . . states that of the number of insane received at that institution during the last year, no less than 32 lost their senses from this cause."[7]

In 1832, a book by a Swiss neurologist named Samuel-August Tissot, *Treatise on the Diseases Produced by Onanism*, was made available in the United States. It had originally been published in French in 1760.[8] To my knowledge, this book was the first medical text to reference the idea that masturbation could be "addictive," which it did in numerous instances,[8] and urged abstinence and thoughts about not getting into Heaven as treatment.[6] (If this sounds at all silly to you, remember that in the year 2200 people may be looking back at whatever we think we know today about human sexuality as similarly preposterous.)

In the United States, masturbation became less stigmatized in the 1970s and 1980s,[9] and the concept of sex addiction emerged. Although the idea that sex could be addictive had been written about in a few books by clinicians between 1951 and 1967,[10] one historian traced its first practical use to an

Alcoholics Anonymous group in Boston that took place in the 1970s.[11] Members of the group substituted the idea of "sex and love addiction" for alcohol addiction and began to develop self-help practical knowledge about addressing it.[11] Following the first peer-reviewed paper outlining a theory of dependence on sex, or hypersexuality, published in 1978,[10] a psychiatrist named Lawrence Hatterer wrote a pop-psychology book about "the addictive process" and food, sex, drugs, alcohol, and work.[12] Soon thereafter, in 1983, the psychologist Patrick Carnes popularized the term "sex addiction" in his book *Out of the Shadows: Understanding Sexual Addiction*.[13]

It is more difficult to pinpoint when the idea that people could be addicted to pornography, specifically, became commonplace. The idea was, in part, promoted to the general public by the US magazine *Christianity Today* in 1982 when it reported that psychologist Victor Cline had spoken at a national conference on the addicting effects of pornography,[14] including that pornography requires escalating use (i.e., over a period of time, the consumer needs increasingly rough materials) and desensitizes viewers, and that there is a strong tendency for users to act out what they see.[14,15] *Christianity Today* also produced an 8-page feature on the "cyberporn invasion" in 1994,[15] and celebrity televangelist James Robison published a book called *Pornography: The Pollution of America* in 1982 that had numerous references to pornography as a drug.[16] One reason that sex-positive activists today tend to be skeptical of porn addiction science may be because the danger of porn addiction was promoted by sex-negative and homophobic ideologues in the 1980s and 1990s.

In the scientific world, the idea that behaviors, and not just substances like alcohol, cocaine, heroin, and tobacco, could be addictive gained prominence in 2001, when the science journalist Constance Holden published an article in *Science* suggesting that the brain's dopamine reward system does not distinguish between chemicals and experiences like gambling, eating, sex or shopping.[17] The idea that sex addiction, called hypersexuality (and formerly called nymphomania), should be included in the *Diagnostic and Statistical Manual of Mental Disorders* (DSM) was proposed just over a decade ago, in 2010, by Martin Kafka.[18] In 2011, the American Society of Addiction Medicine (ASAM) officially changed its definition of addiction to include behaviors, and in the 2010s peer-reviewed papers about pornography addiction began to proliferate. However, in 2013, the DSM excluded hypersexuality disorder and pornography addiction from the 5th edition (DSM-5), as well as Internet-related behaviors like Internet video-gaming and television viewing because there was insufficient peer-reviewed evidence to establish the diagnostic criteria and course descriptions needed to identify these behaviors as mental health disorders.[19]

The Discourse about Problematic Pornography Use: "Addictive" vs. "Compulsive Use Disorder"

Importantly, current debates about whether pornography is addictive mainly center on whether it is addictive versus whether people become compulsive about using it. To be clear, there isn't a faction that argues that pornography is always harmless, or that excessive pornography use never occurs. No matter their stance on how to define and name problematic pornography use, or what causes it, virtually all experts acknowledge that a percentage of people suffer from an inability to stop using pornography, and that those people can experience severe impairment because of it. There is disagreement about whether the individuals experiencing impairment are "addicted" or if they have a "compulsive use disorder." This might sound like a petty argument over semantics. It is reasonable to wonder: why are there such bitter controversies about substituting the word "addiction" for "compulsive use disorder"? One answer is that addictions and compulsions are different phenomena, and their etiology, duration, and appropriate treatments vary. Another answer is that language can influence how people perceive the problem. The word "addiction" may be more powerful, more frightening, and public policy decision-makers may be more easily convinced to ban pornography outright if it sounds as dangerous as opioids or other illegal drugs.

However, the disease or addiction model frame as applied to pornography use may be useful to those who want to shift the focus away from blaming an individual for vice. In public health, we embrace the medical model of addiction as a way to understand alcohol and drug use disorder in part for this very reason—because there is too much stigma associated with drug use disorder, and for too long people blamed those with addictions for making bad choices instead of viewing them as in need of help and support. The idea that alcohol and illicit drugs are addictive and that unhealthy use is not just the result of an individual's choice has helped encourage more compassionate responses to people with substance use disorders. We are more likely to regard those who suffer from these disorders with empathy. In this way, applying the addiction model framework to pornography overuse is consistent with public health. But there are possible drawbacks, as well. People told that they have a pornography "addiction" may feel fatalistic about their prognosis, when it is not clear that problematic pornography use is a lifelong, progressive disorder with no cure.[20] Moreover, people told that they have a pornography addiction might face discrimination and stigmatization that they would not otherwise. However, these drawbacks may prove minimal in comparison to the benefits of destigmatizing problematic pornography use and developing new treatment approaches. Inarguably, the word "addiction" resonates for a subset of affected individuals and they feel strongly in favor of this framework, which is a reason to work with it, and not against it, from a public health perspective.

DSM-5, ICD-11, and Other Authoritative Sources on Pornography Addiction

As of January 2021, you will not find an entry for "pornography addiction" in the DSM-5 or any other international or national handbook for diagnosing disorders and diseases. That does not mean that pornography addiction will never be considered a disorder by these sources. As evidence accrues, there may be advances in how problematic Internet use and other behavioral addictions are understood, and awareness, treatment, and prevention of them may become more highly prioritized. It may be helpful to review what is considered an addictive disorder by these sources in order to contemplate whether and how pornography addiction may (or may not) ever align.

The DSM-5 section on substance-related and addictive disorders describes substance-related disorders for 10 separate classes of drugs and one behavioral addiction—gambling. Other behaviors, such as shopping, eating, and having sex, which may also produce excessive behavioral patterns, are not presently recognized as behavioral addictions due to inadequate supporting evidence for their inclusion. The reason that gambling was added to the DSM-5 category of "Substance-related and Addictive Disorders" is that there was sufficient research that demonstrated clinical, phenomenological, genetic, neurobiological, and other similarities between gambling and substance-use disorders.[19] In other words, for future DSM workgroups to consider pornography addiction for inclusion, pornography addiction would likely have to clear the bar of having clinical, phenomenological, genetic, neurobiological, and other similarities to substance-use disorders.

In the United States, there is no higher authoritative source for mental health diagnoses than the DSM, but there are additional authoritative sources that define diseases, disorders, and addiction. These include the *International Classification of Disease* (ICD), which is now in its 11th edition. Whereas the DSM is intended for use by US mental health providers specifically, the ICD is published by the World Health Organization and is often used for reimbursement for health problems by medical care systems and providers around the world, and 117 countries use ICD codes to record cause of death.[21] "Pornography addiction" does not appear as a diagnosis in the ICD. However, in 2019, for the first time the ICD-11 included compulsive sexual behavior disorder under its impulse control disorders category. This decision generated more public stakeholder comments than any other new diagnosis in the topics of mental, behavioral, and neurodevelopmental disorders, sleep–wake disorders, and conditions related to sexual health.[22] Interestingly, activists on both sides of the porn addiction debate were pleased by the inclusion of compulsive sexual disorder in the ICD-11. On the one hand, those who view pornography as addictive were gratified because it was a step toward formal recognition of excessive sexual behavior as a disorder or disease. On the other hand, pro-pornography activists were pleased that compulsive sexual behavior was listed under the compulsive behavior diagnostic codes and not under the ICD codes for substance use or disorders due to addictive behaviors.

ASAM is the professional society of addiction medicine providers in the United States. It is an influential society that educates physicians and the public, and its members work closely with lawmakers and government administration leaders to set policy and to standardize addiction treatment. Of note, ASAM revised their definition of addiction in 2011 to include behavioral addictions, which was impactful for the field.[23] As a result of the inclusion of behavioral addictions in the scope of addiction medicine, for over a decade now many practitioners and providers have become accustomed to thinking about Internet use, online gaming, sex, and other behaviors—including pornography use—as addictive for practical purposes. However, an analogous professional society for sexuality educators, counselors, and therapists, the American Association for Sexuality Educators, Counselors and Therapists (AASECT), announced in 2016 that it did *not* find "sufficient empirical evidence to support the classification of sex addiction or porn addiction as a mental health disorder," and did not find "the sexual addiction training and treatment methods and educational pedagogies to be adequately informed by accurate human sexuality knowledge."[24] Following AASECT's lead, in 2017, three additional sexuality practitioners' alliance groups also issued position statements declaring that linking problems related to pornography use with the addiction model "cannot be advanced as a standard of practice."[25] In response, the International Institute for Trauma and Addiction Professionals (IITAP) wrote a response to the AASECT position that asserted that there are now more than 20 studies showing that sex can be an addiction and that pointed out that the AASECT-affiliated sexologists may lack familiarity with the neuroscientific evidence on addiction that informed the ASAM definition.[26] In short, scores of dedicated professionals from multiple fields are influencing the discourse on this topic, and speedy resolutions on the points of contention seem unlikely.

Given that additional work is needed on this topic, Table 6.1 provides definitions of key terms that will be germane for future consideration of how the addiction model applies to problematic pornography use. In the table, the DSM-5 definition of mental health disorder is included to draw attention to the fact that sexual behaviors that deviate from societal norms are *not* considered mental disorders unless a clinically significant disturbance is also present. This is important because it means that, simply because an individual prefers to have a lot of sex, or to engage in a lot of pornography viewing or masturbating, they should not be, and cannot be, judged to have a disorder or pathology unless there is evidence that the behavior is causing them a "clinically significant disturbance" in some other way. This is meant to protect people with unconventional sexualities from being persecuted.

Key Studies on the Topic of Problematic Pornography Use

Here I offer a brief summary of some key findings that may help public health professionals consider the state of the evidence, but it is by no means a comprehensive review of the literature. This is also an area of research that may progress rapidly, particularly if new funding is devoted to neurobiological research on Internet addition or the influence of media (sexually explicit or otherwise) on mental health.

To date, researchers and other experts who are engaged in the work of trying to determine if pornography is addictive have investigated several hypotheses about whether and how the brain changes, physiologically, as a result of repeated pornography use. One of the distinguishing features of an addiction, as compared to a compulsion, is that addiction changes the brain either permanently or for an extended period of time even after the substance use (or excessive behavior) has been discontinued.[27] Therefore, the thinking goes that if pornography is addictive, scientists should observe some changes in the brains of those with a pornography addiction. Another distinguishing feature of addiction is that initially users engage in the behavior for pleasure, but eventually when they begin to experience withdrawal, use is motivated by the desire to avoid negative states.[28] In contrast, if people are compulsive about a behavior, they may continue to do it because it always causes pleasure—not because they are

Table 6.1. Definitions of mental health disorder, addiction, and substance use disorder

Concept	Source	Definition
Mental Health Disorder	DSM-5[34]	A mental disorder is a syndrome characterized by clinically significant disturbance in an individual's cognition, emotion regulation, or behavior that reflects a dysfunction in the psychological, biological, or developmental processes underlying mental functioning. Mental disorders are usually associated with significant distress in social, occupational, or other important activities. An expectable or culturally approved response to a common stressor or loss, such as the death of a loved one, is not a mental disorder. Socially deviant behavior (e.g., political, religious, or sexual) and conflicts that are primarily between the individual and society are not mental disorders unless the deviance or conflict results from a dysfunction in the individual, as described above.
Addiction	ASAM[35]	Addiction is a treatable, chronic medical disease involving complex interactions among brain circuits, genetics, the environment, and an individual's life experiences. People with addiction use substances or engage in behaviors that become compulsive and often continue despite harmful consequences. Prevention efforts and treatment approaches for addiction are generally as successful as those for other chronic diseases.
Substance Use Disorder	DSM-5[36]	Over at least the past 12 months, the individual meets $\geq$ 2 criteria: 1. Hazardous use 2. Social/interpersonal problems related to use 3. Neglected major roles to use 4. Legal problems 5. Withdrawal (defined as substance is taken to relieve or avoid withdrawal symptoms) 6. Tolerance (defined as markedly increased amounts of substance to achieve intoxication or desired effect, or markedly diminished effect with continued use of the same amount of substance) 7. Used larger amounts/longer 8. Repeated attempts to quit/control use 9. Much time spent using 10. Physical/psychological problems related to use 11. Activities given up to use
Disorders Due to Substance Use	ICD-11[37]	Disorders due to substance use include single episodes of harmful substance use, substance use disorders (harmful substance use and substance dependence), and substance-induced disorders, such as substance intoxication, substance withdrawal and substance-induced mental disorders, sexual dysfunctions, and sleep–wake disorders.

Table 6.1. *Continued*

Concept	Source	Definition
Disorders Due to Addictive Behaviors	ICD-11[37]	Disorders due to addictive behaviors are recognizable and clinically significant syndromes associated with distress or interference with personal functions that develop as a result of repetitive rewarding behaviors other than the use of dependence-producing substances. Disorders due to addictive behaviors include gambling disorder and gaming disorder, which may involve both online and offline behavior.
Compulsive Sexual Behavior Disorder	ICD-11 (6C72)[38]	Compulsive sexual behavior disorder is characterized by a persistent pattern of failure to control intense, repetitive sexual impulses or urges resulting in repetitive sexual behavior. Symptoms may include repetitive sexual activities becoming a central focus of the person's life to the point of neglecting health and personal care or other interests, activities, and responsibilities; numerous unsuccessful efforts to significantly reduce repetitive sexual behavior; and continued repetitive sexual behavior despite adverse consequences or deriving little or no satisfaction from it. The pattern of failure to control intense sexual impulses or urges and resulting repetitive sexual behavior is manifested over an extended period of time (e.g., 6 months or more) and causes marked distress or significant impairment in personal, family, social, educational, occupational, or other important areas of functioning. Distress that is entirely related to moral judgments and disapproval about sexual impulses, urges, or behaviors is not sufficient to meet this requirement.

avoiding negative states when they discontinue use. To explore whether pornography affects users in ways that resemble addiction to substances, researchers have investigated whether individuals become desensitized to pornography content (meaning that they need more and more, or more extreme content, to achieve an effect); whether individuals crave pornography when they are not watching it, or whether they experience withdrawal when they cannot see pornography (i.e., experience irritability, stress, depression, or illness); and whether people's brains react when they see images of pornography in a manner that suggests what is called sensitization (e.g., when a drug user sees an image of their drug of choice, their brain activates with excitement from the visual cue).

What Is the Evidence Supporting the Idea that Pornography Is Addictive?

One complicated aspect of studying the neuroscience of addiction is that there is no way to look at a brain and simply see addiction there. We can't give someone a blood test, x-ray them, or even examine them with magnetic resonance imaging (MRI), electroencephalography (EEG), or functional magnetic resonance imaging (fMRI) to directly measure if they have an addiction. Instead, in addition to observing behavior and listening to people's self-reports about their own behavior and symptoms, researchers assess other things about how the brain works that tend to be different for people who have otherwise been characterized as living with addictions. These factors include impulsivity, memory, P300 brain wave latencies, gamma oscillation intensity, N400 amplitude, attention, cognition, medial frontal negativity, cognitive rigidity, emotion regulation, and the release of dopamine. When it comes to pornography, neuroscientists have measured, among other things, brain gray matter, cue reactivity (i.e., reacting to being shown short clips of pornography), and subjective craving.[29–31] However, another challenge is that these observable factors could be atypical for a variety of reasons, not just because of addiction—for example, because of head injury or lack of sleep. So while certain measures are generally accepted as proxies for the purpose of studying addiction, they are not direct measures of addiction.

Two studies of this type published in high-impact journals (*PLOS One* and *JAMA Psychiatry*) appear to be among the most widely cited.[29,30] The first study tested the hypothesis that the brains of heterosexual males (recruited from the Internet and from therapists) who think that they have compulsive sexual behavior disorder (CSBD) would show more desire (wanting) when shown pornography, but not more liking of pornography, than healthy volunteers. Specific areas of the brain—the ventral striatum, dACC, and amygdala—were expected to show more activity in the people with CSBD when they saw pornography.[30] The study found that, compared to healthy volunteers, men with CSBD were more likely to report desiring sexually explicit videos, and their brains were activated differently than the brains of healthy volunteers when they viewed pornography clips.[30] The second study tested the hypothesis that in a sample of adult males, frequent pornography use would be associated with the structure and function of certain brain regions.[29] The study found that those who used more pornography had less gray matter volume in the right caudate of the striatum. In addition, the part of the brain called the left putamen was involved in the visual processing of sexual content. The observed results are in line with the hypothesis that intense exposure to pornography stimuli results in a downregulation of the natural neural response to sexual stimuli.

In addition to these two studies, several other studies have also assessed neural reactions to pornography.[32–35] For example, Prause and co-authors (2015) investigated the hypothesis that the brains of people who had a problem regulating their viewing of pornography (called "visual sexual stimuli" (VSS) viewing problems in the article) would react strongly to seeing pornographic images.[32] The idea was that, if cocaine users' and other illegal drug users' brains were more reactive in anticipation of a reward when they see images that cue them about their substance use (i.e., they experience "cue reactivity"), then people addicted to pornography should also experience a small voltage in their brain called an event-related potential (ERP) when they view pornography. The ERP is observable with EEG. In the Prause study, though, the brains of a sample of 55 adult men and women who reported that they did have pornography problems and high sexual desire did not exhibit more late positive potential (LPPs) in response to neutral pictures than the brains of those with lower sexual desire. The authors concluded that their results were inconsistent with addiction models.

A separate study using fMRI to examine brain responses to erotic stimuli in 28 heterosexual adult men who were seeking treatment for problematic pornography use (PPU) found that men with PPU *did* experience increased activation of their ventral striatal response to erotic images, suggesting that there was evidence of cue reactivity.[33] A third study attempted to improve upon some prior research in this area by exploring whether individualizing the pornographic pictures used in these types of studies mattered. The study found that in a sample of 19 adult men, neural responses to preferred pornography pictures were stronger to nonpreferred pictures, and that the neural reactions were stronger among those with higher scores on the Internet addiction test modified for cybersex.[35] A fourth study investigated pornography viewing as a possible predictor of self-reported erectile problems.[34] Prause and Pfaus (2015) conducted a study to investigate if viewing VSS videos influenced sexual arousal or erectile problems with a sexual partner in a sample of 280 men.[34] The idea behind the study was to investigate the hypothesis that watching pornography results in tolerance or desensitization to it, which can be operationalized as decreased sexual arousal when viewing it, and as erectile problems with a real-life sexual partner. If pornography viewing results in tolerance, which is the sixth of 11 criteria for substance use disorder in the DSM-5, that would help make the case that pornography viewing should be viewed through an addiction framework. The study authors found that men who reported viewing more VSS in their own life reported higher sexual arousal to

VSS in the laboratory.[34] Self-reported erectile functioning with a partner was not related to the hours of VSS viewed weekly.

The review given here is not a comprehensive scoping review. It is intended, instead, to relay to the reader the results of a few key studies that have been highly cited and often discussed and debated, and to pique interest in continuing the exploration of the literature in this area. I have learned that this area of pornography research faces several challenges. Brain imaging studies are costly and often time-intensive for both researchers and participants; as a result, the studies commonly use relatively small samples and cross-sectional designs. Another problem is that if the index subjects are frequent pornography consumers, finding comparable samples of infrequent pornography users who are otherwise similar (in religion, culture, relationship status, sexuality, etc.) may be complicated. Therefore, making causal inferences is difficult. One can never be certain if the results of these studies reflect differences in people's brains that are a result of their pornography use or if differences in pornography use are a result of people's being wired differently in the first place. A third possibility is that there are other factors, unmeasured confounders, that are responsible for the differences in how the subjects' brains are working *and* their pornography use (e.g., depression). Another challenge for this body of research more generally is that the specialized conditions in which research participants view pornography (in a lab, connected to a machine that measures brain activity) raises questions about generalizability. But these research limitations are not a reason to disregard the findings. Making causal inferences is often challenging, and in some cases public health professionals decide to move forward based on the best available evidence that has accrued.

How Prevalent Is Compulsive Pornography Use?

A nationally representative US study recently found that as many as 7% of women and 10% of men endorse clinically relevant levels of distress and/ or impairment associated with difficulty controlling sexual feelings, urges, and behaviors,[36] although other studies have found the prevalence of compulsive sexual behavior to be as low as 3% for men and 1% for women.[37–39] One exception was a study of US military veterans that found a prevalence of 17%.[40]

Although studies of the prevalence of pornography addiction have been rare, at least five studies have attempted to estimate the prevalence of pornography addiction, specifically, in samples of Internet-using adults and adolescents. Collectively, the studies have generally found that the prevalence is moderate, between 3% and 16%,[41–45] even when relying on individuals' self-diagnosis rather than any clinical definition or assessment.

Why Might Some People Develop an Excessive Pornography Use Habit?

Current thinking about why and how behavioral addictions form is that they are a consequence of predisposing variables, an individual's response to stimuli—such as a thrill from gambling or an orgasm from pornography—and the individual's ability to control their impulses and to make decisions about a habit. This model of behavioral addictions is called Interaction of Person-Affect-Cognition-Execution (I-PACE).[46] With regard to pornography addiction, specifically, there are a few correlates that may be causal. These include: male gender, being younger, earlier age of pornography use,[43] being introverted,[43] and more frequent daily pornography use.[41,44] A study of Italian adolescents 13 to 18 years old found that compulsive pornography use was associated with sexting, but because the study was cross-sectional, it may not reflect a causal relationship and instead may reflect the fact that individuals with higher libido or more interested in sex, generally, were more likely to both sext and look at pornography.[47]

Another predictor of considering oneself addicted to pornography is having morals or values that are at odds with pornography use behavior, which Grubbs and colleagues refer to as "moral incongruence."[41] Being more religious is also a risk factor for considering oneself addicted to pornography.[44] In other words, people who believe that pornography use is morally wrong are more likely to feel that they have a pornography addiction than people who think that pornography use is healthy, acceptable, or fine.[41] This begs the question: Is it the pornography that is making people sick, or is it that the pornography users' impressions of how society is judging them are making them feel sick about their pornography use, and *that* is the real problem? We need to know more about whether some people who feel anxious, depressed, and out of control about pornography use are reacting to how other people and society make them feel about masturbating and using pornography, or if they would be feeling that bad even in the absence of any social feedback.

What Are the Consequences of Excessive Pornography Use?

The consequences of unhealthy pornography use appear to be similar to other unhealthy behavior compulsions—spending too much time on pornography use; avoiding friends, family, or daily activities to engage in pornography use; feeling preoccupied with pornography; not being able to cut back or quit despite knowing the negative consequences of pornography use; and restlessness or irritability if not able to use pornography.[43,48] In addition to these consequences, there are some that are specific to pornography. Research suggests that people who believe they have a pornography addiction may need more or longer stimulation to reach orgasm,[49] may experience erectile dysfunction,[50] may experience sexual dissatisfaction, and may encounter problems in their romantic relationships.[43] It has been argued that having problems with orgasm or erections could be due to the frequency of masturbation and orgasm and may not be the fault of pornography (i.e., having orgasms frequently for any reason may make it more difficult to sustain erections or have subsequent orgasms).[49]

How Is Pornography Addiction or Compulsive Use Treated, and What Are the Concerns about that?

People who seek treatment for problematic pornography use may be treated with cognitive behavioral therapy, which preliminary evidence suggests is effective for compulsive sexual behavior, although not pornography addiction specifically (as reported by Kraus and Sweeney 2019; Hallberg et al. 2017).[51,52] Other possible treatment approaches for compulsive sexual behavior with preliminary evidence include acceptance commitment therapy[53] and medications, such as paroxetine[54] and naltrexone.[55,56] Eli Coleman, Professor and Director of the Program in Human Sexuality at the University of Minnesota Medical School, as well as editor of the *International Journal of Sexual Health*, suggested using an intensive therapy model that addresses identity development, trauma repair, building self-esteem, and addressing intimacy.[57] Others recommend mindfulness training[58] and spiritual solutions, including prayer.[59]

One difficulty in matching patients to the right treatment is that people with unhealthy or problematic pornography use may have diverse clinical presentations, reasons for seeking help, and underlying needs.[51] For example, for some, the true underlying problem may be loneliness or stress,[60] and so the right treatment might entail addressing social anxiety, social skills, or stress management—not necessarily an impulse disorder. For others, their use of pornography may actually be within their control, but their spouse or partner has demanded that they seek treatment. In such cases, marital or couples counseling may be appropriate.

A Possibly Helpful Reframe from Public Health

The debate about whether pornography *is* or *is not* addictive, as well as the debate about whether pornography overuse is an *addiction* or a *compulsive use disorder*, will likely continue for the next decade. Public health and allied professionals may want to step back from the polarizing and divisive nature of these debates and apply a different frame in order to move forward with an agenda for healthier pornography use. Substance use experts tend to think of a spectrum of use. For example, people may use alcohol with no or minimal risk of harm, and then use it with some harm or risk of harm, and then become dependent and develop an addiction, disorder, or disease. In other words, in the substance use world, it has been helpful for experts to think in terms of use→risky use→harmful use→dependent use→disorder (or something along those lines). It may be helpful for those of us with compassion for people who feel out of control about their pornography use to embrace the idea of an unhealthy use spectrum. It would be clinically useful if researchers were able to determine how to move people from more severe levels of the unhealthy use spectrum to less severe levels.

Conclusions

People may turn to pornography because they have preexisting problems with depression, anxiety, their relationships, or sex. In some cases, their use of pornography may cause them shame and guilt. They may *feel like* they are unable to control their pornography use, or they may become *truly unable* to control their pornography use. People who masturbate to online pornography may alter the physiology of their brain, temporarily, which may be corrected when they stop using online pornography. However, pornography addiction is not presently considered a diagnosable condition according to the DSM. Alternatives to the DSM, such as the ICD-11, also have not subscribed to the addiction model for pornography, though they recognize that people may become compulsive about its use. Going forward, public health professionals can accumulate and study evidence that pornography is causing harms to individuals, families, and communities due to people's inability to control their use and can advocate for evidence-based treatment as the best option for addressing unhealthy pornography use in affected individuals. Collaborating with, and supporting, the networks of people who describe themselves as porn addicted or in recovery from porn addiction is also important for public health practice. Effective health promotion advocacy is inclusive and accommodates diverse viewpoints even on the most hotly debated topics, such as pornography addiction.

References

1. US Department of Justice. 1986. *Attorney General's Commission on Pornography: Final Report*. Washington, DC: US Dept. of Justice.
2. National Decency Coalition. 2020. "PPHC Resolution." https://nationaldecencycoalition. org/wp-content/uploads/2019/11/PPHC-Resolution-2020.pdf
3. Stolberg, M. 2003. "The Crime of Onan and the Laws of Nature: Religious and Medical Discourses on Masturbation in the late Seventeenth and Early Eighteenth Centuries." *Paedagogica Historica* 39, no. 6: 701–717.
4. Capel, R. 1633. *Tentations: Their Nature, Danger, Cure . . . : To which is Added a Briefe Dispute, as Touching Restitution in the Case of Usury*. London: R[ichard] B[adger].
5. Engelhardt, H. 1974. "The Disease of Masturbation: Values and the Concept of Disease." *Bulletin of the History of Medicine* 48, no. 2: 234.
6. Taylor, K. 2019. "Pornography Addiction: The Fabrication of a Transient Sexual Disease." *History of the Human Sciences* 0952695119854624.
7. Deslandes, L. 1839. *A Treatise on the Diseases Produced by Onanism, Masturbation, Self-Pollution and Other Excesses*. Boston: Otis, Broaders, and Company.
8. Tissot, S. A. 1832. *Treatise on the Disease Produced by Onanism*. New York: Collins & Hannay.
9. Stengers, J., and Anne van Neck. 2001. *Masturbation: The History of a Great Terror*. Translated by K. Hoffmann. New York: St. Martin's Press.
10. Orford, J. 1978. "Hypersexuality: Implications for a Theory of Dependence." *The British Journal of Addiction to Alcohol and Other Drugs* 73, no. 3: 299–310.
11. Voros, F. 2009. "The Invention of Addiction to Pornography." *Sexologies* 18, no. 4: 243–246.
12. Hatterer, L. J. 1980. *The Pleasure Addicts: The Addictive Process—Food, Sex, Drugs, Alcohol, Work, and More*. South Brunswick, NJ: Barnes.
13. Carnes, P. 2001. *Out of the Shadows: Understanding Sexual Addiction*. Center City, Minnesota: Hazelden Publishing.
14. Genet, H. 1982. "Why People Don't Fight Porn." *Christianity Today* 26: 52–53.
15. Thomas, J. N. 2016. "The Development and Deployment of the Idea of Pornography Addiction Within American Evangelicalism." *Sexual Addiction & Compulsivity* 23, no. 2–3: 182–195.
16. Robison, J. 1982. *Pornography, the Polluting of America*. Wheaton, IL: Tyndale House Publishers.
17. Holden, C. 2001. "Behavioral Addictions: Do They Exist?" *Science* 294, no. 5544: 980.

18. Kafka, M. P. 2010. "Hypersexual Disorder: A Proposed Diagnosis for DSM-V." *Archives of Sexual Behavior* 39, no. 2: 377–400.

19. Potenza, M. N. 2014. "Non-substance Addictive Behaviors in the Context of DSM-5." *Addictive Behaviors* 39, no. 1: 1–2.

20. Ley, D. 2012. *The Myth of Sex Addiction*. Lanham, MD: Rowman and Littlefield.

21. World Health Organization. 2020. "International Classification of Diseases (ICD) Information Sheet." https://www.who.int/classifications/icd/factsheet/en/

22. Fuss, J., K. Lemay, D. J. Stein, et al. 2019. "Public Stakeholders' Comments on ICD-11 Chapters Related to Mental and Sexual Health." *World Psychiatry* 18, no. 2: 233–235.

23. ASAM. 2011. "ASAM Releases New Definition of Addiction." *ASAM News* 26, no. 3: 1–23.

24. American Association of Sexuality Educators, Counselors, and Therapists. 2017. "AASECT Position on Sex Addiction." www.aasect.org/position-sex-addiction

25. Center for Positive Sexuality TASHRA, and the National Coalition for Sexual Freedom. 2017. "Addiction to Sex and/or Pornography: A Position Statement from the Center for Positive Sexuality (CPS), The Alternative Sexualities Health Research Alliance (TASHRA), and the National Coalition for Sexual Freedom (NCSF)." *Journal of Positive Sexuality* 3, no. 3: 40–43.

26. IITAP. 2019. "Response to AASECT Position Statement." https://cdn.ymaws.com/iitap.com/resource/collection/FB72F3C4-C4D3-41E9-8AB1-A2FE5A9A325A/Response_to_AASECT_Position_Statement.pdf

27. Substance Abuse and Mental Health Services Administration. 2016. "The Neurobiology of Substance Use, Misuse, and Addiction." In *Facing Addiction in America: The Surgeon General's Report on Alcohol, Drugs, and Health*. Washington, DC: US Department of Health and Human Services.

28. Koob, G. F., and M. Le Moal. 2008. "Addiction and the Brain Antireward System." *Annual Review of Psychology* 59: 29–53.

29. Kühn, S., and J. Gallinat. 2014. "Brain Structure and Functional Connectivity Associated with Pornography Consumption: The Brain on Porn." *JAMA Psychiatry* 71, no. 7: 827–834.

30. Voon, V., T. B. Mole, P. Banca, et al. 2014. "Neural Correlates of Sexual Cue Reactivity in Individuals With and Without Compulsive Sexual Behaviours." *PLOS One* 9, no. 7: e102419-e102419.

31. Snagowski, J., E. Wegmann, J. Pekal, C. Laier, and M. Brand. 2015. "Implicit Associations in Cybersex Addiction: Adaption of an Implicit Association Test with Pornographic Pictures." *Addictive Behaviors* 49: 7–12.

32. Prause, N, V. R. Steele, C. Staley, D. Sabatinelli, and G. Hajcak. 2015. "Modulation of Late Positive Potentials by Sexual Images in Problem Users and Controls Inconsistent with 'Porn Addiction.'" *Biological Psychology* 109: 192–199.

33. Gola, M., M. Wordecha, G. Sescousse, et al. 2017. "Can Pornography be Addictive? An fMRI Study of Men Seeking Treatment for Problematic Pornography Use." *Neuropsychopharmacology* 42, no. 10: 2021–2031.

34. Prause, N., and J. Pfaus. 2015. "Viewing Sexual Stimuli Associated with Greater Sexual Responsiveness, Not Erectile Dysfunction." *The Journal of Sexual Medicine* 3, no. 2: 90–98.

35. Brand, M., J. Snagowski, C. Laier, and S. Maderwald. 2016. "Ventral Striatum Activity When Watching Preferred Pornographic Pictures Is Correlated with Symptoms of Internet Pornography Addiction." *NeuroImage* 129: 224–232.

36. Dickenson, J. A., N. Gleason, E. Coleman, and M. H. Miner. 2018. "Prevalence of Distress Associated with Difficulty Controlling Sexual Urges, Feelings, and Behaviors in the United States." *JAMA Network Open* 1, no. 7: e184468–e184468.

37. Kraus, S. W., V. Voon, and M. N. Potenza. 2016. "Should Compulsive Sexual Behavior Be Considered an Addiction?" *Addiction* (Abingdon, England) 111, no. 12: 2097–2106.

38. Reid, R. C., B. N. Carpenter, J. N. Hook, et al. 2012. "Report of Findings in a DSM-5 Field Trial for Hypersexual Disorder." *The Journal of Sexual Medicine* 9, no. 11: 2868–2877.
39. Odlaug, B. L., K. Lust, L. R. Schreiber, et al. 2013. "Compulsive Sexual Behavior in Young Adults." *Annals of Clinical Psychiatry* 25, no. 3: 193–200.
40. Smith, P. H., M. N. Potenza, C. M. Mazure, S. A. McKee, C. L. Park, and R. A. Hoff. 2014. "Compulsive Sexual Behavior Among Male Military Veterans: Prevalence and Associated Clinical Factors." *Journal of Behavioral Addictions* 3, no. 4: 214–222.
41. Grubbs, J. B., J. T. Grant, and J. Engelman. 2018. "Self-identification as a Pornography Addict: Examining the Roles of Pornography Use, Religiousness, and Moral Incongruence." *Sexual Addiction & Compulsivity* 25, no. 4: 269–292.
42. Baranowski, A. M., R. Vogl, and R. Stark. 2019. "Prevalence and Determinants of Problematic Online Pornography Use in a Sample of German Women." *The Journal of Sexual Medicine* 16, no. 8: 1274–1282.
43. Dwulit, AD, Rzymski P. 2019. "Prevalence, Patterns and Self-Perceived Effects of Pornography Consumption in Polish University Students: A Cross-Sectional Study." *International Journal of Environmental Research and Public Health* 16, no. 1861: 1–16.
44. Grubbs, J. B., S. W. Kraus, and S. L. Perry. 2019. "Self-reported Addiction to Pornography in a Nationally Representative Sample: The Roles of Use Habits, Religiousness, and Moral Incongruence." *Journal of Behavioral Addictions* 8, no. 1: 88–93.
45. Twohig, M. P., J. M. Crosby, and J. M. Cox. 2009. "Viewing Internet Pornography: For Whom is it Problematic, How, and Why?" *Sexual Addiction & Compulsivity* 16, no. 4: 253–266.
46. Brand, M., E. Wegmann, R. Stark, et al. 2019. "The Interaction of Person-Affect-Cognition-Execution (I-PACE) Model for Addictive Behaviors: Update, Generalization to Addictive Behaviors Beyond Internet-use Disorders, and Specification of the Process Character of Addictive Behaviors." *Neuroscience & Biobehavioral Reviews* 104: 1–10.
47. Morelli, M., D. Bianchi, R. Baiocco, L. Pezzuti, and A. Chirumbolo. 2017. "Sexting Behaviors and Cyber Pornography Addiction Among Adolescents: The Moderating Role of Alcohol Consumption." *Sexuality Research and Social Policy* 14, no. 2: 113–121.
48. Alavi, S. S., M. Ferdosi, F. Jannatifard, M. Eslami, H. Alaghemandan, and M. Setare. 2012. "Behavioral Addiction versus Substance Addiction: Correspondence of Psychiatric and Psychological Views." *International Journal of Preventive Medicine* 3, no. 4: 290–294.
49. Dwulit, A. D., and P. Rzymski. 2019. "The Potential Associations of Pornography Use with Sexual Dysfunctions: An Integrative Literature Review of Observational Studies." *Journal of Clinical Medicine* 8, no. 7: 1–15.
50. Grubbs, J. B., and M. Gola. 2019. "Is Pornography Use Related to Erectile Functioning? Results from Cross-Sectional and Latent Growth Curve Analyses." *The Journal of Sexual Medicine* 16, no. 1: 111–125.
51. Kraus, S. W., and P. J. Sweeney. 2019. "Hitting the Target: Considerations for Differential Diagnosis When Treating Individuals for Problematic Use of Pornography." *Archives of Sexual Behavior* 48, no. 2: 431–435.
52. Hallberg, J., V. Kaldo, S. Arver, C. Dhejne, and K. G. Öberg. 2017. "A Cognitive-Behavioral Therapy Group Intervention for Hypersexual Disorder: A Feasibility Study." *The Journal of Sexual Medicine* 14, no. 7: 950–958.
53. Crosby, J. M., and M. P. Twohig. 2016. "Acceptance and Commitment Therapy for Problematic Internet Pornography Use: A Randomized Trial." *Behavior Therapy* 47, no. 3: 355–366.
54. Gola, M., and M. N. Potenza. 2016. "Paroxetine Treatment of Problematic Pornography Use: A Case Series." *Journal of Behavioral Addictions* 5, no. 3: 529–532.
55. Kraus, S. W., S. Meshberg-Cohen, S. Martino, L. J. Quinones, and M. N. Potenza. 2015. "Treatment of Compulsive Pornography Use With Naltrexone: A Case Report." *American Journal of Psychiatry* 172, no. 12: 1260–1261.

56. Raymond, N. C., J. E. Grant, and E. Coleman. 2010. "Augmentation with Naltrexone to Treat Compulsive Sexual Behavior: A Case Series." *Annals of Clinical Psychiatry* 22, no. 1: 56–62.

57. Coleman, E., J. A. Dickenson, A. Girard, et al. 2018. "An Integrative Biopsychosocial and Sex Positive Model of Understanding and Treatment of Impulsive/Compulsive Sexual Behavior." *Sexual Addiction & Compulsivity* 25, no. 2/3: 125–152.

58. Fraumeni-McBride, J. 2019. "Addiction and Mindfulness: Pornography Addiction and Mindfulness-Based Therapy ACT." *Sexual Addiction & Compulsivity* 26, no. 1–2: 42–53.

59. Sneck, W. J. 2014. "Overcoming Pornography Addiction: A Spiritual Solution." *The Journal of Theological Studies* 75, no. 2: 465–466.

60. Bőthe, B., I. Tóth-Király, M. N. Potenza, M. D. Griffiths, G. Orosz, and Z. Demetrovics. 2019. "Revisiting the Role of Impulsivity and Compulsivity in Problematic Sexual Behaviors." *The Journal of Sex Research* 56, no. 2: 166–179.

7
Pornography and Intimate Partnerships

In July 2019, the House of Representatives of the State of Ohio became the 15th state legislative body in the United States to pass a resolution declaring pornography a public health hazard. The resolution argued that pornography is a public health problem based on 17 points. One of the points was that pornography use can "lead to difficulty in forming or maintaining positive, intimate relationships."[1] A second point was: "Pornography use is correlated with (1) a decreased desire in young men to marry, pursue intimacy, or engage socially, (2) dissatisfaction in marriage, and (3) infidelity, all of which demonstrate that pornography has a detrimental effect on the family unit."[1]

The idea that pornography is bad for marriage, and that this is a reason to consider it a public health problem, hinges on the idea that *marriage* is good for public health. What's more, the argument hinges on the idea that couples should be having sex with one another—if that is what is meant by "pursuing intimacy." So public health professionals need to know whether marriage and couple relationships are, in fact, fundamental to public health, and if pornography interferes with those relationships. Public health professionals also need to know if pornography use makes it difficult for users to form or maintain relationships. As with so many other empirical questions about pornography, the answer appears to be: *it depends*. To reiterate the theme from prior chapters: it likely matters what type of pornography is being used, by whom, the person's predisposing factors (e.g., propensity to communicate honestly with a partner or not), whether one person in the relationship is being secretive about their use, whether two people in a couple tend to watch pornography together or if the pornography use is a solo activity by one member, and if pornography use is frequent or rare. But before we dig into the research on pornography and relationship health, we should address the question already hinted at above—Is marriage is good for public health? The answer to this question is germane to the premise of the argument that pornography is bad for public health because it might have a negative impact on marriage rates.

Pornography and Public Health. Emily F. Rothman, Oxford University Press. © Oxford University Press 2021.
DOI: 10.1093/oso/9780190075477.003.0007

Is Marriage Good for Public Health?

The history of marriage is fascinating and beyond the scope of this book. However, it is important to acknowledge that marriage was invented at some point in human history—it isn't as natural or essential to our existence as breathing. Anthropologists believe that thousands of years ago hunger-gatherers lived in loose family groups. Evidence suggests that early human societies comprised a mix of monogamous couples and polygynous individuals.[2] The Bible has many references to polygamous marriages. Monogamy may have evolved as the dominant family mode because it made it easier for men to protect their offspring and genetic material, or because it reduced male fighting over mates.[2,3] Historians have documented that marriage was invented for a few different reasons, including to extend family bloodlines in strategic ways, to ensure that land or other things of value remained in a kinship group, and to help people survive economic and other types of hardships.[4] Marriage was also helpful to governing entities because it made people easier to control or rule over. As per the *National Review* in 2013: "The state has an interest in marriage and marital norms because they serve the public good by protecting child well-being, civil society, and limited government."[5] Some argue that the main advantage of societies with stable marriages is that they "produce high-quality children."[6] The idea that people should marry based on love is a relatively modern invention; romance was invented in the 12th century.[7]

So: Are marriages important to public health? Most nations in the world have now spent many centuries structuring society, laws, institutions, cultural norms, and holidays around monogamous marriage. As a result, there are many ways in which marriage now *does* appear to benefit human health. Pooling resources and living communally is less expensive, and for many couples there are benefits of being married when it comes to taxes, health insurance, pensions, social security, disability payments, military and veterans' benefits, or crime victims' recovery benefits, for example. Sharing parenting responsibilities with a spouse can also be beneficial. Children are more likely to experience academic, social, and behavioral difficulties when raised by a divorced parent instead of continuously married parents,[8] although parental divorce is not uniformly detrimental across all types of families.[9] Importantly, historically, the right to marry in the United States was granted only to white, heterosexual people. The federal government recognized marriages between emancipated slaves only after the Civil War,[10] state bans on interracial marriage were not ruled unconstitutional by the Supreme Court until 1967,[11] and same-sex marriage was legalized in all states only as recently as 2015.[12]

For decades, people believed that marriage was important for public health because a number of studies found that married people had lower rates of depression and higher rates of positive health habits, such as going to medical appointments, which subsequently influenced cardiovascular, endocrine, and immune system health.[13] But then researchers discovered that whether the marriages were happy or dysfunctional influenced health-related results, and that race, gender, and class mattered, too.[13,14] Men were found to benefit from marriage whether they were in a functional or dysfunctional relationship. But some studies suggested that, on average, women's mental health suffered if they were married.[15] Among Black men and affluent Black women, the married were more depressed than the unmarried.[14] Marriage also was found to benefit those with more education and income more than it benefited people with less—suggesting that strategic policy efforts to encourage people living in poverty to marry were misguided.[16]

Recently, several studies have called into question the idea that marriage is beneficial to human health more generally. A large Swiss study found that the negative impact of divorce was three times stronger than the benefit of getting married in the first place. The authors concluded that "marriage is primarily linked to a more positive evaluation of one's life rather than better health"(p. 1607). [17]

Certainly, marriage isn't beneficial for all people. Approximately 3% of married women with children are "seriously injured" or are "slapped, kicked, hit with a fist or object, cut, or bruised" by their children's father,[18] and 10% to 14% of US married women report that they are raped during marriage.[19] The sequelae of physical and sexual partner violence can be serious and long-lasting and can include death. But it isn't just physically and sexually violent marriages that may harm, rather than help, health. Even nonviolent but unhappy marriages can cause depression.[20] The results of some studies suggest that being in an unhappy marriage has worse health effects than never getting married to begin with or getting married and divorced.[21]

An increasing number of US youth and youth from other nations are eschewing marriage and, according to some sources, are increasingly eschewing pair-bonding relationships. As of 2018, 51% of 18- to 34-year-olds in the United States reported that they did not have a steady dating partner.[22] This has implications for population growth; as a result, some countries now try to encourage young people to get together, get married, and have babies—because a low birth rate could affect military power or industry.[23] But does *not* having children have negative implications for the individuals who opt out? Will it impair their health if they are not interested in marriage or not interested in relationships? The idea that healthy adulthood necessarily involves marriage, partnership, and child-rearing is becoming outmoded, and in part it's because health, happiness, and well-being are attainable without sexual and romantic partnerships.

Is Having Sex with Other Humans, in Person, Good for Individual or Public Health?

Even if there is no clear indication that marriage is essential for public health, there *is* evidence to suggest that, in general, people function better when they are in sexual and affectionate relationships. At the most basic level, it has been demonstrated that having more social support tends to be better for people.[24,25] Family and friends offer instrumental support, such as giving you a ride to work or cooking you a meal when you need one. Having friends or close family relationships also provides opportunities to give and receive emotional support, which can lower blood pressure[26] and decrease stress, depression, and anxiety,[27] and thus is clearly helpful for population-level health. But what if a person has plenty of family and friends and is asexual or not romantic? Will their health suffer because they choose not to engage in sexual activity or to socialize with potential dating partners? Or what if a person is sexual but in a long-distance relationship and spends an extended period of time masturbating and being sexual with their partner over the Internet, but not with skin-to-skin contact? Will their health suffer? Is it bad for public health if people aren't having enough sex with other people, in person?

Research on the apparent health benefits of having a partner, being married, and having sex may also be confounded. For example, studies that compare rates of health among married people and single people should control for mental health, resources, being perceived as conventionally attractive, or other factors that could be related to both coupling up and health. Researchers are now investigating whether "platonic friendships or kin can serve at least some of the functions of sexual partnerships in adulthood" (p. 139).[28] Research also suggests that, for some people, online sexual activity that doesn't involve in-person contact causes *more* arousal than in-person sex and *better* communication between real-life sex partners.[29] In other words, human connection may be necessary for a variety of reasons but the contentions that we need to have sex with other people in the flesh, or be married, to be healthy as individuals or as a society are far from foregone conclusions. We may need emotional intimacy, and we may benefit from skin-to-skin contact or social touch,[30] from affection, from orgasms, and from the instrumental help of people who care about us—but do those people need to be our marital or sexual partners? Friendships, cuddle buddies (or pets), getting a nonsexual massage, the feeling of belonging one derives from joining an online support group, and the tension reduction of orgasm from masturbation (either solo or with the involvement of the Internet) could, in theory, provide many or all of the same benefits of cohabiting with a partner.

The suggestion that it's a public health crisis, or problem, that young people are losing interest in marriage and relationships is tenuous at best. The state resolutions that lament a national declining interest in marriage or intimate relationships may be wrong on three levels. First, they suppose marriage and intimate relationships are important, and they may not be. Second, the presumption is that pornography influences relationships strongly, but there are likely other factors that are driving national trends in partnerships more strongly. Third, the presumption is that the research on pornography and relationships finds that pornography influences relationships negatively, but not all of it does.

Theoretical Explanations for Pornography's Possible Influence on Relationships

Hypothetically, why might pornography cause relationships to sour? Several theories have been proposed. They include social learning theory, scripting theory, and 3AM theory. Social learning theory is the idea that people learn to behave in certain ways by watching other people.[31] For example, children watch their parents or other adults, their peers, people on TV or in movies, and teachers and observe what kind of behavior elicits good reactions from others. They also notice what behaviors elicit negative consequences. According to social learning theory, we adapt our behavior to fit what we see being rewarded or punished and to be consistent with the norms that we see established in our environments. The application to pornography and relationship behavior is that by watching pornography the viewer may learn that certain sexual behaviors are rewarded and then imitate them. And because one of the ways in which pornography is able to excite viewers is to show transgressive or boundary-crossing and taboo material, it depicts some socially unacceptable behavior as acceptable. For example, the viewer may see a man call a woman a dirty slut and observe that the woman appears to enjoy this language. The viewer may then replicate the behavior with their partner, who actually does not enjoy it and therefore refuses to have sex. The relationship suffers as a result. In this way, viewing pornography might "teach" viewers incorrect social norms or sexual behaviors, which in turn harm relationships.

The second possibility is scripting theory,[32] which rests on the supposition that human sexuality is powered by what are called "scripts" that we internalize. In other words, humans don't have a purely instinctual sex drive. What turns us on, what we think is sexy, and what we want to do sexually are, in part, derived from stories that we tell ourselves. For example, a woman who sees a large, muscular, uniformed man and thinks to herself that he looks sexy is acting out her part of a heteronormative and gender-traditional social script that says that women are supposed to think that athletic men in positions of power are desirable. A man who sees a woman in a black bodysuit, high-heeled boots, and holding a whip and thinks to himself that she looks hot is acting out his part of a different heteronormative social script that says that a woman who defies certain conventions and takes control sexually is desirable. Wright explained sexual scripts in more formal terms. He wrote, "Sexual scripts are socially constructed guidelines for sexual encounters," and went on to explain that our sexual scripts may be influenced by pornography, which might color our perceptions of which other people are desirable, what should happen during a sexual encounter, and how we can expect sexual partners to react to us during sex (p. 318).[33] According to this theory, there is a possibility that pornography could influence a person's sexual script in a way that makes them lose interest in their partner. Alternatively, a person's sexual script could be altered so that they become interested in particular sexual acts, and although they are still aroused by their partner, their new kink or turn-on could be a turn-off to their partner and erode their intimate bond.

A third theory is Wright's 3AM theory, which uses and elaborates on sexual scripting theory.[34] The three *A*'s of the theory are: sexual script acquisition, activation, and application, and the *M* is for model. According to this theory, the way that pornography influences a sexual script is a function of how easily a person comes across the media, how arousing the sex it depicts is to them, how realistic it seems, how it interacts with their existing sexual script, and what they might already know about sex, as well as factors like their gender and age, how well they can recall the pornography, the situation in which they view it, and whether they feel rewarded or punished when they try acting on the script, as well as other factors.[34] The key is that 3AM theory applies the full richness and complexity of theories about how any type of media influences our thoughts and behavior to the question of how pornography may shape our sexual desires. The resulting proposal, as it pertains to pornography and relationship health, is that any attempt to characterize the influence of pornography on relationships is bound to be a gross oversimplification unless it in some way addresses the fact that there are many different factors that influence whether and how pornography influences our sexual wiring.

Does Pornography Cause Divorce?

Without question, there are individuals who argue with their partner about pornography use, and disagreements about it have undoubtedly contributed to the dissolution of some intimate partnerships. But when anti-pornography activists argue that pornography impairs people's ability to form relationships and harms marriages, I think that they are trying to suggest that there is something about watching pornography that changes the psychology of the viewer and that makes them less capable of functioning in a healthy relationship—not merely that partners might squabble over discrepant viewpoints on pornography or how much time is spent on it. It's possible that some people's psychology is altered by their pornography viewing, but whether such a substantial percentage of viewers are affected in this way that the problem rises to the level of being a public health crisis is not at all clear. In this section, I relay research findings about pornography and divorce. There are several studies that have found some type of pornography use to be associated with divorce rates, but the quality of these studies is important to evaluate.

One frequently used citation to support the idea that pornography causes divorce was published in *Sexual Addiction & Compulsivity* in 2006.[35] The article is a review, so it digests and summarizes findings that were originally presented elsewhere. One of the findings about pornography and divorce pertains to survey data that were collected at the November 2002 meeting of the American Academy of Matrimonial Lawyers (AAML) in Chicago, Illinois. The article, and testimony to the US Senate by the article's author on the same data,[36] reported that 62% of 350 attendees of a meeting of the AAML who responded to a poll reported that the Internet had played some role in past-year divorce cases. Of the 62% of lawyers who felt the Internet caused divorce, 56% felt that pornography was to blame. Unfortunately, the lawyers' opinions are now often cited as evidence that pornography causes divorce[37] and—worse—that 56% of divorces are caused by pornography.[38] That isn't an accurate interpretation of the AAML survey findings, which were that only 56% of lawyers who thought that the Internet caused divorce felt that pornography caused the Internet-related divorce issue. More to the point, though, is that the opinions of two-thirds of lawyers who happened to attend one conference in 2002 should probably be recognized as having low validity.

Unfortunately, there are other studies that are similarly problematic but are nevertheless cited as evidence that pornography causes divorce. For example, in one study, 91 women and three men who were in therapy to cope with a partner's Internet involvement were recruited into research by 20 sex addiction therapists.[39] The survey questions posed to these research participants were not specific to pornography. Participants were asked about their partners' "Internet sexual behaviors," which included reading or writing sexually explicit letters and stories, using the Internet to email someone to set up a personal meeting, placing ads to meet sex partners, and visiting sexually oriented chat rooms. But, despite the fact the study wasn't about pornography use and didn't use a comparison group, the fact that 22% of the research participants were divorced or separated has been cited as evidence that pornography use is associated with relationship dissolution. If that seems suspect, even worse are references to a conference presentation (so, not a peer-reviewed paper) that concluded that 10% to 25% of US divorces are caused by pornography, which was inferred by comparing sales of *Playboy* magazine to divorce rates in the 1960s and 1970s.[40] This is a great example of what is likely a correlational fallacy. The availability of pornographic magazines and divorce rates may have increased at the same time, but both could have been attributable to some third variable, such as the availability of birth control and a resulting culture shift toward more sexual partnerships, or perhaps domestic violence, or even marital rape laws, which were introduced in the same era.

More convincing evidence about pornography and divorce come from a series of longitudinal studies by Samuel Perry and co-authors.[41–43] There is also cross-sectional evidence from an analysis of the General Social Survey (GSS), a US-representative survey of adults 18 to 64 years old that found that men who reported any pornography use had 40% increased odds of also being divorced, as compared to men without pornography use.[44] For women, the odds of being divorced increased 10%.[44] But the authors conceded that they were unable to determine if pornography use preceded the divorce or if the order was the other way around. Perry and Schleifer (2017) also used the GSS but studied the same respondents at three separate times. They found that the probability of divorce within 2 years roughly doubled for men and women subsequent to the initiation of pornography use.[41] That is, among men, about 10% of porn users and 5% of non-porn users got divorced within 2 years. Among women, 16% of porn users and 6% of non-porn users got divorced within 2 years. Quitting pornography use at some point was also associated with a lower probability of divorce in future, but only for women. There remains a possibility that those who were already on a trajectory to divorce started using porn because of existing relationship problems, or that both the pornography use and the divorce could be related to a third factor (e.g., a lack of sex in marriage).

Perry and Davis (2017) used the Portraits of American Life Study (PALS) to examine romantic breakups among pornography users and non-users over time.[42] PALS is a nationally representative data set, and two waves of data were studied (2006 and 2012). Pornography use at Time 1 was associated with 86% increased odds of breakup 6 years later. Those who never viewed pornography had a 13% breakup rate, while those who viewed at some point in 2006 had a 23% breakup rate. The authors concluded that habitual pornography use may cause porn users to devalue monogamy or to have unrealistic sexual expectations of their partner, or that pornography use may upset partners and cause a rift in the relationship. The other possibility is that those who use pornography may be more prone to breaking up for some other reason (i.e., confounding).

Perry (2018) contributed a third study, also using PALS, and found that those who viewed pornography in 2006 were twice as likely as nonviewers to experience a marital separation by 2012, even controlling for marital happiness, sexual satisfaction, and other demographic variables.[43] However, the surprising aspect of the findings was that there was an inverted U-shaped relationship between frequency of pornography use and separation. Those who never or only sometimes used pornography had lower rates of separation, while those who used two to three times a month had higher separation rates. But, the people who used pornography the most often had separation rates even lower than those who said that they never used pornography. One possible explanation for these findings offered by the author is that the negative association between pornography use and marital stability may attenuate over time—meaning that as pornography use becomes more commonplace, couples may not think it's such a big deal if one or the other uses pornography, and it may not cause conflict.

Does Pornography Cause Infidelity?

A recent study found that 10% of young adults in the United States and 13% of young adults in Spain believe that the act of watching pornography counts as being unfaithful to one's partner.[45] In short, to them, watching pornography *is* infidelity, which creates a bit of a tautological problem for those wondering if pornography *causes* infidelity. So perhaps a better way to phrase this section's question is: Does watching pornography cause people to have sexual experiences outside their committed sexual and romantic partnerships?

There are at least six research studies that have looked at the relationship between pornography use and infidelity.[44,46–50] Most studies that have examined pornography use and infidelity have found that they are positively associated, but there are several reasons why an association between pornography use and infidelity may exist. One reason could be that watching pornography affects people's brains and psychology in such a way that it changes who they are, what they value, and how they want to conduct themselves. However, other reasons for the association could be that people who are unhappy in their relationships turn to both pornography and extradyadic encounters in order to try to feel better. It is also possible that there is a recursive relationship, where people who are curious about infidelity and perhaps are going to engage in infidelity start by checking out pornography, and the pornography affirms their interest in extradyadic sex. By way of example, a person might have a vague interest in baking and because of that decide to watch a reality show about baking, which solidifies their intention and inspires them to bake something right away. Did the baking show cause the baking? Maybe, but did the person's interest in baking cause them to watch the baking show, and all along their baking was inevitable? Disentangling whether watching influences doing can be tricky, because predilections also shape watching choices.

That said, it's helpful to have the facts handy, so here is a brief review of the six studies that support the relationship between pornography and infidelity. In a cross-sectional study of data from the GSS, year 2000, Stack et al. (2004) found that those who reported that they had visited a pornography website in the past month also had threefold increased odds of reporting that they engaged in adultery.[46] Similarly, Maddox et al. (2011) studied infidelity in a randomly selected sample of 1,291 unmarried adults in relationships and also found that couples who viewed pornography together had higher rates of infidelity than couples where neither person viewed pornography.[47] Using GSS data from 2000, 2002, and 2004, Wright and Randall (2012) also found that having used Internet pornography in the past month was associated with 65% higher odds of ever having had sex with someone other than one's spouse while married.[48] Doran and Price's 2014 study using GSS data found that for men, pornography use was associated with double the odds of having had an extramarital affair as compared to men who did not report pornography use (OR 2.08), and for women, the OR was 1.95.[44] While the study controlled for whether the respondents had children, whether they were religious, and their attitudes about pornography, it's simply not possible to know from cross-sectional studies if those who had a higher sex drive and were simply more sexually active people were more likely to use pornography and also more likely to seek out extradyadic sex, or if the pornography caused them to engage in infidelity. Either, or both, is possible.

Two experimental studies provide possibly somewhat more compelling data. Lambert and colleagues (2012) conducted an analysis of data from 240 undergraduate students who participated in the research study to earn course credit in a psychology class.[49] The students were asked: "Approximately how many times in the past 30 days have you viewed pornographic material (website, magazine, video)?" The researchers also asked the students if they were in a relationship, how long they'd been in that relationship, and how many people they had hooked up with in the past year. Anyone who said that they were in a relationship but had hooked up with more than one person was classified as a cheater (i.e., the researchers did not consider consensual non-monogamy a possibility). Students were also asked if they had done anything in the past 2 months that the thought counted as physically unfaithful, or that their partner might think would count as physically unfaithful. There was a minor association between pornography use and being unfaithful, which was mediated by a how committed the student felt to their relationship. Because pornography use was associated with decreased commitment, which was in turn associated with increased infidelity, the authors concluded that there is a relationship cost associated with pornography consumption. However, the idea that pornography use, extradyadic sex, and low commitment might be normative for some college students was not explored. A similar study by Gwinn and colleagues (2013) of 74 undergraduate students who participated in a pornography experiment for course credit found that students who saw pornography were more likely to report, 12 weeks later, that they had kissed or had sex with someone other than their partner, controlling for baseline extradyadic behavior, relationship length and satisfaction, and other factors.[50] Again, consensual non-monogamy was not considered by the researchers, although the authors did concede that college students are "typically engaged in relatively young 'fledgling' relationships."

Does Pornography Cause Sexual or Relationship Dissatisfaction?

By my count, there are more than 40 unique studies that have examined pornography use and relationship satisfaction, sexual satisfaction in a relationship, or both. Rather than describe the design and results of each, a summary observation is that there is heterogeneity in their findings. One of the key takeaways from this body of literature is that the gender of the pornography user matters, as well as whether the relationship was a satisfying one to begin with, and whether the pornography is used by one partner in secret, or not in secret but alone instead of in tandem with their partner, or sometimes in tandem with a partner, or always with their partner. One study even found that the individuals' body weight mattered: pornography use was more likely to cause relationship problems for overweight people than for non-overweight people.[51] In short, the context of pornography use and the underlying dynamic between the people in the relationship can influence how the use of pornography affects them. In the same way that buying a new car could increase relationship satisfaction for some couples, who are excited to take road trips together, and might decrease satisfaction in other couples if one partner spent money that the other didn't want expended on a vehicle—pornography, too, might cause either increased or decreased satisfaction in relationships depending on what is watched, how often, by whom, with whom, and for what purpose; whether the relationship or individuals were secure or anxious to begin with; and how they communicate about the pornography use. In the words of one researcher: "The impact of pornography consumption on sexual satisfaction is almost zero in secure [individuals], negative in anxious or avoidant individuals, [and] positive in fearful individuals" (p. 176).[52] Thus, the condemnation of all pornography as elevating risk for relationship harm among all types of people doesn't square with the research evidence.

Wright and colleagues conducted a meta-analysis of this literature relatively recently (2017).[33] They found, across 50 studies from 10 countries and involving more than 50,000 individuals, that there was no association between women's pornography use and relationship satisfaction, but that there was one for men. Acknowledging that the causal relationships between pornography use and satisfaction, if extant, may be bidirectional or reciprocal, Wright and colleagues summed up by suggesting that "the convergence of results across cross-sectional survey, longitudinal survey, and experimental results points to an overall negative effect of pornography on men's sexual and relational satisfaction" (p. 336).[33] One limitation of meta-analysis is that it is only as sound as the underlying studies that go into it. In this case, the underlying studies analyzed by Wright and colleagues had fundamental limitations, such as potential confounding, that weren't resolved by the meta-analytic techniques.

Does Pornography Cause Women in Relationships to Feel Inadequate?

One of the hypotheses about why pornography may harm relationships is that it causes women to feel inadequate as sexual partners or that they are unattractive. The logic goes like this: heterosexual, partnered men watch pornography, they like the women that they see in pornography and the sex that they see, so this causes them to compare their partners to the women in pornography and to disfavor their partners, the women perceive that they are being compared to women in pornography and have been found lacking, and this causes women to feel inadequate. The feelings of inadequacy harm the relationship stability and quality. Another hypothesis is that men become excited by the supernormal stimuli they see in pornography—extra-large breasts, for example—and lose interest in normal stimuli.[53] Both hypotheses sound plausible, but are they supported by evidence? There is little doubt that some heterosexual, partnered men watch pornography, and there is evidence that men who watch pornography may compare their intimate partners unfavorably to the women in pornography (see Zillmann and Bryant 1988).[54] But perhaps surprisingly, early research on this topic found that pornography might *enhance* men's sexual desire for their partner, not lessen it.

In 1978, Dermer and Pyszczynski became the first researchers to study the effects of pornography on men's responses to women they love.[55] In a randomized laboratory study, 51 undergraduate college men with intimate partners were asked to read an erotic story or a control condition article about herring gulls mating and then complete a survey about their intimate partner. Those who were exposed to the erotic stories were more likely to endorse more loving statements about their partners. The researchers concluded that being in an aroused sexual state enhanced romantic, amorous feelings toward a partner. These findings fit neatly into the body of research that was developing at that time on excitation transfer theory, which is the idea that becoming emotionally aroused by one experience can intensify other emotional moments that follow. For example, riding a roller coaster might intensify feelings of sexual attraction.[56] In this case, reading erotic material got the subjects worked up, and that feeling transferred into amorous feelings toward their partners. A key aspect of the Dermer and Pyszczynski study was that the erotic material was text, not images, and perhaps that is what made the difference. Because the next subsequent study on this topic, by Zillmann and Bryant (1988), used 7-minute pornographic video clips and non-pornographic video clips as a control, and they found something different.[55] Subjects who were assigned to view pornography were subsequently more likely to rate their intimate partners as *less* attractive and *less* sexually proficient than control subjects who had not been primed with pornography. Excitation transfer theory was cast aside to make room for a newer and better hypothesis: pornography use by men caused them to lose interest in their partners because they were hyperstimulated by pornography and subsequently unable to feel stimulated by live sexual encounters. The presumption was that if men were feeling less stimulated by live sexual encounters, then their female partners were likely blaming themselves, and therefore were suffering from low self-esteem and feelings of inadequacy as a direct result.

In the dozen studies that followed, researchers used various study designs and methods and drew different conclusions about whether pornography viewing did make women feel inadequate. Some researchers used convenience samples of women who were known to be upset about their partners' pornography use and recorded their thoughts and feelings, which was then cited as evidence by other researchers that pornography harms relationships. For example, Bergner and Bridges analyzed 100 letters posted to Internet message boards by women who perceived their partners to be heavy pornography users,[57] Bridges et al. (2003) solicited survey participants from Internet message boards geared toward women and romantic relationship advice,[58] Zitzman and Butler recruited couples who were seeing therapists because of problematic pornography use by one member of the couple,[59] and Schneider solicited comments from women who had sought relationship counseling due to problems in their relationships caused by their partner's Internet use.[39] Stewart and Szymanski (2012) did not relay how they recruited participants, nor did they describe their sampling frame or response rate.[60] In any case, the designs of these five studies do not permit inferences about how widespread the problem of women feeling inadequate because of partners' pornography use may be.

Researchers who used more representative samples, such as Daneback and colleagues' study of 398 heterosexual Norwegian couples who were part of a standing panel, found that women who did not use pornography but had partners who did tended to have a worse self-perception than women whose partners did not use pornography. They also found that couples in which both people used pornography tended to have fewer sexual and mental perception problems than those where neither used pornography.[61] But the survey response rate was 20%, and the women with an axe to grind about pornography may have been more likely to respond to the survey than women who were content.

The most recent research findings suggest that whether women in couples feel inadequate because of pornography depends on the pattern of use within the couple, and whether pornography use is concealed. In other words, is there "concordance" in use—meaning that both people use pornography, whether separately or in tandem—or is there discordance, meaning that one person is using alone with or without informing their partner.[29,62] And are partners honest with each other about pornography?[63] Women in couples that share pornography use style, and where partners are honest about pornography use, tend to feel better about themselves and the relationships than women in couples where there is no concordance, or where one person is concealing use from the other.[29,62,63] So the takeaway is that because individuals and couples are diverse, and there is tremendous variety in the content of pornography, it is not possible to conclude that if someone in a couple watches pornography, the woman is going to feel terrible about herself, and the relationship is headed somewhere awful. That unhappy chain of events might happen in some relationships, and it might not happen in others. What's more, and adding to uncertainty about the application of research findings to the present moment, the relationship between pornography use in couples and women's self-esteem may be changing rapidly over time. For example, today's youth grew up with a President who referenced the size of his penis during a nationally televised debate and had a well-publicized affair with a porn actress that came to light while he was in office. These cultural events, or other changing norms related to Internet sex, may be influencing how young people interpret a partner's pornography use—and it may be causing either less, or more, insecurity than it did even a decade ago.

Does Pornography Lessen the Desire to Marry?

One of the points made in the state resolutions that pornography is a public health crisis is that the availability of pornography is lessening young men's desire to marry. This specific complaint about pornography may reflect a finding from a study that came out in 2016. Malcolm and Naufal (2016) analyzed GSS data from 2000, 2002, and 2004, limited to men 18 to 35 years old (i.e., young men).[6] They found that the more hours that individuals used the Internet to look at finance, news, education, health, or sports websites, the less likely they were to be married, though looking at religious websites was positively associated with marriage. For pornography consumption, each 1% increase in looking at pornography one or more times in the past month was associated with a 0.6% decrease in likelihood that the respondent would also report being married. Malcolm and Naufal therefore concluded that Internet pornography was *causing* young men to lose their motivation for forming marital unions. However, the authors did not interpret their finding that Internet use in general was associated with decreased likelihood of being married. Moreover, the results may actually reflect the influence of a third, unmeasured variable. For example, perhaps people who prefer solitude and consider dating relationships boring are also more likely to find browsing the Internet fun, but the Internet didn't cause them to find relationships boring. The evidence to support the contention that Internet pornography is causing people to lose interest in marriage is limited.

Is Pornography Good for a Couple's Sex Life?

While numerous studies have reported on the likelihood of relationship problems, breakups, divorce, and low self-esteem as a potential result of pornography use, a handful of studies have also found that pornography can have some positive effects on some relationships. Collectively, these studies have found that pornography use can bolster communication,[64] encourage sexual experimentation (which decreases sexual boredom),[65] facilitate discussion of sexuality, increase intimacy, and increase arousal.[66] But, because there is such variety in pornography content, and between couples, and because none of these studies have been carried out on representative samples, it's impossible to know how common it is for couples to find pornography use helpful. Complicating the matter further, even within one couple, dynamics or practicalities may change over time, so pornography use may help the couple communicate one month, but cause problems the next.

Conclusions

Most studies that have examined pornography use and infidelity have found that they are positively associated. Frustratingly, however, there is no clear evidence that the relationship is causal (nor clear evidence that it is *not* causal). There have also been multiple studies of pornography use and relationship satisfaction, and a meta-analysis found that men's pornography use is associated with less sexual and relational satisfaction. But, men who are unhappy in their relationships may turn to pornography to solve their sexual satisfaction problems, so the possibility of bidirectional and reciprocal causality is strong. If pornography does influence relationship health, the influence is likely weak—because measures of association across studies are small, and because there is variation in the association between pornography and relationships by gender, attachment style, relationship functionality, and other factors. Existing evidence does not support the conclusion that the existence of pornography in society, or the use of pornography by adult viewers, is jeopardizing population health by virtue of a negative influence on marriages, relationships, sexual satisfaction, or women's self-esteem. Pornography causes problems for some individuals and in some relationships, but evidence does not support the conclusion that this is a threat to human health.

References

1. State of Ohio. 2019. "A Resolution to Declare Pornography Is a Public Health Hazard with Statewide and National Public Health Impacts Leading to a Broad Spectrum of Individual and Societal Harms." *H.R. No. 180,* 133rd General Assembly Regular Session. https://www.ccv.org/wp-content/uploads/House-Resolution-180_Rep-Powell.pdf

2. Chapais, B. 2011. "The Evolutionary History of Pair-bonding and Parental Collaboration." In *The Oxford Handbook of Evolutionary Family Psychology*, edited by T. Shackelford and C. Salmon. New York: Oxford University Press.

3. Gavrilets, S. 2012. "Human Origins and the Transition from Promiscuity to Pair-bonding." *Proceedings of the National Academy of Sciences USA* 109, no. 25: 9923–9928.

4. Graff, E. J. 1999. *What is Marriage For?* Boston, MA: Beacon Press.

5. Lopez, K. J. 2013. "Why Is Government Involved with Marriage Anyway?" *National Review* https://www.nationalreview.com/corner/why-government-involved-with-marriage-anyway-kathryn-jean-lopez/

6. Malcolm, M., and G. Naufal. 2016. "Are Pornography and Marriage Substitutes for Young Men?" *Eastern Economic Journal* 42, no. 3: 317–334.

7. Bloch, R. H. 1991. *Medieval Misogyny and the Invention of Western Romantic Love.* Chicago: University of Chicago Press.

8. Amato, P. R. 2001. "Children of Divorce in the 1990s: An Update of the Amato and Keith (1991) Meta-analysis." *Journal of Family Psychology* 15, no. 3: 355–370.

9. Brand, J. E., R. Moore, X. Song, and Y. Xie. 2019. "Parental Divorce Is Not Uniformly Disruptive to Children's Educational Attainment." *Proceedings of the National Academy of Sciences USA* 116, no. 15: 7266–7271.

10. Goring, D. 2006. "The History of Slave Marriage in the United States." *LSU Law Digital Commons* 262: 299–347.

11. Loving v. Virginia, 388 U.S. 1 (U.S. Supreme Court 1967).

12. US Department of Justice. 2015. "Attorney General Lynch Announces Federal Marriage Benefits Available to Same-Sex Couples Nationwide." https://www.justice.gov/opa/pr/attorney-general-lynch-announces-federal-marriage-benefits-available-same-sex-couples

13. Kiecolt-Glaser, J. K., and T. L. Newton. 2001. "Marriage and Health: His and Hers." *Psychological Bulletin* 127, no. 4: 472–503.

14. Roxburgh, S. 2014. "Race, Class, and Gender Differences in the Marriage-Health Relationship." *Race, Gender & Class* 21, no. 3/4: 7–31.

15. Gove, W. R. 1972. "The Relationship Between Sex Roles, Marital Status, and Mental Illness." *Social Forces* 51, no. 1: 34–44.

16. Choi, H., and N. F. Marks. 2013. "Marital Quality, Socioeconomic Status, and Physical Health." *Journal of Marriage and Family* 75, no. 4: 903–919.

17. Kalmijn, M. 2017. "The Ambiguous Link between Marriage and Health: A Dynamic Reanalysis of Loss and Gain Effects." *Social Forces* 95, no. 4: 1607–1636.

18. DeKlyen, M., J. Brooks-Gunn, S. McLanahan, and J. Knab. 2006. "The Mental Health of Married, Cohabiting, and Non-coresident Parents with Infants." *American Journal of Public Health* 96, no. 10: 1836–1841.

19. Russell, D. E. H. 1990. *Rape in Marriage.* Bloomington: Indiana University Press.

20. Woods, S. B., J. B. Priest, T. L. Signs, and C. A. Maier. 2019. "In Sickness and in Health: The Longitudinal Associations Between Marital Dissatisfaction, Depression and Spousal Health." *Journal of Family Therapy* 41, no. 1: 102–125.

21. Williams, K. 2003. "Has the Future of Marriage Arrived? A Contemporary Examination of Gender, Marriage, and Psychological Well-being." *Journal of Health and Social Behavior* 44, no. 4: 470–487.

22. Bosos, L., and E. Guskin. "It's Not Just You: New Data Shows More Than Half of Young People in America Don't Have a Romantic Partner." *The Washington Post* March 21, 2019.

23. Howe, N. 2019. "Nations Labor to Raise Their Birthrates." https://www.forbes.com/sites/neilhowe/2019/03/29/nations-labor-to-raise-their-birthrates/

24. Cohen, S. 2004. "Social Relationships and Health." *American Psychologist* 59, no. 8: 676–684.

25. Uchino, B. N., J. T. Cacioppo, and J. K. KiecoltGlaser. 1996. "The Relationship Between Social Support and Physiological Processes: A Review with Emphasis on Underlying Mechanisms and Implications for Health." *Psychological Bulletin* 119, no. 3: 488–531.

26. Coulon, S. M, and D. K. Wilson. 2015. "Social Support Buffering of the Relation Between Low Income and Elevated Blood Pressure in At-Risk African-American Adults." *Journal of Behavioral Medicine* 38, no. 5: 830–834.

27. Ozbay, F., D. C. Johnson, E. Dimoulas, C. A. Morgan, D. Charney, and S. Southwick. 2007. "Social Support and Resilience to Stress: From Neurobiology to Clinical Practice." *Psychiatry* (Edgmont) 4, no. 5: 35–40.

28. Zeifman, D. M. 2019. "Attachment Theory Grows Up: A Developmental Approach to Pair Bonds." *Current Opinion in Psychology* 25: 139–143.

29. Grov, C., B. J. Gillespie, T. Royce, and J. Lever. 2011. "Perceived Consequences of Casual Online Sexual Activities on Heterosexual Relationships: A U.S. Online Survey." *Archives of Sexual Behavior* 40, no. 2: 429–439.

30. Cascio, C. J., D. Moore, and F. McGlone. 2019. "Social Touch and Human Development." *Developmental Cognitive Neuroscience* 35: 5–11.

31. Bandura, A. 1973. *Aggression: A Social Learning Analysis.* Englewood Cliffs, NJ: Prentice Hall.

32. Simon, W., and J. H. Gagnon. 1984. "Sexual Scripts." *Society* 22, no. 1: 53–60.

33. Wright, P. J., R. S. Tokunaga, A. Kraus, and E. Klann. 2017. "Pornography Consumption and Satisfaction: A Meta-Analysis." *Human Communication Research* 43, no. 3: 315–343.

34. Wright, P. J. 2011. "Mass Media Effects on Youth Sexual Behavior: Assessing the Claim for Causality." *Annals of the International Communication Association* 35, no. 1: 343–385.

35. Manning, J. C. 2006. "The Impact of Internet Pornography on Marriage and the Family: A Review of the Research." *Sexual Addiction & Compulsivity* 13, no. 2–3: 131–165.

36. *Hearing on Pornography's Impact on Marriage and the Family, Before the Subcommittee on the Constitution, Civil Rights, and Property Rights, Committee on the Judiciary* (2005) (testimony of J. Manning).

37. Larson, V. 2011. "Does Porn Watching Lead to Divorce?" *Huffpost* https://www.huffpost.com/entry/porn-and-divorce_b_861987

38. Skinner, K. 2011. "Is Porn Really Destroying 500,000 Marriages Annually?" https://www.psychologytoday.com/us/blog/inside-porn-addiction/201112/is-porn-really-destroying-500000-marriages-annually

39. Schneider, J. P. 2000. "Effects of Cybersex Addiction on the Family: Results of a Survey." *Sexual Addiction & Compulsivity* 7, no. 1–2: 31–58.

40. Shumway, T., and R. Daines. June 4, 2012. "Pornography and Divorce." *7th Annual Conference on Empirical Legal Studies Paper.* Available at SSRN: https://ssrn.com/abstract=2112435 or http://dx.doi.org/10.2139/ssrn.2112435

41. Perry, S. L., and C. Schleifer. 2018. "Till Porn Do Us Part? A Longitudinal Examination of Pornography Use and Divorce." *Journal of Sex Research* 55, no. 3: 284–296.

42. Perry, S., and J. Davis. 2017. "Are Pornography Users More Likely to Experience A Romantic Breakup? Evidence from Longitudinal Data." *Sexuality & Culture* 21, no. 4: 1157–1176.

43. Perry, S. L. 2018. "Pornography Use and Marital Quality: Testing the Moral Incongruence Hypothesis." *Personal Relationships* 25, no. 2: 233–248.

44. Doran, K., and J. Price. 2014. "Pornography and Marriage." *Journal of Family and Economic Issues* 35, no. 4: 489–498.

45. Negy, C., D. Plaza, A. Reig-Ferrer, and M. D. Fernandez-Pascual. 2018. "Is Viewing Sexually Explicit Material Cheating on Your Partner? A Comparison Between the United States and Spain." *Archives of Sexual Behavior* 47, no. 3: 737–745.

46. Stack, S., I. Wasserman, and R. Kern. 2004. "Adult Social Bonds and Use of Internet Pornography." *Social Science Quarterly* 85, no. 1: 75–88.

47. Maddox, A. M., G. K. Rhoades, and H. J. Markman. 2011. "Viewing Sexually-Explicit Materials Alone or Together: Associations with Relationship Quality." *Archives of Sexual Behavior* 40, no. 2: 441–448.

48. Wright, P., and A. Randall. 2012. "Internet Pornography Exposure and Risky Sexual Behavior Among Adult Males in the United States." *Computers in Human Behavior* 28: 1410–1416.

49. Lambert, N. M., S. Negash, T. F. Stillman, S. B. Olmstead, and F. D. Fincham. 2012. "A Love That Doesn't Last: Pornography Consumption and Weakened Commitment to One's Romantic Partner." *Journal of Social and Clinical Psychology* 31, no. 4: 410–438.

50. Gwinn, A. M., N. M. Lambert, F. D. Fincham, and J. K. Maner. 2013. "Pornography, Relationship Alternatives, and Intimate Extradyadic Behavior." *Social Psychological and Personality Science* 4, no. 6: 699–704.

51. Dwulit, A. D., and P. Rzymski. 2019. "Prevalence, Patterns and Self-Perceived Effects of Pornography Consumption in Polish University Students: A Cross-Sectional Study." *International Journal of Environmental Research and Public Health* 16, no. 10, 1–16.

52. Gouvernet, B., T. Rebelo, F. Sebbe, et al. 2017. "Is Pornography Pathogen by Itself? Study of the Role of Attachment Profiles on the Relationship Between Pornography and Sexual Satisfaction." *Sexologies* 26, no. 3: 176–185.

53. Gottman, J., and J. Gottman. 2016. "An Open Letter on Porn." https://www.gottman.com/blog/an-open-letter-on-porn/ Accessed August 4, 2020.

54. Zillmann, D., and J. Bryant. 1988. "Pornography Impact on Sexual Satisfaction." *Journal of Applied Social Psychology* 18, no. 5: 438–453.

55. Dermer, M., and T. A. Pyszczynski. 1978. "Effects of Erotica Upon Men's Loving and Liking Responses for Women They Love." *Journal of Personality and Social Psychology* 36, no. 11: 1302–1309.

56. Meston, C. M., and P. F. Frohlich. 2003. "Love at First Fright: Partner Salience Moderates Roller-Coaster-Induced Excitation Transfer." *Archives of Sexual Behavior* 32, no. 6: 537–544.

57. Bergner, R. M., and A. J. Bridges. 2002. "The Significance of Heavy Pornography Involvement for Romantic Partners: Research and Clinical Implications." *Journal of Sex & Marital Therapy* 28, no. 3: 193–206.

58. Bridges, A. J., R. M. Bergner, and M. Hesson-Mcinnis. 2003. "Romantic Partners Use of Pornography: Its Significance for Women." *Journal of Sex & Marital Therapy* 29, no. 1: 1–14.

59. Zitzman, S. T., and M. H. Butler. 2009. "Wives' Experience of Husbands' Pornography Use and Concomitant Deception as an Attachment Threat in the Adult Pair-Bond Relationship." *Sexual Addiction & Compulsivity* 16, no. 3: 210–240.

60. Stewart, D. N., and D. M. Szymanski. 2012. "Young Adult Women's Reports of Their Male Romantic Partner's Pornography Use as a Correlate of Their Self-Esteem, Relationship Quality, and Sexual Satisfaction." *Sex Roles* 67, no. 5–6: 257–271.

61. Daneback, K., B. Traen, and S-A. Mansson. 2009. "Use of Pornography in a Random Sample of Norwegian Heterosexual Couples." *Archives of Sexual Behavior* 38, no. 5: 746–753.

62. Kohut, T., R. N. Balzarini, W. A. Fisher, and L. Campbell. 2018. "Pornography's Associations with Open Sexual Communication and Relationship Closeness Vary as a Function of

Dyadic Patterns of Pornography Use Within Heterosexual Relationships." *Journal of Social and Personal Relationships* 35, no. 4: 655–676.

63. Carroll, J. S., D. M. Busby, B. J. Willoughby, and C. C. Brown. 2017. "The Porn Gap: Differences in Men's and Women's Pornography Patterns in Couple Relationships." *Journal of Couple & Relationship Therapy* 16, no. 2: 146–163.

64. Grov, C., B. J. Gillespie, T. Royce, and J. Lever. 2011. "Perceived Consequences of Casual Online Sexual Activities on Heterosexual Relationships: A U.S. Online Survey." *Archives of Sexual Behavior* 40, no. 2: 129–139.

65. McCormack, M., and L. Wignall. 2016. "Enjoyment, Exploration and Education: Understanding the Consumption of Pornography among Young Men with Non-Exclusive Sexual Orientations." *Sociology* 51, no. 5: 975–991.

66. McNabney, S. M., K. Heves, and D. L. Rowland. 2020. "Effects of Pornography Use and Demographic Parameters on Sexual Response during Masturbation and Partnered Sex in Women." *International Journal of Environmental Research and Public Health* 17, no. 9: 16.

8

The Effects of Pornography on Youth

As unimaginable as it might seem today, comic books were once declared a public health crisis.[1] In the 1940s, comic books of all varieties became popular with children and adolescents. The US Senate held televised hearings on the violence and sex depicted in comic books and whether it might be influencing pre-teen behavior problems.[1] In the wake of the Senate hearings, bills prohibiting the distribution of comics depicting illicit sex, physical torture, or physical violence were passed, as well as restrictions on the sale of "lurid" comic books to those younger than 18 years old.[2] And a regulatory group, the Comics Code Authority, was established to "enforce strict guidelines of morality, decency, and good prevailing over evil."[3] Today, the idea that comic books could cause an epidemic of violence and crime might strike most people as implausible. But there are lessons to be learned from the moral panics of prior eras with regard to how we approach present-day concerns over youth exposure to the content of video games, Internet and entertainment content, and pornography.[4]

The bulk of the evidence on the influence of mainstream online pornography on youth suggests that there is, on average, a negative effect, and that there may be particular reasons for concern if youth have little other health-promoting information or few caring adults in conversation with them about sex to offset what they see. The job of public health professionals, therefore, is to determine how best to safeguard underage youth from the potential harms of pornography while pushing back against nonscientific claims about its effects.

Is It Illegal for Youth to See Pornography?

In the United States, according to federal law, it is illegal to show pornography to people younger than 16 years old.[5] There may also be state laws that layer on additional prohibitions, such as in the state of California, where it is not legal to send sexually explicit material to a person less than 18 years old.[6] Importantly, according to federal law, if someone younger than 16 years old

Pornography and Public Health. Emily F. Rothman, Oxford University Press. © Oxford University Press 2021.
DOI: 10.1093/oso/9780190075477.003.0008

sees pornography, the one in the wrong is the person or entity that showed the pornography to the child—not the child.

Prevalence of Use

In 2016, Peter and Valkenburg published a review of 20 years of research on adolescents and pornography.[7] Contained within the review is a table presenting 43 research studies conducted with samples of youth from 19 nations, including the United States, Taiwan, Korea, Italy, the Netherlands, Australia, Israel, Nigeria, Sweden, Greece, Switzerland, Hong Kong, China, Morocco, Belgium, Ethiopia, Malaysia, the Czech Republic, and Cambodia. The rates range from a low of 1% of Swiss girls 16 to 20 years old having experienced intentional Internet pornography use in the past month (see Luder et al. 2011),[8] to 98% of 16- to 19-year-old German boys ever having seen a pornographic video or film (see Weber et al. 2012).[9] For the United States, rates ranged from a low of 7% of a nationally representative sample of 10- to 17-year-old youth intentionally viewing pornography in non-Internet media in the past year,[10] to 83% of high school boys in California ever having seen a pornographic video.[11] The problem with research on the prevalence of adolescents' pornography use or exposure is that inconsistent definitions of pornography, use, the ages of youth in the sample, and the time period of the research mean that estimates vary widely.

To characterize the prevalence of pornography "exposure" (i.e., viewing) among younger children, one probability-based nationally representative estimate is available from the Youth Internet Safety Survey (YISS), a nationally representative study of children 10 to 17 years old who used the Internet.[10] In 2000, 15% of this sample reported that they had purposely sought out and seen pornography, either on the Internet or in offline sources like magazines, in the past year.[10] The same survey was repeated in 2005 and 2010.[12] In 2010, 13% of US youth 10 to 17 years old reported Internet pornography exposure in the past year.[12] This study also found that there was a modest increase in the percentage of youth who reported internet pornography exposure between 2000 and 2010, and virtually all of the increase took place in the first 5 years.[12] Interestingly, the increases were primarily among youth 16 to 17 years old. In 2010, only 2% of youth 10 to 11 years old reported having seen pornography in the past year.[12]

A different nationally representative study that collected data in 2010–2011 from 14- to 21-year-old youth found that, among those who had used the

Internet in the past 6 months, 37% reported seeing pornography in the past year, where pornography was defined as an X-rated movie, magazine, or "adult" website.[13] Of those who had seen pornography, 85% had seen nonviolent pornography and 15% had seen violent pornography, defined as a movie, magazine, or adult website that showed a person being physically hurt by another person while they were doing something sexual.[13] Overall, only 5% of this nationally representative sample of youth had seen violent pornography in the past year.[13] This same study found that those who had seen violent pornography were at substantially increased risk for having perpetrated forced sexual contact or coerced sex, as well—in fact, those who saw violent pornography were five times more likely than those who had not to report any sexual violence perpetration.[13]

Importantly, youth may be as likely to see sexual content in nonpornographic TV shows and movies as they are to see it on the Internet. The Growing Up with Media Study collected data from 1,058 youth 14 to 21 years old in 2010 to 2012.[14] Exposure to sexual media was elicited via five separate questions covering TV and movies, music, video games, and websites that show cartoons and real people. Youth were asked to report on media that showed people "kissing, fondling, or having sex." The study revealed that 32% of youth reported that many, almost all, or all of the TV shows and movies they watched contained sexual content, whereas 5% of the youth said that many, almost all, or all of the websites they visited depicted sexual scenes. This study tells us that if we are worried about youth exposure to sexual content in media, focusing only on pornography, pornography-specific websites, or the pornography industry isn't consistent with a public health approach.

The percentage of adolescents who have viewed sexually explicit media online in the past year may be increasing because of the ever-widening availability of Internet-connected devices and high-speed Internet. It makes intuitive sense that more and more youth have access to unrestricted time on the Internet—but it's an assumption, and as of yet, largely untested. For what it's worth, as long ago as 1971, a survey of US college students found that 95% of males and 43% of females reported that they at least sometimes (or fairly or very often) looked at pornographic photos, suggesting that looking at sexually explicit media was a common youth behavior long before the advent of the Internet.[15,16]

The Age of First Exposure to Pornography

People worry that the younger a person is when he or she first sees pornography, the more harm that is done to them. The idea is that the younger a person is, the less capable they are of understanding what they are seeing, and the more likely they are to be traumatized or to develop unhealthy sexual scripts.[17] A number of studies have investigated the average age of children's first exposure to pornography. Taken together, it seems that most have found that the average age of first pornography exposure tends to be between 10 and 15 years old for most teenagers, and several studies support the idea that the average age of first pornography exposure is now 11 to 12 years old (see Table 8.1). Given that the average age of heterosexual sexual intercourse debut for US adolescents is 16 to 17 years old, the fact that 11- to 12-year-old youth are seeking out information about sex and sexual images makes sense from a developmental perspective (see Table 8.1).[18]

Table 8.1. Studies that provide estimates of the age of first pornography exposure

Author and Date	Sample and Year That Data Were Collected	Average Age of First Exposure to Pornography (Years)
Wilson and Abelson 1973 (as reported by Bryant and Brown 1989[16])	National probability sample of 2,486 US adults, ages 21 years and older, 1970–1971	Boys: 17 Girls: 20
Sabina et al. 2008[78]	College students in New England, 2006	Boys: 14.3 Girls: 14.8
Romito and Beltramini 2011[42]	Northeastern Italian high school students and young adults, 2007	Boys: 43% ages 13 to 15 Girls: 35% ages 13 to 15
Sinković et al. 2013[79]	Croatian young adults, 2010	Boys: 11.5 Girls: 13.5
Sun et al. 2017[80]	German female college students 18 years old and older, 2011–2012	Girls: 31.5% between the ages of 10 and 12, and 31% between the ages of 13 and 15
Wright and Štulhofer 2019[81]	Study of 16-year-olds in Croatia, 2015	Boys: 11.45 Girls: 12.45
Lim et al. 2017[46]	Australian youth 15 to 29 years old, 2015	Boys: 13 Girls: 16
Nelson et al. 2019[82]	Convenience sample of gay youth in the United States, 14 to 17 years old, 2017	Boys: 12
Laemmle-Ruff et al. 2019[83]	Convenience sample of people who used health and fitness social media, 19 to 30 years old, 2016	All: 16
Herbenick et al. 2020[84]	US probability sample of adults 18 to 60 years old, 2016	Boys: 13.8 Girls: 17.8

What Do Adolescents See When They Are Exposed to Pornography?

Because online pornography sites like Pornhub do not require age or identity verification, and because pornography may be embedded in other platforms to which youth have access (e.g., Twitter), underage youth can see any genre of pornography. What they are most likely to see by chance, or what they choose to see, is a question of interest that a handful of studies have investigated. For example, in the United States, a cross-sectional study of a convenience sample of 72 US-based, urban-residing, economically disadvantaged, and primarily Black and Hispanic youth found that youth were most likely to report watching porn with the tags lesbian/bisexual (44%), big butt/big tits (43%), Ebony/Latina (39%), Blowjob (21%), Threesome (16%), Teen (13%), and Group sex (11%).[19] An anonymous online survey study of young, heterosexual, Australian youth found that 97% of the sample reported seeing "men's pleasure" in pornography they had seen in the past year, 91% reported seeing men being dominant, and 77% had seen violence in pornography. In addition, 89% reported they had seen romance and/or affection in pornography, 96% reported seeing a focus on women's pleasure, and 74% had seen women portrayed as dominant. Approximately 43% had seen violence or aggression toward a woman that appeared nonconsensual, and 18% had seen violence or aggression toward a man that appeared nonconsensual.[20]

A longitudinal study of Dutch adolescents 13 to 17 years old, conducted in 2013–2014, found that 20% of the sample had encountered "affection-themed" and "dominance-themed" pornography, while 10% indicated that they had seen "violence-themed" pornography.[21] Older adolescents in the sample were more likely to have been exposed to dominance-themed pornography, while younger adolescents were more likely to have been exposed to affection-themed pornography.[21] Adolescents who had a hyper gender orientation (i.e., adhered strongly to hypermasculine or hyperfeminine norms related to gender) were more likely to choose to watch violence-themed pornography.[21]

Risk Factors for the Use of Sexually Explicit Media in Adolescence

Numerous studies, both cross-sectional and longitudinal, have identified risk factors and some protective factors for adolescent and young adult pornography consumption. These have been summarized in multiple review articles, including those by Koletić (2017) and Peter and Valkenburg (2016).[7,22] Public health practitioners and researchers often array risk and protective factors according to the "levels" of the social-ecological model.[23] The levels represent spheres of influence on a person's development, and the fact that each is nested inside the next is a reminder that there are synergistic and dynamic connections between factors across the levels. When it comes to what makes certain youth more or less likely to use pornography, there are factors that will affect their likelihood of use at the level of their own individual biology or psychology, factors that pertain to their family of origin, factors related to peers, and factors related to their connection to school. There are also, of course, factors related to the neighborhood, society, and culture in which they live—but these are more difficult to study and have not, to my knowledge, been studied relative to youth pornography use yet (see Figure 8.1).

Many of the risk factors for pornography use are similar to risk factors for what are commonly called other "adolescent problem behaviors" (see Figure 8.1).[24] Research has confirmed that there is a constellation of behaviors that includes problem drinking, cannabis use, delinquent-type behavior, and precocious sexual intercourse that tend to predict adolescent health problems.[25] Adolescent health

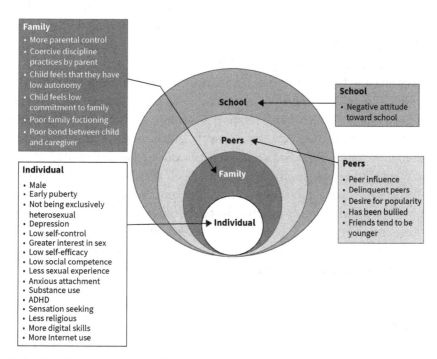

Figure 8.1. Risk factors for youth pornography use according to four levels of the social-ecological model.

researchers have noted that there are some common precursors to all of these adolescent problem behaviors, and many of them also appear to be associated with adolescent pornography use (Figure 8.1). These include being male,[10,26–29] experiencing early puberty,[30–33] depression,[10] low self-control,[34] greater interest in sex,[35,36] low self-efficacy,[37,38] low social competence,[38] having less sexual experience,[39,40] anxious attachment,[41] substance use,[10,42] being less religious,[43] having more digital (online) skills,[44] being a more frequent Internet user,[40] being a rule-breaker,[29] not being exclusively heterosexual,[45,46] and sensation seeking.[8,32] A study of adults found that there may also be an association between ADHD and problematic pornography use.[47] Household functioning,[38] including parenting style (i.e., coercive discipline practices),[10] parental monitoring of the child's activities,[33] the child's feeling less autonomy because of parenting practices,[29] the relationship between parent or guardian and the child,[10,48,49] and parent-to-child abuse[42] matter for most adolescent problem behaviors and for pornography use, as well. When one is an adolescent, what one's peers do, say, or think also tends to be highly influential and can have a strong influence on behavior,[9] as well as on what one perceives one should do to be more popular among peers.[50] Being engaged in school activities and generally positively bonded with one's school is also associated with healthier behavior[48,51] or less pornography use. One caveat to this presentation of risk and protective factors is that there are also some factors about which they are conflicting findings regarding pornography. For example, some studies find that religiosity is protective against pornography use,[43] while others have found no influence of religiosity.[21,31]

Considering the risk and protective factors for youth pornography use that have been identified, and their similarity to risk and protective factors for other adolescent problem behaviors, is it possible to identify a profile of an underage pornography user? One could say that, on average, an adolescent male with high sexual interest, with good online skills and access to the Internet, who is not getting along well with parents or feels overly controlled by parents, and who isn't involved in school activities is more likely to be viewing pornography than adolescents in general—but because the relative risks for each of these correlates tends to be small, the profile isn't precise. And much of the information that we have about so-called risk factors is actually derived from cross-sectional studies, so causality isn't certain.

Consequences

Many people want to know how pornography use affects youth. The best available evidence suggests that it matters who the youth are in terms of their predisposing risk factors, what they are watching, how much they are watching, why they are watching it, in what context (with a partner, with friends, or alone), how they feel about watching it (e.g., guilty, curious, aroused, bored), and what other sources of information they have about sex, sexuality, and relationships—in other words, are their parents communicating with them (and about what), are they getting comprehensive sex education in school, what other kinds of media do they consume, and what are the messages that they are getting from that?

I like to organize what we know from the research literature in a table that keeps track of each outcome that has been assessed as a possible correlate (either cross-sectional or longitudinal) of pornography use in people 11 to 24 years old. The table can get complicated quickly because in some research studies the authors have found support for a particular variable only for a subset of their respondents (e.g., girls but not boys, or young boys but not older boys), or only in certain situations (e.g., only if parental monitoring is absent, or only if they had preexisting violent tendencies). In some cases, authors have examined a particular outcome relative to pornography use and not found support for the association at all (see Table 8.2).

Table 8.2 lacks details about findings. For example, at least one study has found that the association between pornography exposure and interpersonal aggression is stronger when youth were using violent (but not nonviolent) pornography: Ybarra and Thompson (2018) found that exposure to violent pornography was associated with a fourfold increased odds of sexual violence perpetration by youth.[52] It is also important to note that there are some outcomes for which there are mixed results. Take, for example, academic achievement. One longitudinal research study found that pornography use was associated with less academic achievement, but a second study did not find any association.[32,53] On the whole, the study of the impact of pornography use on youth remains an emerging science, and what is known remains in a nascent stage.

As frustrating as it is to journalists, activists, and parents, it's genuinely hard to know, conclusively, exactly what pornography is doing to kids who see it, and whether the risks can be offset with helpful supports like parent–child conversations about sex or school-based education. That said, if we had to draw inferences based on what we do know, all signs point to the idea that mainstream online pornography appears to negatively influence youth in several ways. There is longitudinal evidence—suggestive of a causal relationship—that pornography may negatively influence attitudes toward women,[30] that it may increase the tendency of youth to view women as sex objects,[54] and that it may cause depression,[55–57] anxiety,[57,58] decreases in well-being,[57] reduced

Table 8.2. Selected studies that provide information about correlates of adolescent pornography consumption, by study design

Factor	Cross-Sectional Evidence	Longitudinal Evidence
Attitudes		
Rape myth acceptance	Maas and Dewey 2018[85]	—
Resistance to the #MeToo movement	Maes et al. 2019[86]	—
Attitudes toward women or gender attitudes	Stanley et al. 2018[87]	Brown and L'Engle 2009[30] Peter and Valkenburg 2011[88,a]
Self-objectification	Vandenbosch and Eggermont 2013[63,c]	—
Viewing women as sex objects	Peter and Valkenburg 2007[89]	Peter and Valkenburg 2009a[90]
Depression	—	Ma 2019[55] Mattebo et al. 2018[56] Kohut and Štulhofer 2018[57,b]
Well-being		Kohut and Štulhofer 2018[57,b]
Mental health problems	Lim et al. 2017[46]	
Anxiety	Morrison et al. 2004[91,d]	Kohut and Štulhofer 2018[57,c]
Self-esteem	Morrison et al. 2004[91,d]	Doornwaard et al. 2014[58] Kohut and Štulhofer, 2018[57,b,d]
More intense sexual performance orientation	—	Vandenbosch et al. 2018[59]
Less sexual satisfaction	—	Milas et al. 2019[92,a] Peter and Valkenburg 2009b[93] Doornwaard et al. 2014[58,c]
Sexual uncertainty	—	van Oosten (2016)[94] Peter and Valkenburg 2010[95]
More permissive sexual norms	Lo and Wei 2005[26] Braun-Courville and Rojas 2009[96] Peter and Valkenburg 2006[27] Peter and Valkenburg 2008[62]	Brown and L'Engle 2009[30,c] Doornwaard et al. 2015[97,c] Ma 2019[55] Baams et al. 2015[68]
Perceiving pornography to be realistic and/or unrealistic attitudes about sex	Tsitsika et al. 2009[28] Peter and Valkenburg 2006[31]	Peter and Valkenburg 2010b[98]
Sexual preoccupancy	Donevan and Mattebo 2017[99]	Peter and Valkenburg 2008[62]
Behaviors		
Sexual behaviors		
Sexual debut	Svedin et al. 2011[100,c] Lim et al. 2017[46]	Vandenbosch and Eggermont 2013[63] Cheng et al. 2014[64] Brown and L'Engle 2009[30]
Condom non-use	Nelson et al. 2019[82] Wright et al. 2019[101]	—

Table 8.2. *Continued*

Factor	Cross-Sectional Evidence	Longitudinal Evidence
HIV risk behaviors, including condom non-use, use of intravenous drugs, sex with a bisexual partner, multiple concurrent partners	Sinković et al. 2013[79] Lim et al. 2017[46,a]	Maas et al. 2019[65] Peter and Valkenburg 2011a[88,a]
Sexting	Tomić et al. 2017[102] Stanley et al. 2018[87]	—
Sexual behavior	Mattebo et al. 2014[103] Martyniuk et al. 2019[104] Rothman and Adhia 2016[19]	Doornwaard et al. 2015[58] Hennessy et al. 2009[105]
Group sex	Haggstron-Nordin et al. 2005[106,c] Rothman et al. 2012[107,b]	—
Anal sex	Mattebo et al. 2016[108,b] Haggstron-Nordin et al. 2005[106,c] Lim et al. 2017[46]	—
Number of sexual partners	Maas and Dewey 2018[85] Morrison et al. 2004[91,b]	—
Casual sex and one-night stands	Mattebo et al. 2013[40,c]	—
More or compulsive pornography use	Donevan and Mattebo 2017[99]	Peter and Valkenburg 2009[54] Doornwaard et al. 2016[109] Mattebo et al. 2018[56]
Aggressive behaviors		
Physical dating violence victimization	Rostad et al. 2019[110,c] Rothman et al. 2012[107,b] Rothman and Adhia 2016[19]	Maas et al. 2019[65]
Physical dating violence perpetration	Rostad et al. 2019[110,b]	—
Sexual violence victimization	Rostad et al. 2019[110]	Maas et al. 2019[65]
Sexual aggression or harassment perpetration	Mikorski & Szymanski 2017[111] Tomić et al. 2017[102,a] Rostad et al. 2019[110,c] Svedin et al. 2011[100,c]	Ybarra and Thompson 2018[52] Brown and L'Engle 2009[30,c] Dawson et al. 2019[112,a] Ybarra et al. 2011[66]
Other behaviors		
Body monitoring	Maas and Dewey 2018[85]	Doornwaard et al. 2014[58]
Evaluating women's bodies	Mikorski and Szymanski 2017[111]	
Less academic achievement	—	Beyens et al. 2015[32] Šević et al. 2019[53,a]
Problems with peers	Mattebo et al. 2013[40,c]	—

Continued

Table 8.2. *Continued*

Factor	Cross-Sectional Evidence	Longitudinal Evidence
School truancy	Mattebo et al. 2013[40],[c] Svedin et al. 2011[100],[c]	—
Obesity	Mattebo et al. 2013[40],[c]	—
Use of oral tobacco	Mattebo et al. 2013[40],[c]	—
Use of alcohol	Mattebo et al. 2013[40],[c] Svedin et al. 2011[100],[c] Rothman and Adhia 2016[19]	—
Use of cannabis	Svedin et al. 2011[100],[c] Rothman and Adhia 2016[19]	—

[a] Study found no support for an association with pornography use.

[b] Association was for girls only.

[c] Association was for boys only.

[d] Pornography use was associated with better self-esteem or less anxiety.

self-esteem,[57],[58] a tendency to "perform" sex instead of engage in it authentically in real life,[59] a tendency to experience less sexual satisfaction in real life,[58],[60] a tendency to develop the incorrect perception that pornography is realistic,[61] a tendency to become preoccupied with thought of sex,[62] a likelihood to initiate sexual activity earlier in life than one might have otherwise,[30],[63],[64] a tendency to engage in riskier sexual behaviors (such as condom non-use),[30],[63–65] a likelihood to experience unhealthy dating relationships,[65] a tendency to perpetrate and/or experience sexual violence,[30],[52],[65],[66] and concern about one body's not being good enough.[58] There is also evidence to suggest that more frequent pornography viewing may be associated with what researchers have called more permissive sexual attitudes.[30],[55],[67],[68]

Sexting and So-Called Self-Produced Child Pornography

One concern that has emerged recently has been called self-produced child pornography (also called self-porn). When someone younger than 18 years old engages in sexting, or the production and/or dissemination of sexually explicit images of themselves, they are technically guilty of creating child pornography, since the subject of the imagery is a person under the legal age for consenting to be in pornography.[69] Specifically, Section 2256 of Title 18, United States Code, defines child pornography as any visual depiction of sexually explicit conduct involving someone less than 18 years old. The nonprofit

National Center for Missing and Exploited Children works with law enforcement on the Child Victim Identification Project, which entails reviewing sexually explicit images of children that are seized from sexual offenders in order to locate the victimized children. They have reported that a small but significant percentage of images seized from those collecting or trading child pornography were originally created by the minors themselves (14%), and that the percentage is increasing.[70,71]

Sexting appears to be prevalent among US adolescents. A national survey found that in 2010–2011, 7% of youth 13 to 18 years old reported sending or showing someone sexual pictures of themselves during the past year in which they were nude or nearly nude.[72] A recent meta-analysis found, on average, that 14.8% of adolescents had sent a sext, whereas 27.4% reported receiving sexts.[73,74] The prevalence may be even higher among nonheterosexual adolescents.[75] A separate probability study of US adults 18 to 24 years old found that 47% of men and 48% of women in this age group had ever received nude or seminude of photos of someone.[76] There is recognition that consensual sexting may be an expected and even normative part of adolescent development, given that much romantic and sexual communication now happens on electronic devices, but there is recognition that it nevertheless may not be safe. Negative consequences can result from sexting, including that the images can be disseminated widely and without the consent of the adolescent who originally sent them.[73] Some research suggests that sexting is associated with stress and anxiety, although it is not clear if sexting causes stress and anxiety.[77] It might also be true that people who feel more stressed and anxious engage in more sexting for various reasons—perhaps to try to relieve stress, or in an anxious attempt to connect socially with others. Either way, paying increased attention to bolstering the mental health of those who sext is warranted.

Conclusions

It is not easy to disentangle the effects of pornography on youth from other types of sexual media, and without question any effects that have been identified are moderated by the type of pornography consumed, the frequency of exposure, predisposing factors in the youth exposed, and other situational factors. Nevertheless, there is a growing body of literature supporting the contention that youth online pornography exposure is associated, longitudinally, with a range of negative consequences. While it is not easy to prove causality, because even longitudinal associations may be confounded by other factors, the preponderance of evidence supports the idea that adolescent sexual development can be altered by the adolescent's pornography viewing experiences and may require offsets, such as parental communication about pornography, comprehensive sex education in school, or other helpful interventions. Public health professionals have a reason to be concerned about the impact of pornography on children, adolescents, and young adults, and they have reason to take considered action.

References

1. *Juvenile Delinquency (Comic Books): Hearings before the United States Senate Committee on the Judiciary, Subcommittee to Investigate Juvenile Delinquency,* 83rd Congress, second session on April 21–22 to June 4, 1954. Washington, DC: US Government Printing Office.
2. Comic Book Legal Defense Fund. 2019. *History of Comics Censorship, Part 1.* http://cbldf. org/resources/history-of-comics-censorship/history-of-comics-censorship-part-1/
3. Senate Committee on the Judiciary. 1955. *Comic Books and Juvenile Delinquency,* Interim Report, 1955. Washington, DC: United States Government Printing Office.
4. Springhall, J. 1998. "'Horror Comic' Panic: Campaigning Against Comic Books in the 1940s and 1950s." In *Youth, Popular Culture and Moral Panics: Penny Gaffs to Gangsta-Rap, 1830–1996,* edited by J. Springhall, 121–146. London: Macmillan Education UK.
5. US Department of Justice. 2020. "Obscenity." https://www.justice.gov/criminal-ceos/ obscenity
6. California Penal Code Section 288.2. http://leginfo.legislature.ca.gov/faces/codes_ displaySection.xhtml?lawCode=PEN&sectionNum=288.2
7. Peter, J., and P. M. Valkenburg. 2016. "Adolescents and Pornography: A Review of 20 Years of Research." *The Journal of Sex Research* 53, no. 4-5: 509–531.
8. Luder, M-T., I. Pittet, A. Berchtold, C. Akré, P-A. Michaud, and J-C. Surís. 2011. "Associations Between Online Pornography and Sexual Behavior Among Adolescents: Myth or Reality?" *Archives of Sexual Behavior* 40, no. 5: 1027–1035.
9. Weber, M., O. Quiring, and G. Daschmann. 2012. "Peers, Parents and Pornography: Exploring Adolescents' Exposure to Sexually Explicit Material and Its Developmental Correlates." *Sexuality & Culture* 16, no. 4: 408–427.
10. Ybarra, M. L., and K. J. Mitchell. 2005. "Exposure to Internet Pornography Among Children and Adolescents: A National Survey." *Cyberpsychology & Behavior* 8, no. 5: 473–486.
11. Cowan, G., and R. R. Campbell. 1995. "Rape Causal Attitudes Among Adolescents." *The Journal of Sex Research* 32, no. 2: 145–153.
12. Rothman, E. F., and K. J. Mitchell. "A Trend Analysis of U.S. Adolescents' Intentional Pornography Exposure on the Internet, 2000–2010" (unpublished). http://sites.bu.edu/ rothmanlab/files/2019/09/porn-trends-report-version.pdf
13. Ybarra, M. L., and K. J. Mitchell. 2013. "Prevalence Rates of Male and Female Sexual Violence Perpetrators in a National Sample of Adolescents." *JAMA Pediatrics* 167, no. 12: 1125.
14. Ybarra, M. L., V. C. Strasburger, and K. J. Mitchell. 2014. "Sexual Media Exposure, Sexual Behavior, and Sexual Violence Victimization in Adolescence." *Clinical Pediatrics* 53, no. 13: 1239–1247.
15. Berger, A. S., W. Simon, and J. H. Gagnon. 1973. "Youth and Pornography in Social Context." *Archives of Sexual Behavior* 2, no. 4: 279–308.

16. Bryant, J., and D. Brown. 1989. "Uses of Pornography." In *Pornography: Research Advances and Policy Considerations*, edited by D. Zillmann and J. Bryant. Mahwah, New Jersey: Lawrence Erlbaum Associates.

17. Rothman, E. F., J. Paruk, A. Espensen, J. R. Temple, and K. Adams. 2017. "A Qualitative Study of What US Parents Say and Do When Their Young Children See Pornography." *Academic Pediatrics* 17, no. 8: 844–849.

18. Cavazos-Rehg, P. A., M. J. Krauss, E. L. Spitznagel, et al. 2009. "Age of Sexual Debut Among US Adolescents." *Contraception* 80, no. 2: 158 162.

19. Rothman, E. F., and A. Adhia. 2016. "Adolescent Pornography Use and Dating Violence Among a Sample of Primarily Black and Hispanic, Urban-Residing, Underage Youth." *Behavioral Sciences* 6, no. 1: 1.

20. Davis, A. C., E. R. Carrotte, M. E. Hellard, and M. S. C. Lim. 2018. "What Behaviors Do Young Heterosexual Australians See in Pornography? A Cross-Sectional Study." *The Journal of Sex Research* 55, no. 3: 310–319.

21. Vandenbosch, L. 2015. "Antecedents of Adolescents' Exposure to Different Types of Sexually Explicit Internet Material: A Longitudinal Study." *Computers in Human Behavior* 50: 439–448.

22. Koletić, G. 2017. "Longitudinal Associations Between the Use of Sexually Explicit Material and Adolescents' Attitudes and Behaviors: A Narrative Review of Studies." *Journal of Adolescence* 57: 119–133.

23. Bronfenbrenner, U. 1979. *The Ecology of Human Development: Experiments by Nature and Design*. Cambridge, MA: Harvard University Press.

24. Jessor, R., and S. Jessor. 1977. *Problem Behavior and Psychosocial Development: A Longitudinal Study of Youth*. New York: Academic Press.

25. Donovan, J. E., R. Jessor, and F. M. Costa. 1988. "Syndrome of Problem Behavior in Adolescence: A Replication." *Journal of Consulting and Clinical Psychology* 56, no. 5: 762–765.

26. Lo, V-H., and R. Wei. 2005. "Exposure to Internet Pornography and Taiwanese Adolescents' Sexual Attitudes and Behavior." *Journal of Broadcasting & Electronic Media* 49, no. 2: 221–237.

27. Peter, J., and P. M. Valkenburg. 2006. "Adolescents' Exposure to Sexually Explicit Online Material and Recreational Attitudes Toward Sex." *Journal of Communication* 56, no. 4: 639–660.

28. Tsitsika, A., E. Critselis, G. Kormas, E. Konstantoulaki, A. Constantopoulos, and D. Kafetzis. 2009. "Adolescent Pornographic Internet Site Use: A Multivariate Regression Analysis of the Predictive Factors of Use and Psychosocial Implications." *Cyberpsychology & Behavior* 12: 545–550.

29. Wolak, J., K. Mitchell, and D. Finkelhor. 2007. "Unwanted and Wanted Exposure to Online Pornography in a National Sample of Youth Internet Users." *Pediatrics* 119, no. 2: 247–257.

30. Brown, J. D., and K. L. L'Engle. 2009. "X-Rated: Sexual Attitudes and Behaviors Associated with U.S. Early Adolescents' Exposure to Sexually Explicit Media." *Communication Research* 36, no. 1: 129–151.

31. Peter, J., and P. M. Valkenburg. 2006. "Adolescents' Exposure to Sexually Explicit Material on the Internet." *Communication Research* 33, no. 2: 178–204.

32. Beyens, I., L. Vandenbosch, and S. Eggermont. 2015. "Early Adolescent Boys' Exposure to Internet Pornography: Relationships to Pubertal Timing, Sensation Seeking, and Academic Performance." *The Journal of Early Adolescence* 35, no. 8: 1045–1068.

33. Nieh, H. P., L. Y. Chang, H. Y. Chang, T. L. Chiang, and L. L. Yen. 2020. "Pubertal Timing, Parenting Style, and Trajectories of Pornography Use in Adolescence: Peer Pornography Use as the Mediator." *The Journal of Sex Research* 57, no. 1: 29–41.

34. Holt, T. J., A. M. Bossler, and D. C. May. 2012. "Low Self-Control, Deviant Peer Associations, and Juvenile Cyberdeviance." *American Journal of Criminal Justice* 37, no. 3: 378–395.

35. Doornwaard, S. M., R. J. van den Eijnden, G. Overbeek, and T. F. ter Bogt. 2015. "Differential Developmental Profiles of Adolescents Using Sexually Explicit Internet Material." *The Journal of Sex Research* 52, no. 3: 269–281.

36. Doornwaard, S. M., D. S. Bickham, M. Rich, T. F. M. ter Bogt, and R. J. M. van den Eijnden. 2015. "Adolescents' Use of Sexually Explicit Internet Material and Their Sexual Attitudes and Behavior: Parallel Development and Directional Effects." *Developmental Psychology* 51, no. 10: 1476–1488.

37. Kim, Y. 2011. "Adolescents' Health Behaviour and Its Associations with Psychological Variables." *Central European Journal of Public Health* 19, no. 4: 205–209.

38. Shek, Daniel T. L., and Cecilia M. S. Ma. 2014. "Using Structural Equation Modeling to Examine Consumption of Pornographic Materials in Chinese Adolescents in Hong Kong." *International Journal on Disability and Human Development* 13, no. 2: 239–245.

39. Bleakley, A., M. Hennessy, M. Fishbein, and A. Jordan. 2008. "It Works Both Ways: The Relationship Between Exposure to Sexual Content in the Media and Adolescent Sexual Behavior." *Media Psychology* 11, no. 4: 443–461.

40. Mattebo, M., T. Tyden, E. Haggstrom-Nordin, K. W. Nilsson, and M. Larsson. 2013. "Pornography Consumption, Sexual Experiences, Lifestyles, and Self-Rated Health Among Male Adolescents in Sweden." *Journal of Developmental and Behavioral Pediatrics: JDBP* 34, no. 7: 460–468.

41. Efrati, Y., and Y. Amichai-Hamburger. 2018. "The Use of Online Pornography as Compensation for Loneliness and Lack of Social Ties Among Israeli Adolescents." *Psychological Reports* 122, no. 5: 1865–1882.

42. Romito, P., and L. Beltramini. 2011. "Watching Pornography: Gender Differences, Violence and Victimization. An Exploratory Study in Italy." *Violence Against Women* 17, no. 10: 1313–1326.

43. Hardy, S. A., M. A. Steelman, S. M. Coyne, and R. D. Ridge. 2013. "Adolescent Religiousness as a Protective Factor Against Pornography Use." *Journal of Applied Developmental Psychology* 34, no. 3: 131–139.

44. Sevcikova, A., J. Šerek, M. Barbovschi, and K. Daneback. 2014. "The Roles of Individual Characteristics and Liberalism in Intentional and Unintentional Exposure to Online Sexual Material Among European Youth: A Multilevel Approach." *Sexuality Research and Social Policy* 11, no. 2: 104–115.

45. Peter, J., and P. M. Valkenburg. 2011. "The Use of Sexually Explicit Internet Material and Its Antecedents: A Longitudinal Comparison of Adolescents and Adults." *Archives of Sexual Behavior* 40, no. 5: 1015–1025.

46. Lim, M. S. C., P. A. Agius, E. R. Carrotte, A. M. Vella, and M. E. Hellard. 2017. "Young Australians' Use of Pornography and Associations with Sexual Risk Behaviours." *Australian and New Zealand Journal of Public Health* 41, no. 4: 438–443.

47. Bothe, B., M. Koos, I. Toth-Kiraly, G. Orosz, and Z. Demetrovics. 2019. "Investigating the Associations of Adult ADHD Symptoms, Hypersexuality, and Problematic Pornography Use Among Men and Women on a Largescale, Non-Clinical Sample." *The Journal of Sexual Medicine* 16, no. 4: 489–499.

48. Mesch, G. S. 2009. "Social Bonds and Internet Pornographic Exposure Among Adolescents." *Journal of Adolescence* 32, no. 3: 601–618.

49. Astle, S., N. Leonhardt, and B. Willoughby. 2020. "Home Base: Family of Origin Factors and the Debut of Vaginal Sex, Anal Sex, Oral Sex, Masturbation, and Pornography Use in a National Sample of Adolescents." *The Journal of Sex Research* 57, no. 9: 1089–1099.

50. Vanden Abeele, M., S. W. Campbell, S. Eggermont, and K. Roe. 2014. "Sexting, Mobile Porn Use, and Peer Group Dynamics: Boys' and Girls' Self-Perceived Popularity, Need for Popularity, and Perceived Peer Pressure." *Media Psychology* 17, no. 1: 6–33.

51. Mesch, G., and T. Maman. 2009. "Intentional Online Pornographic Exposure Among Adolescents: Is the Internet to Blame?" *Verhaltenstherapie & Verhaltensmedizin* 30, no. 3: 352–367.

52. Ybarra, M. L., and R. E. Thompson. 2018. "Predicting the Emergence of Sexual Violence in Adolescence." *Prevention Science* 19, no. 1: 103–115.

53. Šević, S., J. Mehulić, and A. Štulhofer. 2020. "Is Pornography a Risk for Adolescent Academic Achievement? Findings from Two Longitudinal Studies of Male Adolescents." *European Journal of Developmental Psychology* 17, no. 2: 275–292.

54. Peter, J., and P. M. Valkenburg. 2009. "Adolescents' Exposure to Sexually Explicit Internet Materials and Notions of Women as Sex Objects: Assessing Causality and Underlying Processes." *Journal of Communication* 59, no. 3: 407–433.

55. Ma, C. M. S. 2019. "Relationships Between Exposure to Online Pornography, Psychological Well-Being and Sexual Permissiveness Among Hong Kong Chinese Adolescents: A Three-Wave Longitudinal Study." *Applied Research in Quality of Life* 14, no. 2: 423–439.

56. Mattebo, M., T. Tyden, E. Haggstrom-Nordin, K. W. Nilsson, and M. Larsson. 2018. "Pornography Consumption and Psychosomatic and Depressive Symptoms Among Swedish Adolescents: A Longitudinal Study." *Upsala Journal of Medical Sciences* 123, no. 4: 237–246.

57. Kohut, T., and A. Štulhofer. 2018. "Is Pornography Use a Risk for Adolescent Well-Being? An Examination of Temporal Relationships in Two Independent Panel Samples." *PLOS One* 13, no. 8: e0202048–e0202048.

58. Doornwaard, S., D. Bickham, M. Rich, I. Vanwesenbeeck, R. Eijnden, and T. Bogt. 2014. "Sex-Related Online Behaviors and Adolescents' Body and Sexual Self-Perceptions." *Pediatrics* 134, no. 6: 1103–1110.

59. Vandenbosch, L., J. M. F. van Oosten, and J. Peter. 2018. "Sexually Explicit Internet Material and Adolescents' Sexual Performance Orientation: The Mediating Roles of Enjoyment and Perceived Utility." *Media Psychology* 21, no. 1: 50–74.

60. Peter, J., and P. M. Valkenburg. 2009. "Adolescents' Exposure to Sexually Explicit Internet Material and Sexual Satisfaction: A Longitudinal Study." *Human Communication Research* 35, no. 2: 171–194.

61. Peter, J., and P. Valkenburg. 2010. "Processes Underlying the Effects of Adolescents' Use of Sexually Explicit Internet Material: The Role of Perceived Realism." *Communication Research* 37: 375–399.

62. Peter, J., and P. Valkenburg. 2008. "Adolescents' Exposure to Sexually Explicit Internet Material, Sexual Uncertainty, and Attitudes Toward Uncommitted Sexual Exploration—Is There a Link?" *Communication Research* 35, no. 5: 579–601.

63. Vandenbosch, L., and S. Eggermont. 2013. "Sexually Explicit Websites and Sexual Initiation: Reciprocal Relationships and the Moderating Role of Pubertal Status." *Journal of Research on Adolescence* 23, no. 4: 621–634.

64. Cheng, S., J. Ma, and S. Missari. 2014. "The Effects of Internet Use on Adolescents' First Romantic and Sexual Relationships in Taiwan." *International Sociology* 29, no. 4: 324–347.

65. Maas, M. K., B. C. Bray, and J. G. Noll. 2019. "Online Sexual Experiences Predict Subsequent Sexual Health and Victimization Outcomes Among Female Adolescents: A Latent Class Analysis." *Journal of Youth and Adolescence* 48, no. 5: 837–849.

66. Ybarra, M. L., K. J. Mitchell, M. Hamburger, M. Diener-West, and P. J. Leaf. 2011. "X-rated Material and Perpetration of Sexually Aggressive Behavior Among Children and Adolescents: Is There a Link?" *Aggressive Behavior* 37, no. 1: 1–18.

67. Doornwaard, S. M., D. S. Bickham, M. Rich, T. F. ter Bogt, and R. J. van den Eijnden. 2015. "Adolescents' Use of Sexually Explicit Internet Material and Their Sexual Attitudes and Behavior: Parallel Development and Directional Effects." *Developmental Psychology* 51, no. 10: 1476–1488.

68. Baams, L., G. Overbeek, J. S. Dubas, S. M. Doornwaard, E. Rommes, and M. A. G. van Aken. 2015. "Perceived Realism Moderates the Relation Between Sexualized Media Consumption and Permissive Sexual Attitudes in Dutch Adolescents." *Archives of Sexual Behavior* 44, no. 3: 743–754.

69. Leary, M. 2010. "Sexting or Self-Produced Child Pornography? The Dialogue Continues— Structured Prosecutorial Discretion Within a Multidisciplinary Response." *Virginia Journal of Social Policy & the Law* 17, no. 3: 487–566, Spring 2010, CUA Columbus School of Law Legal Studies Research Paper No. 2010-31, Available at SSRN: https://ssrn.com/ abstract=1657007.

70. Collins, M. 2012. Federal child pornography offenses. Testimony of Michelle Collins. National Center for Missing & Exploited Children. https://www.ussc.gov/sites/default/ files/pdf/amendment-process/public-hearings-and-meetings/20120215-16/Testimony_ 15_Collins.pdf

71. Seto, M. C., C. Buckman, R. G. Dwyer, and National Center for Missing & Exploited Children. 2018. "Production and Active Trading of Child Sexual Exploitation Images Depicting Identified Victims." https://www.missingkids.org/content/dam/missingkids/ pdfs/ncmec-analysis/Production%20and%20Active%20Trading%20of%20CSAM_ FullReport_FINAL.pdf

72. Ybarra, M. L., and K. J. Mitchell. 2014. "Sexting" and Its Relation to Sexual Activity and Sexual Risk Behavior in a National Survey of Adolescents." *The Journal of Adolescent Health* 55, no. 6: 757–764.

73. Shafer, A. 2019. "Advancing Research on Adolescent Sexting." *The Journal of Adolescent Health* 65, no. 6: 711–712.

74. Madigan, S., A. Ly, C. L. Rash, J. Van Ouytsel, and J. R. Temple. 2018. "Prevalence of Multiple Forms of Sexting Behavior Among Youth: A Systematic Review and Meta-analysis." *JAMA Pediatrics* 172, no. 4: 327–335.

75. Van Ouytsel, J., M. Walrave, and K. Ponnet. 2019. "An Exploratory Study of Sexting Behaviors Among Heterosexual and Sexual Minority Early Adolescents." *The Journal of Adolescent Health* 65, no. 5: 621–626.

76. Herbenick, D., J. Bowling, T-C. J. Fu, B. Dodge, L. Guerra-Reyes, and S. Sanders. 2017. "Sexual Diversity in the United States: Results from a Nationally Representative Probability Sample of Adult Women and Men." *PLOS One* 12, no. 7: e0181198–e0181198.

77. Dodaj, A., K. Sesar, and S. Jerinic. 2020. "A Prospective Study of High-School Adolescent Sexting Behavior and Psychological Distress." *The Journal of Psychology* 154, no. 2: 111–128.

78. Sabina, C., J. Wolak, and D. Finkelhor. 2008. "The Nature and Dynamics of Internet Pornography Exposure for Youth." *Cyberpsychology & Behavior* 11, no. 6: 691–693. https:// doi.org/10.1089/cpb.2007.0179

79. Sinković, M., A. Štulhofer, and J. Božić. 2013. "Revisiting the Association between Pornography Use and Risky Sexual Behaviors: The Role of Early Exposure to Pornography and Sexual Sensation Seeking." *The Journal of Sex Research* 50, no. 7: 633–641.

80. Sun, C. F., P. Wright, and N. Steffen. March 2017. "German Heterosexual Women's Pornography Consumption and Sexual Behavior." *Sexualization, Media, & Society.*

81. Wright, P. J., and A. Štulhofer. 2019. "Adolescent Pornography Use and the Dynamics of Perceived Pornography Realism: Does Seeing More Make it More Realistic?" *Computers in Human Behavior* 95: 37–47.

82. Nelson, K. M., N. S. Perry, and M. P. Carey. 2019. "Sexually Explicit Media Use Among 14–17-Year-Old Sexual Minority Males in the U.S." *Archives of Sexual Behavior* 48, no. 8: 2345–2355.

83. Laemmle-Ruff, I. L., M. Raggatt, C. J. C. Wright, E. R. Carrotte, A. Davis, R. Jenkinson, and M. S. C. Lim. 2019. "Personal and Reported Partner Pornography Viewing by Australian Women, and Association with Mental Health and Body Image." *Sex Health* 16, no. 1, 75–79.

84. Herbenick, D., T. C. Fu, P. Wright, B. Paul, R. Gradus, J. Bauer, and R. Jones. 2020. "Diverse Sexual Behaviors and Pornography Use: Findings From a Nationally Representative Probability Survey of Americans Aged 18 to 60 Years." *The Journal of Sex Research* 17, no. 4: 623–633.

85. Maas, M. K., and S. Dewey. April 2018. "Internet Pornography Use Among Collegiate Women: Gender Attitudes, Body Monitoring, and Sexual Behavior." *SAGE Open.* https://doi.org/10.1177/2158244018786640

86. Maes, C., L. Schreurs, J. M. F. Van Oosten, and L. Vandenbosch. 2019. "#(Me)too Much? The Role of Sexualizing Online Media in Adolescents' resistance Towards the Metoo-Movement and Acceptance of Rape Myths. *Journal of Adolescence* 77: 59–69. https://doi.org/10.1016/j.adolescence.2019.10.005

87. Stanley, N., C. Barter, M. Wood, N. Aghtaie, C. Larkins, A. Lanau, and C. Överlien. 2018. "Pornography, Sexual Coercion and Abuse and Sexting in Young People's Intimate Relationships: A European Study." *Journal of Interpersonal Violence* 33, no. 19: 2919–2944.

88. Peter, J., and P. M. Valkenburg. 2011. "The Influence of Sexually Explicit Internetmaterial and Peers on Stereotypical Beliefs about Women's Sexual Roles: Similarities and Differences Between Adolescents and Adults." *Cyberpsychology, Behavior, and Social Networking*, 14: 511–517.

89. Peter, J., and P. M. Valkenburg. 2007. "Adolescents' Exposure to a Sexualized Media Environment and Their Notions of Women as Sex Objects." *Sex Roles* 56: 381–395. https://doi.org/10.1007/s11199-006-9176-y

90. Peter, J., and P. M. Valkenburg. 2009a. "Adolescents' Exposure to Sexually Explicit Internet Material and Notions of Women as Sex Objects: Assessing Causality and Underlying Processes." *Journal of Communication* 59: 407–433. http://dx.doi.org/10.1111/j.1460-2466.2009.01422.x

91. Morrison, T. G., R. Harriman, M. A. Morrison, A. Bearden, and S. R. Ellis. 2004. "Correlates of Exposure to Sexually Explicit Material Among Canadian Post-Secondary Students." *Canadian Journal of Human Sexuality* 13, no. 3–4: 143–156.

92. Milas, G., P. Wright, and A. Štulhofer. 2020. "Longitudinal Assessment of the Association Between Pornography Use and Sexual Satisfaction in Adolescence." *The Journal of Sex Research* 57, no. 1: 16–28.

93. Peter, J., and P. M. Valkenburg. 2009. "Adolescents' Exposure to Sexually Explicit Internet Material and Sexual Satisfaction: A Longitudinal Study." *Human Communication Research* 35, no. 2: 171–194.

94. van Oosten, J. M. F. 2016. "Sexually Explicit Internet Material and Adolescents' Sexual Uncertainty: The Role of Disposition-Content Congruency." *Archives of Sexual Behavior* 45: 1011–1022. https://doi.org/10.1007/s10508-015-0594-1

95. Peter, J., and P. M. Valkenburg. 2010. "Adolescents' Use of Sexually Explicit Internet Material and Sexual Uncertainty: The Role of Involvement and Gender." *Communication Monographs* 77, no. 3: 357–375. https://doi.org/10.1080/03637751.2010.498791

96. Braun-Courville, D. K., and M. Rojas. 2009. "Exposure to Sexually Explicit Web Sites and Adolescent Sexual Attitudes and Behaviors." *The Journal of Adolescent Health* 45, no. 2: 156–162.

97. Doornwaard, S. M., T. F. ter Bogt, E. Reitz, and R. J. van den Eijnden. 2015. "Sex-Related Online Behaviors, Perceived Peer Norms and Adolescents' Experience with Sexual Behavior: Testing an Integrative Model." *PLoS One* 10, no. 6: e0127787.

98. Peter, J., and P. M. Valkenburg. 2010. "Processes Underlying the Effects of Adolescents' Use of Sexually Explicit Internet Material: The Role of Perceived Realism." *Communication Research* 37, no. 3: 375–399.

99. Donevan, M., and M. Mattebo. 2017. "The Relationship Between Frequent Pornography Consumption, Behaviours, and Sexual Preoccupancy Among Male Adolescents in Sweden." *Sexual and Reproductive Healthcare* 12: 82–87.

100. Svedin, C. G., I. Åkerman, and G. Priebe. 2011. "Frequent Users of Pornography. A Population Based Epidemiological Study of Swedish Male Adolescents." *The Journal of Adolescent Health* 34, no. 4: 779–788.

101. Wright, P. J., C. Sun, A. Bridges, J. A. Johnson, and M. B. Ezzell. 2019. "Condom Use, Pornography Consumption, and Perceptions of Pornography as Sexual Information in a Sample of Adult U.S. Males." *Journal of Health Communication* 24, no. 9: 693–699.

102. Tomić, I., J. Burić, and A. Štulhofer. 2018. "Associations Between Croatian Adolescents' Use of Sexually Explicit Material and Sexual Behavior: Does Parental Monitoring Play a Role?" *Archives of Sexual Behavior* 47, no. 6: 1881–1893.

103. Mattebo, M., T. Tydén, E. Häggström-Nordin, K. W. Nilsson, and M. Larsson. 2014. "Pornography and Sexual Experiences Among High School Students in Sweden." *Journal of Developmental and Behavioral Pediatrics* 35, no. 3: 179–188.

104. Martyniuk, U., L. Okolski, and A. Dekker. 2019. "Pornographic Content and Real-Life Sexual Experiences: Findings From a Survey of German University Students." *Journal of Sex & Marital Therapy* 45, no. 5: 370–377.

105. Hennessy, M., A. Bleakley, M. Fishbein, and A. Jordan. 2009. "Estimating the Longitudinal Association Between Adolescent Sexual Behavior and Exposure to Sexual Media Content." *Journal of Sex Research* 46: 586–596.

106. Häggström-Nordin, E., U. Hanson, and T. Tydén. 2005. "Associations Between Pornography Consumption and Sexual Practices Among Adolescents in Sweden." *International Journal of STD & AIDS* 16, no. 2: 102–107.

107. Rothman, E. F., M. R. Decker, E. Miller, E. Reed, A. Raj, and J. G. Silverman. 2012. "Multi-Person Sex Among a Sample of Adolescent Female Urban Health Clinic Patients." *Journal of Urban Health* 89, no. 1: 129–137.

108. Mattebo, M., T. Tydén, E. Häggström-Nordin, K. W. Nilsson, and M. Larsson. 2016. "Pornography Consumption Among Adolescent Girls in Sweden." *The European Journal of Contraception & Reproductive Health Care* 21, no. 4: 295–302.

109. Doornwaard, S. M., R. J. van den Eijnden, L. Baams, I. Vanwesenbeeck, and T. F. ter Bogt. 2016. "Lower Psychological Well-Being and Excessive Sexual Interest Predict Symptoms of Compulsive Use of Sexually Explicit Internet Material Among Adolescent Boys." *Journal of Youth and Adolescence* 45, no. 1: 73–84.

110. Rostad, W. L., D. Gittins-Stone, C. Huntington, C. J. Rizzo, D. Pearlman, and L. Orchowski. 2019. "The Association Between Exposure to Violent Pornography and Teen Dating Violence in Grade 10 High School Students." *Archives of Sexual Behavior* 48, no. 7: 2137–2147.

111. Mikorski, R., and D. M. Szymanski. 2017. "Masculine Norms, Peer Group, Pornography, Facebook, and Men's Sexual Objectification of Women." *Psychology of Men & Masculinity* 18, no. 4: 257–267.

112. Dawson, K., A. Tafro, and A. Štulhofer. 2019. "Adolescent Sexual Aggressiveness and Pornography Use: A Longitudinal Assessment." *Aggressive Behavior* 45, no. 6: 587–597.

9
Pornography and Body Image

Most people alter their appearance in order to look more attractive to others. Whether it's using makeup, dieting, bulking up, choosing clothes that flatter one's body size and shape, coloring or styling one's hair, adorning oneself with feathers, beads, or other ornaments, wearing a corset or Spanx or shoulder pads, or engaging in piercing, tattooing, hair removal, or scarring—throughout history humans have expended energy and money to appear in a way that they believe will make them more beautiful to others. This makes good sense, because being perceived as beautiful and sexually attractive confers benefits. People who are perceived to be more attractive tend to achieve more education, are less likely to be seen as culpable when they commit a crime, are more likely to be offered jobs, earn more money on average over a lifetime, and tend to have more options for romantic and mating partners—and these advantages may extend longevity.[1–4]

But where do people get their ideas about what will make them more beautiful to others? On the one hand, scientific research supports biological explanations that suggest that what humans tend to perceive as beautiful are indicators of good health and high likelihood of reproductive success. We enjoy looking at faces that are symmetrical,[4] and we tend to find signs of good health attractive—such as even-colored skin.[4] Humans also enjoy looking at things that are familiar to them, so "average" faces—that is, faces that have features that are statistically closer to the norm, tend to be perceived as more visually pleasing.[4] But in addition to these basic and biologically based drivers of attraction, we are also influenced by social factors. If we were not, beauty ideals would not change over time and would have been perfectly fixed since the beginning of human history, but there is no question that what is considered beautiful evolves. For example, among white people in the Victorian era in Europe and the United States, being pale and plump was considered beautiful—reportedly, in part, because it was difficult for the average person to afford the luxury of staying out of the sun and getting enough to eat to attain these ideals. Other beauty ideals for women throughout history and across cultures have included the unibrow (in Ancient Greece), reshaped eyebrows (ancient India), blackened teeth (7th century Japan), a large lower lip or elongated neck (Africa), a high forehead (Renaissance Italy), and a double chin

Pornography and Public Health. Emily F. Rothman, Oxford University Press. © Oxford University Press 2021.
DOI: 10.1093/oso/9780190075477.003.0009

(18th century France).[5] Evidence of rapidly shifting beauty ideals in the United States was demonstrated through an analysis of images of women in the magazines *Vogue* and *Ladies Home Journal* between 1901 and the 1960s. The analysis found that the bust-to-waist ratio decreased by approximately 60% between 1901 and 1925, increased again by one third between 1925 and 1940, and returned to ultrathin by the late 1960s.[6]

Some people are worried that the bodies and faces that are shown to us in sexually explicit media are changing what we think is beautiful, are making us anxious and depressed, and even are pushing us to engage in self-harmful behavior.[7] In this chapter, I present information about ways in which porn performers' bodies may differ from the average viewer's, describe theories that guide research on pornography and body image-related outcomes, and summarize the research findings.

What Kinds of Bodies Do Porn Performers Have?

Many commentators make the assumption that the bodies featured in pornography are atypical—that men and women are thinner than average, with much larger penises and breasts, respectively, than average people. In fact, there is too little documentation of what types of bodies, and beauty or sexual ideals, are being promoted through mainstream online (and other forms of) pornography. We also lack information about how porn performers' bodies may have changed over the decades. For example, perhaps the average mainstream porn performer of today tends to be 10 to 20 pounds heavier than the average porn performer from the year 2000; if so, research about the impact of pornography on body image might become dated quickly, depending on whether porn performers' bodies consistently represent generally unattainable ideals.

To my knowledge, there is one source of information that helps us understand what viewers see when they view performers' bodies in pornography: the Internet Adult Film Database (IAFD.com), which was founded by a Dutch man named Peter van Aarle. Van Aarle started taking notes on pornography performers and films on index cards in 1981—not for any entrepreneurial reason, but just for fun.[8] Eventually, he joined forces with another pornography aficionado and they published their combined files online in 1995. Today, the database has information on more than 200,604 performers and 490,038 films.[9] Users can search for performers by nationality, ethnicity, hair color, tattoos, and sex acts in which they have engaged.

In 2013, a journalist (Millward) extracted thousands of IAFD records with porn performers' self-reported height, weight, waist, hip, and bust measurements and calculated averages in order to make comparisons with average Americans' data available from the US Centers for Disease Control and Prevention website.[8] Millward found that the average male and female porn performers were the same height as the average American man and woman: 5'10" and 5'5", respectively. He also found that the average female performer weighed 48 pounds less than the national average for women, and the average male performer weighed 27 pounds less than the national average for men. In terms of measurements, the most common for women was 34-24-34, or an average of a 34B bra size. The majority of female porn stars also reported being brunette, 43% have a body piercing (as compared to 30% of Americans in general), and 46% have a tattoo (as compared to 37% of Americans in general). The IAFD data have limitations—data were self-reported by eager-to-be-hired and eager-to-please pornography performers, or perhaps imputed by the viewers (it isn't clear from the website or Millward's report), and Millward calculated average height, weight, and other measurements using data from all entries without regard to year, which might mask acute differences in average performer weight over time. Nevertheless, Millward's estimates are at least one data point that suggest that porn performers' bodies are not typical or average American bodies.

My understanding is that claims that pornography performers' penis lengths or breast sizes are larger than average men and women cannot be substantiated. It is likely true—after all, pornography is first and foremost a competitive, money-making enterprise, and performers with exceptional body parts are paid more,[10] which is an indicator that, taken together, pornography likely features performers who do not resemble average adults. But the assumption that on the whole pornography promotes unrealistic, idealistic, unnatural, or outlier bodies and body parts is an assumption that ideally should be confirmed with data before the public health community takes seriously the idea that the public is being harmed because of the bodies featured in pornography. It is also possible that the bodies featured in pornography are atypical but are also representative of bodies featured in entertainment media more generally—so, if one were to assess breast size, for example, across performers in pornography and non-sexually-explicit films, TV shows, music videos, etc., pornography performers may not be outliers compared to other types of entertainment media professionals. That's relevant because the body image problems that may be associated with pornography use could reflect the use of entertainment media in general, and not be specific to pornography.

Theory

Why should the media images of pornography performers harm people's health? There are three theories that provide a framework for understanding why and how this might happen. First, there is objectification theory. Objectification theory posits that the reason that girls and women may be disproportionately affected by eating disorders, as well as experience some forms of depression and sexual dysfunction, is because they are taught to always look at their own bodies as an evaluating stranger might and to feel shame and anxiety about their natural bodies.[11] This theory suggests that viewing pornography might increase people's sense that there is something wrong with their bodies unless they look camera-ready, so that they develop neuroses and other health problems because they feel so bad about themselves and continually take action to enhance their physical attractiveness.[11]

Second, there is the tripartite model of body image. This is a more recent theoretical model that proposes that peers, parents, and media factors work together to influence how people think that they should look to be attractive, and that it can lead to body dissatisfaction and eating disturbances because individuals engage in ongoing comparison of themselves to the ideal.[12] When it comes to pornography, the tripartite model suggests that a combination of what we see in pornography as beauty ideals and feedback and commentary from peers and parents when we are young influence how we think we should look—and how bad we should feel if we have failed to live up to the ideal. Third, social comparison theory asserts that individuals are always trying to figure out their place in the world relative to others, and in their drive to understand who they are, they compare their opinions, abilities, and themselves to those around them whom they perceive as similar.[13] According to this theory, if a young female views pornography featuring a young female, she is likely to make comparisons between the performer's body, genitalia, face, hair, skin, and other features and her own— and the same would be true for young men and nonbinary individuals, as well. In short, according to these theories, we are likely to compare our bodies to the bodies that we see in pornography, and, in theory, we will feel bad about discrepancies, assume that the explanation for discrepancies is that we are inferior and lacking, and feel anxious and depressed because of it.

The Female Viewer Paradox

In just a few paragraphs, I will review what we know from the research literature on pornography and body image and show that some studies have found that there is an association between viewing pornography and negative body self-esteem. But there is also a paradoxical finding in the literature that is simply too interesting not to reveal first: across studies, the association between pornography viewing and negative body self-image appears to be stronger and more consistent for men than it is for women. On the basis of objectification theory and anti-pornography advocacy claims that pornography objectifies and disproportionately harms women, one would assume that women who view thin, large-breasted, waxed, cosmetically enhanced women in pornography would compare themselves to those images, make note of the ways in which they do not live up to the ideal being presented, and internalize a sense of shame and self-doubt that manifests in unhealthy eating behaviors and the pursuit of aesthetic surgery. Certainly, there are women who have this experience. But what the evidence suggests is that it is much more likely that *men* who view pornography are the ones who end up feeling like they don't measure up—several studies have found that women's body image or body self-esteem is relatively unaffected by viewing pornography.[14-16] How could this be? While no one knows for sure, one strong possibility is that most women already feel low because of their exposure to everyday media, so that layering on top of it the additional exposure to sexually explicit media is more like a drop in the bucket when it comes to ruining their self-esteem. In other words, women's body images are already in such bad shape from regular media that viewing pornography doesn't make things much worse. This has relevance for public health advocates because the idea that pornography, specifically, is contributing to eating disorders or poor mental health of women can be questioned in light of the existing research findings.

The Possibility of Confounding for Younger Cohorts of Viewers

There is one other point of interest worth mentioning before the review of the literature. The existing literature on pornography and body image treats pornography as though it is monolithic. My review did not identify any studies that were able to parse out possible differences in the association of pornography viewing with negative body image when pornography was stratified by subtype. But subtype may matter. Of course, there are genres of pornography that purposefully feature diverse body sizes—some of them do so out of a sense of ethics or social justice, while others fetishize larger-sized people. But there are also on average differences in the body shapes and sizes of people featured in professional pornography versus the amateur category.

Amateur pornography is pornography that is supposed to feature "real-life" or everyday people—amateurs, people who are performing in pornography either for fun or as a part-time hobby, but not because they are making a career out of it. In reality, a lot of so-called amateur pornography is actually created by people who are full-time or professional pornography performers, or by people who are hoping that their amateur video attracts enough attention that they will be able to convert to a lucrative career as a professional. But whether they are actually amateurs or not, the bodies of the performers in pornography marketed as amateur may tend to be more statistically average than the bodies of performers in professionally produced pornography.[16] This matters because research suggests that, in comparison to older pornography consumers, younger audiences disproportionately prefer amateur pornography.[17] In other words, there could be a cohort effect. The extent to which younger audiences are viewing amateur pornography or porn featuring more average-looking bodies is unknown, but if a substantial percentage of younger audiences are choosing to view amateur and perhaps exclusively amateur pornography, and the bodies featured in amateur pornography are systematically different than the bodies featured in professionally produced pornography, that means that any observed associations between pornography viewing and body image that do not take into account the age of the cohort or the percentage of amateur pornography watched might bias results. In other words, it's possible that young people are choosing to watch pornography that features average-looking bodies more than their elders did or do, and that whatever we think we know about how watching pornography affects body image should not be applied to the younger generation.

Pubic Hair Removal

Pubic hair doesn't serve much purpose. It's believed to serve as a visual signal that a human is of reproductive age, and it functions as an "olfactory trap"—communicating our reproductive readiness and state via scents.[18] Some people have postulated that pubic hair may also reduce friction during intercourse and protect vaginas from pathogens, but pubic hair can actually increase pathogen transmission in women.[18] Modern humans are not the first to engage in pubic hair removal. Evidence from art and some artifacts suggests that in ancient Egypt and Greece, adult women removed their pubic hair and that hairless or groomed vulvas were considered beautiful.[19]

For the past decade, some of my feminist acquaintances have been repeating one particular narrative about pubic hair grooming and removal: almost all women under age 35 shave their pubic hair, and the reason that they do it is because of pornography, and the reason that pornography features women without pubic hair is in order to make adult women look like pre-pubescent children. The unstated subtext is: *Isn't that disgusting*? Well, yes. The idea that most pornography viewers are not interested in adults and would prefer to masturbate to images that remind them of underage girls upsets me. But there are a number of assumptions built into this argument that deserve consideration. First, is it true that hair removal is really that prevalent, and that there is an age cohort effect? Second, is it true that women who remove their pubic hair do so because of pornography? And third, is it true that the reason that female pornography performers tend to have no pubic hair is in order to resemble children?

It is estimated that 70% to 80% of adults worldwide engage in pubic hair grooming.[20] A 2010 study of 2,451 adult US women 18 to 64 years old found that almost 60% of US women ages 18 to 24 sometimes or always shave all of their pubic hair, and that 50% of women 25 to 29 years old report the same.[21] These results are consistent with those found in other western nations. As reported by Craigh and Gray (2019), data from the United States, United Kingdom, New Zealand, and Southern Australia have found that 65% to 89% of women and 65% to 82% of men engage in some type of pubic hair removal, and that women are more likely than men to remove all of their pubic hair.[18] A 2011 study of Northern Belgian adults found that 30% of women and 18% of men had at some point completely removed their pubic hair. This study also found that men were substantially more likely to remove pubic hair if their partner also engaged in pubic hair removal, and that women tended to feel more inclined to have sex after they groomed.[22] A study that collected data in 2015–2016 from a sample of adult Saudi women found that 100% had either completely or partially removed their pubic hair, and that the average age of first pubic hair removal was 13 years old.[23]

Is pubic hair removal more popular now that it was in a prior era? Unfortunately, this is hard to know because it was not systematically tracked or evaluated in any population-based sample, and using photographs of pornography models or artists' rendering of women over time is dicey—it could be that models have always been outliers, are more likely to have engaged in pubic grooming, and are not representative of the average person in their time. That said, one 1968 study of adult women belonging to an Australian nudist club found that only 10% had completely removed their pubic hair, and two separate studies of *Playboy* magazine centerfolds from 1953 to 2007 both demonstrated that a far greater proportion of centerfolds in issues dated 2000–2007 had little or no pubic hair compared to the centerfolds from older issues.[21,24,25] Whether these data may be taken as evidence that pubic hair removal is now vastly more prevalent among the general public than it was 50 years ago is debatable, but as of 2020 it was commonly accepted that pubic hair removal was a substantially more common behavior than it was in the last century.

Frustrated that the majority of the research on pubic hair removal was limited to Western nations, one team undertook an analysis of documentation related to grooming practices in 31 societies across the globe from 1910 to 1991, including for example Native American Blackfoot, Cherokee, and Navajo tribes, African Zulu, Middle Eastern Kurds, South American Ticuna, Caribbean Aztecs and Tzeltal, Asian Yakut, and others.[18] They found that people in 100% of the cultures engaged in either partial or complete pubic hair removal, and that the main reason people in these cultures did so was for hygiene and comfort reasons—pornography was referenced in 0% of the ethnographic accounts that described the reasons for pubic hair removal.[18]

So while pornography may be one reason that people remove pubic hair today, there are numerous possible reasons why throughout history people have selected to groom pubic hair, including perceptions that it is more hygienic, because it feels more comfortable, makes it easier to receive cunnilingus, and may appeal sexually to a partner, as well as because of pressure from family or friends to participate in hair removal practices. Women's bathing suits and underwear have also changed markedly in the past three decades, and pubic hair grooming may have become more prevalent when styles changed. The trend in public hair removal may also reflect the fact that hair removal of all types (i.e., from legs, arms, and underarms) has increased in popularity.[26]

It is possible that pornography producers seek performers with no pubic hair or ask them to remove pubic hair because they are hoping to make women's genitals appear juvenile. But there are other possibilities to consider. First, women's genitals may be more easily seen if pubic hair is removed. If the purpose of pornography is to show genitals, and intercourse, removing pubic hair may simply be advantageous. Second, evidence suggests that pubic lice have been reduced because of pubic hair removal,[20] so for reasons pertaining to public health or the perception that hygiene is improved due to pubic hair removal, it may be the norm on pornography sets. Third, some performers may find it more physically comfortable to remove their pubic hair or may find it more sexually stimulating to engage in sex acts without pubic hair. In other words, it may be their preference to perform without pubic hair. Still, the possibility remains that even if performers are not conscious that the reason why it originally became the norm on porn sets for performers to have removed hair is so that they would resemble pre-pubescent children, it is nevertheless true. Some have argued that if pornographers' goal is to make adult women look pre-pubescent, it is not clear why progressively larger breasts have also been the trend.[27] At best, public health advocates should be aware that there are multiple possible explanations for why performers may have removed pubic hair and should avoid leaping to the conclusion that there is a single explanation for the phenomenon.

Let's assume, for a moment, that pornography is responsible for a massive uptick in pubic hair removal—and that the vast majority of adults and adolescents in the United States are now grooming their pubic hair as a direct result of pornography. After all, one qualitative research study quoted an 18-year-old girl as saying that pornography "makes me feel like my stomach, thighs and arms are too fat and that I need to wax all of my pubic hair," so for argument's sake let's presume for a moment that her comment is emblematic of a real trend.[28] Is this a public health concern? Pubic hair grooming is generally considered safe, although it can results in ingrown hairs, skin abrasions, folliculitis, vulvitis, contact dermatitis, and postinflammatory hyperpigmentation.[23] It is unlikely to result in increased transmission of sexually transmitted infections.[18] Given that the potential adverse consequences of pubic hair removal are not acute or severe, may be relatively uncommon, and are generally easily remedied, pubic hair removal—even if attributable to pornography—should not be considered a public health crisis.

Labiaplasty and Vulva Acceptance

Women are increasingly pursuing surgical modification of the vulva for cosmetic reasons. Popular procedures include reduction of the labia minora and clitoral hood, tightening of the vagina, "plumping" of the labia majora, liposuction of the mons pubis, and collagen injections of the G-spot.[25] Between 2011 and 2018, the number of labiaplasty cases in the United States grew 600%, from 2,124 surgeries to 12,756.[29] But are women pursuing these surgeries because of pornography, or for other reasons? And is it a public health problem that people are pursuing genital aesthetic surgeries?

The popular press has run numerous articles suggesting that pornography is to blame for the increase in labiaplasty.[30,31] However, the results of a study of labiaplasty patients in the United States suggest that pornography alone may not be responsible for labiaplasty increases. The study collected data from 124 US women in 2016 to 2018 who were seeking labiaplasty and 50 who were seeking cosmetic surgery other than labiaplasty. It found that only 11% of those seeking labiaplasty reported that pornography had an influence on their decision, and 4% of those in the cosmetic surgery control group reported the same.[29] However, the number one reason women gave for seeking labiaplasty was feeling self-conscious about how they looked, and 65% reported feeling less attractive because of their labia—so a fair question is why they should have felt self-conscious or less attractive because of their labia. In an indirect way, perhaps pornography contributed to a beauty ideal that made them consider the aesthetics of their labia. But there is another piece of evidence to consider: to date, no study has documented that there is a uniform or ideal labia look in pornography. In fact, it is equally possible that mainstream online pornography features a wide diversity of labia—some pornography performers and directors attest to this.[32] Just as Millward's analysis of the IAFD data set found that the average female pornography performer was not blonde and not a DD bra cup size (they are, on average, brunette with a 34B cup), the idea that performers' labia all tend to look one particular way is, as of now, rumor that needs empirical confirmation.[8] This may be why studies of women's pornography use have tended to find no association with dissatisfaction with one's genitals.[16,33]

The findings of at least one research study support the idea that women may become more satisfied with their own vulvar appearance because of pornography. A study published in 2017 found that 346 primarily low-income and racial minority female US hospital patients 18 to 44 years old were more satisfied with their vulvar appearance than their counterparts 45 years old and older.[34] The participants "who learned about genitalia from the Internet or any type of pornography" were *more likely* to report that they felt that they had normal-appearing vulvas than those not exposed to media (96.7% vs. 90.8%, respectively). The study also found that among the small subset who reported that they had considered vulvar surgery, 74% had been exposed to Internet media, but more than a quarter of them (26%) had no media exposure. An additional cross-sectional study of 393 US young adults surveyed using MTurk found no association between women's pornography use and genital self-image, and also found that women who frequently viewed pornography felt more comfortable being nude.[16]

How is it possible that seeing pornography could make some women feel better about their vulvas or naked bodies? Unlike men, who arguably may have the opportunity to see a variety of other men's penises in locker rooms and bathrooms because male genitalia are external, adult women may lack experience seeing inside vulvas—even their own. By observing the variety in shape, size, and coloration in pornography, some women may get a sense that their own body parts are within the norm. Indeed, contrary to the researchers' expectations, one recent study found that, in a sample of Canadians 15 to

58 years old, an increased frequency of pornography use predicted more accurate knowledge of anatomy, physiology, and sexual behavior.[35]

Pornography and Men's Genital Dissatisfaction

To my knowledge, there have been no studies of the average penis size of pornography performers. However, reportedly, pornography producers typically hire male performers who have penises 7 inches or longer when erect.[36]
Given that the average adult man's penis is slightly longer than 5 inches when
erect,[37] it is reasonable to conclude that on average pornography likely tends
to feature larger-than-average penises in both length and girth. Qualitative research findings suggest that pornography provides an unrealistic standard for
penis size, and that Internet pornography influences how men who undergo
penile augmentation surgery feel about their genitals.[38] Consistent with these
results, at least four studies of Canadian undergraduate college students, and
of adult men, respectively, found that men's dissatisfaction with their genitals
was associated with frequency of pornography use.[15,33,39] However, a longitudinal 2014 study of Dutch men found that frequent online pornography use
did not increase dissatisfaction with penis size, although it did affect men's
body dissatisfaction more generally,[14] and a study of 1,274 Norwegian and
Swedish university students found that more frequent pornography viewing
predicted better satisfaction with one's penis.[40] A 2019 study of US MTurk
survey users found that men's pornography use was not associated with men's
genital self-image,[16] and a survey of sexual minority males in Australia and
New Zealand found the same.[41] In sum, the research on pornography and
men's genital dissatisfaction is inconclusive at this time, although there is
more evidence to suggest that pornography influences men's genital dissatisfaction than there is evidence about women's genital dissatisfaction.

Satisfaction with Body Shape and Size

More than two thirds of US adults are either overweight or obese.[42] Body acceptance advocates assert that the negative health consequences of obesity have
been exaggerated.[43] However, the US Centers for Disease Control and World
Health Organization consider the prevalence of overweight and obesity to be a
serious public health problem because overweight and obesity are risk factors
for multiple chronic diseases.[44,45]Whether it's for health or aesthetic reasons, too
many people are unhappy with their bodies. A recent meta-analysis found that

between 11% and 72% of US women and 8% and 61% of US men experience "body dissatisfaction."[46] Body dissatisfaction is its own public health problem. It does not predict participating in exercise or healthful eating; instead, it can actually inhibit these healthy behaviors and is associated with problematic social and sexual functioning, depression, and anxiety.[47] Is pornography contributing to the current epidemic of body dissatisfaction?

Qualitative research suggests that it's not only women who feel less confidence about their bodies when comparing themselves to celebrities and pornography performers—it happens to men, too.[48] And several quantitative studies support the idea that pornography consumption may be associated with internalizing unrealistic body ideals[49] and body dissatisfaction in men.[16,49] However, a recent meta-analysis found that across 16 studies, men's pornography use was not associated with body satisfaction.[50] Some research also suggests that women who use Internet pornography are more likely than those who do not to engage in body monitoring (i.e., worrying about how one's body looks all the time)[51] and to have more concerns about their body,[15] although the relationship between pornography use and negative body image is far less consistent in samples of women than it is in men.[16,28,52] As described in the section on the female paradox, above, one possible explanation for this is that women already experience self-objectification and suffer negative body image effects from media in general, so sexually explicit media do not pile on that much more negativity. Another explanation could be that the women in pornography are more likely to resemble average women than antipornography activists presume, and so, as the data suggest, some women may feel better about themselves after viewing pornography, rather than worse. In the words of one 16-year-old girl quoted in a qualitative research study on the impact of pornography on body image: "Not all the women [in pornography] are 'skinny skinny' and it reminds me there are normal-sized girls."[28] The takeaway for public health advocates is, again, that the literature on pornography and body image is conflicted and sparse—but if there is an influence of pornography on body image, it should be viewed as part of the overarching problem, which is the influence of media on body image more generally. It does not appear to be the case that pornography alone, or in particular, is eroding men's or women's positive, confident feelings about their bodies.

Self-Esteem and Sexual Confidence

Another way in which pornography could affect people's satisfaction with themselves is by negatively influencing their sexual self-esteem or self-confidence, or their self-esteem overall. What's more, being preoc-cupied and distracted thinking about whether one's body or sexual tech-nique is good enough, compared to pornography, might make it difficult for people to focus on having sex in real time when they have the opportu-nity and thus for them to feel less satisfied with their sex lives. On the one hand, there are isolated cross-sectional studies that have found that in some samples, women's and men's self-esteem is negatively associated with their pornography use.[16,39] On the other hand, at least two studies have found that frequent Internet pornography viewing and a belief in the realism of pornography were related to a higher level of sexual self-esteem in hetero-sexual, gay, and bisexual men (although not in women).[40,53] A meta-analysis of nine studies assessing the relationship between pornography use and self-esteem or sexual self-esteem found that there was no relationship.[50] Because the meta-analysis also took into account the year that studies were published, the results also suggest that any change in pornography content over time toward what some have called "more violent and dehumanizing content preferences" has not altered the lack of association between por-nography use and body and self-satisfaction.[50] This is important because it counters two arguments made by anti-pornography activists, which are: (1) that pornography causes body dissatisfaction, and (2) that the increasingly extreme content of pornography means that health-related outcomes are becoming worse and worse.[54,55] The takeaway for public health advocates is not that there is nothing to worry about when it comes to pornography and self-esteem. Pornography may damage the sexual confidence and self-esteem of some viewers, and there may be subgroups of people who are par-ticularly vulnerable to that harm. The issue is that whether this is true, and for which subgroups, remains undetermined.

Expectations of Partners' Bodies

Thus far, this chapter has explored how one's own pornography use may affect body image or eating-related behavior. Researchers have also studied whether one's partner's use of pornography influences one's behavior, or if one's use of pornography use influences how one appraises one's partner. In other words, even if you never see pornography, but your partner does, you might start competing with the images you assume that they are seeing and engage in unhealthy dieting or weight-control practices. And if you are a pornography user, it's possible that you will start to see your partner in a new, less favorable light because of it.

The first experiment on pornography and sexual satisfaction with one's partner was conducted by Zillman and Bryant (1988).[56] In this experiment, 160 young adults were assigned to either view television comedy videos or nonviolent pornography for 1 hour per week for six consecutive weeks. For both men and women, being in the pornography condition was associated with diminished satisfaction with their sexual partner's affection, physical appearance, sexual curiosity, and sexual performance. [56] Subsequently, Weaver et al. (1984) and Kenrick et al. (1989) found that men who were exposed to photographs of attractive nude women subsequently rated their own sexual partners as less attractive.[57,58]

Several non-experimental studies have also found that one's partner's use of pornography may influence one's perception of oneself. For example, a study of 409 US women 18 to 64 years old using the MTurk online survey system found that perceived current and previous partner pornography use was associated with dieting, preoccupation with body fat, extreme eating-related guilt, and vomiting after eating.[59] Perceived previous (but not current) partner pornography use was also associated with women's bulimia/food preoccupation and binge eating.[59] The study was cross-sectional, so it's possible that male partners who watch pornography were more likely to seek partners who were already preoccupied with being thin. A study of Australian women also found that the frequency of one's partner's pornography use was associated with an increased desire to be muscular, although 85% of the women in the study reported that they were happy with their partner's pornography use and their partners' pornography use was not associated with body image or mental health other than the drive for muscularity.[28] In addition, a cross-sectional survey study of Canadian undergraduates found that women who viewed pornography had higher expectations of their partners' sexual performance than women who were nonviewers, and that for men, pornography viewing was associated with "body- and performance-related cognitive distractions during sexual activity"—meaning that pornography interfered with their ability to give real-life sex their full attention.[15]

Research in this area is sparse but seems to coalesce around the idea that viewing pornography could encourage people to compare their partners unfavorably with pornography performers, and that if women know their partners are viewing pornography, they may compare themselves unfavorably or feel that they have to compete with what they imagine to be pornographic ideals. The idea that women's bulimia and food preoccupation may be associated with partners' use of pornography is particularly worrisome from a public health perspective and should be investigated through longitudinal research.

Men Who Have Sex with Men

Gay and bisexual men are particularly vulnerable to body dissatisfaction, and some data suggest that they may also be particularly vulnerable to media influence related to body ideals.[60,61] This would amount to a perfect storm for acute vulnerability to body dissatisfaction related to pornography use except for one thing. Some have argued that gay and bisexual men may use pornography differently than heterosexual men and women.[62] They argue, on the basis of qualitative research, that gay and bisexual men may view pornography as a utilitarian masturbatory aid, and may be less likely than heterosexual people to change their sexual behavior because of what they see depicted in it.[62] Still, research findings on the impact of pornography on gay and bisexual men's body image are diverse. On the one hand, qualitative and some cross-sectional survey studies have found that men who have sex with men (MSM) report that pornography sets unreasonably high expectations for body ideals and influences their body satisfaction negatively.[41,63,64] On the other hand, several studies have found either no effect of pornography on body image and related constructs, such as drive for muscularity,[39,65] or positive effects.[53] For example, data collected in 2012 from 529 Norwegian MSM found that gay and bisexual men had more confidence in their sexual skills if they watched pornography in longer sessions, which the authors hypothesized stemmed from a sense of erotic empowerment derived from watching pornography.[53] In part, this may be because MSM often choose to watch pornography that does not feature pornography performers with ideal bodies, but choose to watch pornography with performers whose bodies resemble their own.[53] Thus, there is mixed evidence for an association between pornography viewing and negative body image or body-related self-esteem even in MSM, who may be at heightened risk for experiencing these adverse consequences of pornography use.

Conclusions

Sexually explicit media are part of the spectrum of all media through which humans communicate about beauty. Sexually explicit media, like other media, reflect back to people what they find aesthetically pleasing and have selected to see and promote beauty ideals by offering exaggerated images. Like all other forms of media, pornography invites comparisons between the self and the performers and between one's sexual partners and the performers and appears to cause some people to self-objectify and to objectify others. Furthermore, pornography appears to cause people to develop feelings of body dissatisfaction and preoccupation with their appearance or food and eating, and some people may engage in unhealthful dieting or body modification as a result. But there is no clear evidence that pornography, apart from other forms of media, is particularly to blame for these possible negative outcomes. And there is some evidence, although not much, that pornography may in fact reassure some individuals that their genitals are normal and that their body is acceptable and might be desirable to others. In the end, the literature on pornography and body image is mixed. To conclude that this means there is no negative impact of pornography on body image or people's health would be wrong, and it would also be wrong to conclude that there is only negative impact or that negative impact is widespread and acute. The appropriate conclusion based on the literature at this time is that pornography likely harms some people's self-image, and for a minority of those who are harmed it drives them to extreme behaviors and terrible negative mental health consequences. For the majority, pornography either has no effect on how they feel about their bodies, improves how they feel about their bodies, or merely underscores the body-related attitudes that they have already acquired from non-sexually-explicit media.

References

1. Ryabov, I. 2019. "How Much Does Physical Attractiveness Matter for Blacks? Linking Skin Color, Physical Attractiveness, and Black Status Attainment." *Race and Social Problems* 11, no. 1: 68–79.
2. Bauldry, S., M. J. Shanahan, R. Russo, B. W. Roberts, and R. Damian. 2016. "Attractiveness Compensates for Low Status Background in the Prediction of Educational Attainment." *PLOS One* 11, no. 6: 15.
3. Morris, R. D., and J. A. Morris. 2004. "Sexual Selection, Redundancy and Survival of the Most Beautiful." *Journal of Biosciences* 29, no. 3: 359–366.
4. Little, A. C., B. C. Jones, and L. M. DeBruine. 2011. "Facial Attractiveness: Evolutionary Based Research." *Philosophical Transactions of the Royal Society B: Biological Sciences*. 366, no. 1571: 1638–1659.
5. Cooper, A. D. 2019. *Patriarchy and the Politics of Beauty*. Lanham, Maryland: Lexington Books.
6. Silverstein, B., L. Perdue, B. Peterson, and E. Kelly. 1986. "The Role of the Mass Media in Promoting a Thin Standard of Bodily Attractiveness for Women." *Sex Roles* 14, no. 9: 519–532.
7. Kaye, P. 2019. "The True Toll of Porn: Girls Who Hate Their Bodies and Young Men Who Can't Perform in Relationships, by a GP Who's Seen the Harm It Does to Teens." https://www.dailymail.co.uk/femail/article-6831573/The-true-toll-porn-Pretty-girls-hate-bodies-young-men-perform.html Accessed December 22, 2019.
8. Millward, J. 2013. "Deep Inside: A Study of 10,000 Porn Stars and Their Careers." https://jonmillward.com/blog/studies/deep-inside-a-study-of-10000-porn-stars/   Accessed December 20, 2019.

9. IAFD.com. 2020. "IAFD Home Page." http://www.iafd.com/ Accessed August 28, 2020.
10. Snow, A. 2019. "The Porn Stars Who Regret Getting Breast Implants: 'Don't Do It.'" *The Daily Beast*. https://www.thedailybeast.com/the-porn-stars-who-regret-getting-breast-implants-dont-do-it
11. Fredrickson, B. L., and T-A. Roberts. 1997. "Objectification Theory: Toward Understanding Women's Lived Experiences and Mental Health Risks." *Psychology of Women Quarterly* 21, no. 2: 173–206.
12. Shroff, H., and J. K. Thompson. 2006. "The Tripartite Influence Model of Body Image and Eating Disturbance: A Replication with Adolescent Girls." *Body Image* 3, no. 1: 17–23.
13. Morrison, T. G., R. Kalin, and M. A. Morrison. 2004. "Body-image Evaluation and Body-image Investment Among Adolescents: A Test of Sociocultural and Social Comparison Theories." *Adolescence* 39, no. 155: 571–592.
14. Peter, J., and P. M. Valkenburg. 2014. "Does Exposure to Sexually Explicit Internet Material Increase Body Dissatisfaction? A Longitudinal Study." *Computers in Human Behavior* 36: 297–307.
15. Goldsmith, K., C. R. Dunkley, S. S. Dang, and B. B. Gorzalka. 2017. "Pornography Consumption and Its Association with Sexual Concerns and Expectations Among Young Men and Women." *The Canadian Journal of Human Sexuality* 26, no. 2: 151–162.
16. Vogels, E. A. 2019. "Loving Oneself: The Associations Among Sexually Explicit Media, Body Image, and Perceived Realism." *The Journal of Sex Research* 56, no. 6: 778–790.
17. Hald, G. M., and A. Štulhofer. 2016. "What Types of Pornography Do People Find Arousing and Do They Cluster? Assessing Types and Categories of Pornography in a Large-Scale Online Sample." *The Journal of Sex Research* 53, no. 7: 849–859.
18. Craig, L. K., and P. B. Gray. 2019. "Pubic Hair Removal Practices in Cross-Cultural Perspective." *Cross-Cultural Research* 53, no. 2: 215–237.
19. Kilmer, M. 2013. "Genital Phobia and Depilation." *The Journal of Hellenic Studies* 102: 104–112.
20. Dholakia, S., J. Buckler, J. P. Jeans, A. Pillai, N. Eagles, and S. Dholakia. 2014. "Pubic Lice: An Endangered Species?" *Sexually Transmitted Diseases* 41, no. 6: 388–391.
21. Herbenick, D., V. Schick, M. Reece, S. Sanders, and J. D. Fortenberry. 2010. "Pubic Hair Removal Among Women in the United States: Prevalence, Methods, and Characteristics." *The Journal of Sexual Medicine* 7, no. 10: 3322–3330.
22. Enzlin, P., K. Bollen, S. Prekatsounaki, L. Hidalgo, L. Aerts, and J. Deprest. 2019. "'To Shave or Not to Shave': Pubic Hair Removal and Its Association with Relational and Sexual Satisfaction in Women and Men." *The Journal of Sexual Medicine* 16, no. 7: 954–962.
23. Rouzi, A. A., R. C. Berg, J. Turkistani, et al. 2018. "Practices and Complications of Pubic Hair Removal Among Saudi Women." *BMC Women's Health* 18: 6.
24. Schick, V. R., B. N. Rima, and S. K. Calabrese. 2011. "Evulvalution: The Portrayal of Women's External Genitalia and Physique Across Time and the Current Barbie Doll Ideals." *The Journal of Sex Research* 48, no. 1: 74–81.
25. Mowat, H., K. McDonald, A. S. Dobson, J. Fisher, and M. Kirkman. 2015. "The Contribution of Online Content to the Promotion and Normalisation of Female Genital Cosmetic Surgery: A Systematic Review of the Literature." *BMC Women's Health* 15: 110.
26. Tiggemann, M., and S. Hodgson. 2008. "The Hairlessness Norm Extended: Reasons for and Predictors of Women's Body Hair Removal at Different Body Sites." *Sex Roles* 59, no. 11–12: 889–897.
27. Placik, O. J., and J. P. Arkins. 2014. "Plastic Surgery Trends Parallel *Playboy* Magazine: The Pudenda Preoccupation." *Aesthetic Surgery Journal* 34, no. 7: 1083–1090.
28. Laemmle-Ruff, I. L., M. Raggatt, C. J. C. Wright, et al. 2019. "Personal and Reported Partner Pornography Viewing by Australian Women, and Association with Mental Health and Body Image." *Sexual Health* 16, no. 1: 75–79.

29. Sorice-Virk, S., A. Y. Li, F. L. Canales, and H. J. Furnas. 2019. "The Role of Pornography, Physical Symptoms, and Appearance in Labiaplasty Interest." *Aesthetic Surgery Journal* 40, no. 8: 876–883.

30. Davis, R. 2011. "Labiaplasty Surgery Increase Blamed on Pornography." https://www.theguardian.com/lifeandstyle/2011/feb/27/labiaplasty-surgery-labia-vagina-pornography

31. Mackenzie, J. 2017. "Vagina Surgery 'Sought by Girls as Young as Nine.'" https://www.bbc.com/news/health-40410459 Accessed August 28, 2020.

32. Alpatrum, L. "5 Porn Stars Debunk the Myth of the Perfect 'Porn Pussy.'" 2018. https://www.refinery29.com/en-us/2016/06/113241/porn-pussy-perfect-vagina-myth

33. Skoda, K., and C. L. Pedersen. 2019. "Size Matters After All: Experimental Evidence that SEM Consumption Influences Genital and Body Esteem in Men." *SAGE Open* 9, no. 2: 1–11.

34. Truong, C., S. Amaya, and T. Yazdany. 2017. "Women's Perception of Their Vulvar Appearance in a Predominantly Low-Income, Minority Population." *Female Pelvic Medicine & Reconstructive Surgery* 23, no. 6: 417–419.

35. Hesse, C., and C. Pedersen. 2017. "Porn Sex Versus Real Sex: How Sexually Explicit Material Shapes Our Understanding of Sexual Anatomy, Physiology, and Behaviour." *Sexuality & Culture* 21: 754–775.

36. Wong, B. 2019. "All the Ways Porn Lied to You, According to Actual Porn Stars." https://www.huffpost.com/entry/porn-lies-sex_l_5cc1ffeee4b066119de3a45c

37. Veale, D., S. Miles, S. Bramley, G. Muir, and J. Hodsoll. 2015. "Am I Normal? A Systematic Review and Construction of Nomograms for Flaccid and Erect Penis Length and Circumference in up to 15,521 Men." *BJU International* 115, no. 6: 978–986.

38. Sharp, G., and J. Oates. 2019. "Sociocultural Influences on Men's Penis Size Perceptions and Decisions to Undergo Penile Augmentation: A Qualitative Study." *Aesthetic Surgery Journal* 39, no. 11: 1253–1259.

39. Morrison, T. G., S. R. Ellis, M. A. Morrison, A. Bearden, and R. L. Harriman. 2006. "Exposure to Sexually Explicit Material and Variations in Body Esteem, Genital Attitudes, and Sexual Esteem Among a Sample of Canadian Men." *The Journal of Men's Studies* 14, no. 2: 209–222.

40. Kvalem, I. L., B. Træen, B. Lewin, and A. Štulhofer. 2014. "Self-perceived Effects of Internet Pornography Use, Genital Appearance Satisfaction, and Sexual Self-Esteem Among Young Scandinavian Adults." *Cyberpsychology: Journal of Psychosocial Research on Cyberspace* 8, no. 4. Article 4. https://doi.org/10.5817/CP2014-4-4

41. Griffiths, S., D. Mitchison, S. B. Murray, and J. M. Mond. 2018. "Pornography Use in Sexual Minority Males: Associations with Body Dissatisfaction, Eating Disorder Symptoms, Thoughts About Using Anabolic Steroids and Quality of Life." *The Australian and New Zealand Journal of Psychiatry* 52, no. 4: 339–348.

42 Yang, L., and G. A. Colditz. 2015. "Prevalence of Overweight and Obesity in the United States, 2007–2012." *JAMA Internal Medicine* 175, no. 8: 1412–1413.

43. Basham, P., and J. Luik. 2008. "Is the Obesity Epidemic Exaggerated? Yes." *BMJ* 336, no. 7638: 245.

44. World Health Organization. 2020. "Obesity and Overweight." https://www.who.int/news-room/fact-sheets/detail/obesity-and-overweight

45. US Centers for Disease Control and Prevention. 2020. "Overweight and Obesity." https://www.cdc.gov/obesity/index.html

46. Fiske, L., E. A. Fallon, B. Blissmer, and C. A. Redding. 2014. "Prevalence of Body Dissatisfaction Among United States Adults: Review and Recommendations for Future Research." *Eating Behaviors* 15, no. 3: 357–365.

47. Davison, T. E., and M. P. McCabe. 2005. "Relationships Between Men's and Women's Body Image and Their Psychological, Social, and Sexual Functioning." *Sex Roles* 52, no. 7: 463–475.

48. Elder, W. B., G. R. Brooks, and S. L. Morrow. 2012. "Sexual Self-Schemas of Heterosexual Men." *Psychology of Men & Masculinity* 13, no. 2: 166–179.

49. Tylka, T. L. 2015. "No Harm in Looking, Right? Men's Pornography Consumption, Body Image, and Well-Being." *Psychology of Men & Masculinity* 16, no. 1: 97–107.

50. Wright, P. J., R. S. Tokunaga, A. Kraus, and E. Klann. 2017. "Pornography Consumption and Satisfaction: A Meta-Analysis." *Human Communication Research* 43, no. 3: 315–343.

51. Maas, M. K., and S. Dewey. 2018. "Internet Pornography Use Among Collegiate Women: Gender Attitudes, Body Monitoring, and Sexual Behavior." *SAGE Open* 8, no. 2: 2158244018786640.

52. Borgogna, N. C., E. C. Lathan, and A. Mitchell. 2018. "Is Women's Problematic Pornography Viewing Related to Body Image or Relationship Satisfaction?" *Sexual Addiction & Compulsivity* 25, no. 4: 345–366.

53. Kvalem, I. L., B. Træen, and A. Iantaffi. 2016. "Internet Pornography Use, Body Ideals, and Sexual Self-Esteem in Norwegian Gay and Bisexual Men." *Journal of Homosexuality* 63, no. 4: 522–540.

54. Fight The New Drug. 2019. "4 Ways Porn Warps the Way Women View Themselves." https://fightthenewdrug.org/4-ways-porn-warps-the-way-women-view-themselves/

55. Fight The New Drug. 2019. "Porn is Inspiring Teen Girls to Undergo This Invasive and Painful Cosmetic Surgery." https://fightthenewdrug.org/growing-trend-of-porn-inspired-plastic-surgery-for-teens/

56. Zillmann, D., and J. Bryant. 1988. "Pornography's Impact on Sexual Satisfaction." *Journal of Applied Social Psychology* 18, no. 5: 438–453.

57. Kenrick, D. T., S. E. Gutierres, and L. L. Goldberg. 1989. "Influence of Popular Erotica on Judgments of Strangers and Mates." *Journal of Experimental Social Psychology* 25, no. 2: 159–167.

58. Weaver, J. B., J. L. Masland, and D. Zillmann. 1984. "Effect of Erotica on Young Men's Aesthetic Perception of Their Female Sexual Partners." *Perceptual and Motor Skills* 58, no. 3: 929–930.

59. Tylka, T. L., and R. M. Calogero. 2019. "Perceptions of Male Partner Pressure To Be Thin and Pornography Use: Associations with Eating Disorder Symptomatology in a Community Sample of Adult Women." *International Journal of Eating Disorders* 52, no. 2: 189–194.

60. Frederick, D. A., and J. H. Essayli. 2016. "Male Body Image: The Roles of Sexual Orientation and Body Mass Index Across Five National U.S. Studies." *Psychology of Men & Masculinity* 17, no. 4: 336–351.

61. Carper, T. L. M., C. Negy, and S. Tantleff-Dunn. 2010. "Relations Among Media Influence, Body Image, Eating Concerns, and Sexual Orientation in Men: A Preliminary Investigation." *Body Image* 7, no. 4: 301–309.

62. Morrison, T. G. 2004. " 'He was treating me like trash, and I was loving it . . .' Perspectives on gay male pornography." *Journal of Homosexuality* 47, no. 3–4: 167–183.

63. Leickly, E., K. Nelson, and J. Simoni. 2017. "Sexually Explicit Online Media, Body Satisfaction, and Partner Expectations Among Men who have Sex with Men: A Qualitative Study." *Sexuality Research and Social Policy* 14, no. 3: 270–274.

64. Whitfield, T. H. F., H. J. Rendina, C. Grov, and J. T. Parsons. 2018. "Viewing Sexually Explicit Media and Its Association with Mental Health Among Gay and Bisexual Men Across the U.S." *Archives of Sexual Behavior* 47, no. 4: 1163–1172.

65. Gleason, N., and E. Sprankle. 2019. "The Effects of Pornography on Sexual Minority Men's Body Image: An Experimental Study." *Psychology & Sexuality* 10, no. 4: 301–315.

10

Child Sexual Abuse Imagery

Child pornography, also called "child sexual abuse imagery" and "child exploitation material," is a serious public health problem for two reasons. First, each instance of child pornography that involves a minor younger than the age of sexual consent is a depiction of a sexual or violent crime that took place. In addition, the production of the image is a separate crime. Children may be psychologically, physically, or sexually abused in order to produce the pornography. Some argue that new damage is done to a child each time the images of their abuse are viewed, because it causes fresh humiliation and pain to know that people are deriving pleasure from their exploitation. In other words, the harms to reputation, privacy, and mental health can be lifelong.[1] Second, child pornography may encourage some people to perpetrate child sexual abuse.[2] Not everyone who views child pornography is pedophilic,[3] and not everyone who perpetrates child sexual abuse is pedophilic.[4] And research suggests that it is rare that healthy adults with no pedophilic interest become pedophilic only because of viewing child pornography—research on the etiology of pedophilia suggests it is influenced by genetics, stressful life events, specific learning processes, and other factors.[4] But for the small subset of people who have antisocial tendencies or pedophilic interests, viewing child pornography may be an aggravator that influences the likelihood that they will commit what is called a "hands-on" or "direct contact" sexual crime against a child.[2] There are no two ways about it: child sexual abuse imagery causes harm and is a serious public health problem.

What Counts as Child Pornography?

Laws pertaining to child pornography vary by country. One nation-by-nation law review published in 2010 found that of 196 countries, almost half ($N = 89$) lacked child pornography laws.[5] In the United States, the first federal law against producing child pornography was passed in 1977,[6] and the first laws pertaining to computers and child pornography were passed in 1988.[7] Today, US federal law defines child pornography "as any visual depiction of sexually explicit conduct involving a minor (persons less than 18 years

Pornography and Public Health. Emily F. Rothman, Oxford University Press. © Oxford University Press 2021.
DOI: 10.1093/oso/9780190075477.003.0010

old)."[8] The crimes of possession, receipt, and trafficking of child pornography are presented in chapters 71 and 110 of U.S.C. Title 18 (18 U.S.C. §§ 2252, 2252A, 2260(b)). Child pornography images may be digitally generated or drawn and may not have involved a human child during production, although digitally generated and drawn images have to be found obscene in order to count as child pornography (18 U.S.C. § 1466A). If not legally obscene, digital and drawn images are protected under the First Amendment. However, any image of a seminude or nude child may count as child pornography if it can be viewed as sexually suggestive.

How can one determine if an image of a child is sexually suggestive? The six-factor Dost test guideline was established in 1986 pursuant to a US district court case that involved nude and seminude photos of girls who were 10 to 14 years old.[9] Not all the criteria need to be met for an image to count as child pornography, and it isn't necessarily true that meeting a sole criterion means that the image is definitely pornographic. In other words, that photo of you naked in the bathtub as an infant probably would not be considered child pornography by a court, but there's no guarantee. The Dost test criteria are: (1) whether the focal point of the visual depiction is the child's genitalia or pubic area; (2) whether the setting of the visual depiction is sexually suggestive, i.e., in a place or pose generally associated with sexual activity; (3) whether the child is depicted in an unnatural pose, or in inappropriate attire, considering the age of the child; (4) whether the child is fully or partially clothed, or nude; (5) whether the visual depiction suggests sexual coyness or a willingness to engage in sexual activity; and (6) whether the visual depiction is intended or designed to elicit a sexual response in the viewer.[10]

Importantly, the production, distribution, import, reception, or possession of any image of child pornography is a federal crime—which has implications for adolescents who take or send others nude selfies (i.e., sexting). There are gradations in the severity of child pornography offenses based on factors like how old the children in the images are and what is happening to them. Punishments for child pornography offenses may include lifetime imprisonment. First-time offenders who produce child pornography can receive sentences of 15 to 30 years in federal prison and a requirement to register as a sex offender.

How Common Is Child Pornography?

Because child pornography is illicit and people tend to hide that they've created it, downloaded it, or possess it, it's difficult to estimate the prevalence of intentional child pornography viewing in the general population. However, one study of Swedish men 17 to 20 years old found that 4.2% reported having ever viewed child pornography.[11] In a 2015 study of 8,718 adult German men, 2.4% reported ever having used child pornography.[12] A nonrepresentative study of adult Internet pornography users in the United States found that as many as 12.5% of male respondents and 3.4% of female respondents had ever sought child pornography on the Internet intentionally.[13]

An international study of child pornography sharing across peer-to-peer file-sharing networks like BitTorrent found that there were over 840,000 individuals sharing child pornography in December 2014.[14] Approximately 56% of the installations of the sharing network software occurred in just four countries: China, Brazil, Mexico, and the United States. The study authors were able to estimate that approximately 2 in 10,000 Internet users in the United States were sharing child pornography in 2011 to 2014.[14] Of the nations studied, the rate was highest in Argentina, where 13 in 10,000 Internet users shared child pornography, and the rate was also high in Mexico (12 in 10,000) and in Spain (11 in 10,000).[14]

In the United States, as reported by the *New York Times* and the National Center for Missing and Exploited Children (NCMEC), in 1998 there were over 3,000 reports of child sexual abuse imagery made to law enforcement.[15] In 2014, there were 1 million reports to NCMEC's cyber tipline. In 2018, there were 18.4 million reports, which pertained to more than 45 million images and videos. Unfortunately, while reports of child pornography have increased steadily between 2010 and 2018, the arrest rate has increased only slightly, and federal funding for investigation and prosecution has remained flat.[15] In addition to advocating for more funding of investigation of child pornography cases, public health advocates could help raise awareness of the fact that federal law enforcement is unable to work with state-of-the-art equipment. Some reports suggest that they use technology outdated by 20 years in order to try to catch criminals who may be using the latest machines. What's more, the personnel who work on child pornography cases and have to contemplate the horrible crimes and abuses perpetrated against the child victims often experience severe secondary trauma and can burn out quickly, causing personnel shortages.

Production: How Is Child Pornography Made?

Warning: this section may be particularly difficult to read. Remember that you have a choice to skip to the next section or even to the next chapter if you need to.

Child exploitation material can be made in a number of ways. Adults may use force, fraud, or coercion to make a child pose for pornography. In some cases, parents or other child pornography producers sedate children with benzodiazepines or other substances.[16] Alternatively, they may use flattery, persuasion, gifts, payments, other inducements, or their position of authority to make the child pose. In some cases, producers of child pornography may take photographs or video of a child when the child is not aware that they are being filmed—such as when they are in a fitting room at a store, or in the shower. Now that most underage children have access to cellular phones or other devices with cameras, some child pornography is actually "self-produced," or created by children and adolescents themselves—although apparently the percentage of child porn cases that involve self-produced porn is very low—it was reportedly 14% in 2014.[17,18] Children may be photographed or filmed solo in various states of undress, while masturbating, while having sexual contact with an animal or another person, or while experiencing a violent assault.

People may produce child pornography for any number of reasons. They may be looking to make money, and because children are coerced or forced to participate in sexual exploitation images, the cost to produce child pornography, as compared to other media, is low. Because some child pornography-sharing platforms and systems require that users submit their own original child pornography images to gain entrance, to ensure that the user can be trusted by the other criminals, some people may produce the images in order to join the sharing networks. Still others produce the images for their own personal use or create the images for other people. The have been numerous cases of adult women who were imprisoned for producing child pornography of their own children to share with their boyfriends, because they were threatened or forced to do so, or for other reasons.[19] Finally, and as mentioned above, some adolescents are now self-producing sexual images that count as child pornography when they "sext" or take nude or seminude selfies. In some cases, they do so under duress—such as coercion by someone else who wants to receive the images. Other adolescents believe that they are sharing nude images with a trusted dating partner and are shocked when the image that they believed was private or deleted is shared on peer-to-peer child pornography networks.

One important question about the content of child pornography is what percentage of it is less severe, in that it depicts a child solo or engaged in nonsexual activity, and what percentage features sexual contact with another child or adult, or sadistic acts. Even though there is a team affiliated with the US government that reviews child pornography when it is seized or reported and classifies it, it is difficult to generalize that team's findings back to the universe of child pornography in existence because the amount of child pornography that is undiscovered remains unknown. In any case, using data from what is known, in the United States in 2009, 53% of arrests for child pornography production included pornography that featured a contact sexual offense—that is, when offenders pressure, flatter, or otherwise persuade a child to participate in sexual contact with someone else in the creation of the explicit images.[20] In 2009, of the arrests made for child pornography production that did include a contact sexual offense, the majority (approximately 80%) involved a penetrative offense, and approximately 10% involved a violent sexual assault.[20]

Dissemination: How Is Child Pornography Shared?

In the United States, the first federal law criminalizing the commercial dissemination of pornography in which the producer had knowingly used a minor (a person < 16 years old) in obscene depictions of sexually explicit content was passed in 1977.[21] In 1984, the Child Protection Act increased the age of protection to 18 years old.[22] In the 1970s, there were reportedly more than 250 print magazines in circulation, produced primarily in Europe, that published child pornography (p. 43).[23] For example, the magazine *Lolita* was published monthly in the Netherlands during the 1970s and reportedly included images of children as young as 3 years old engaged in sex acts with adults.[22] There were also child pornography books and 8-mm films available for legal trade or purchase.

After the passage of a series of federal laws, including the 2003 PROTECT Act, which among other things made it illegal to download Japanese anime style porn or computer-generated images of children engaged in sex acts, people who wanted to view child pornography primarily turned to online peer-to-peer networks. A peer-to-peer network is when two or more computers are connected and share files or folders directly, rather than going through a central server. Peer-to-peer networking, and peer-to-peer protocols like BitTorrent, can share large files fast and sometimes anonymously. There is also a network of cryptographically hidden websites called the "darknet" or the "dark web" that can be accessed through anonymizing browsers like Tor. One study of the dark web found that in 2015, approximately 5% of dark websites were illegitimate pornography.[24]

Who Looks at Child Pornography?

People who use child pornography are heterogeneous and their motivations for use varies. Some people look at child pornography because they have pedophilic interests and would commit hands-on or contact sexual crimes against a child if they had an opportunity. Others would not, and do not, commit contact sexual crimes but view child pornography for sexual self-gratification or arousal. A third group may view child pornography out of curiosity but not feel sexually aroused by it (NB: it is illegal to view child pornography even if one is motivated by curiosity). Then, of course, there are adolescents who technically view child pornography when they take nude selfies or receive them.

What is known about people who use child pornography is based on data from people who are caught. That said, and not including adolescents who sext, the typical profile of a child pornography use offender is male, older than the average offender, white, unmarried/single, without biological children, employed, and with more education than other offenders.[25] One reason that offenders may be more likely to be employed and have more education than other offenders is that, at least historically, employed and more highly educated people were more likely to have a computer—and having a computer facilitates child pornography offenses. There also appear to be early childhood and family factors that are risk markers for perpetration. A case-control study involving Swedish men convicted of child pornography offenses between 1988 and 2009 found that having a father who was younger than 25 years old when the person was born, parents with less education, fewer older brothers, congenital malformations, and parents who had been convicted of a violent crime were predictors of child pornography use.[26]

The psychological profile of child pornography use offenders differs from that of contact child sexual abuse offenders. The child pornography-only offenders tend to be less assertive, have poorer social skills, and are less able to manage their emotions than contact sexual offenders.[25] Some have deficits in empathy for victims, and some exhibit "cognitive distortions" (or warped thinking) about children and sex, including that minors are capable of making their own decisions about sexual activity with an adult.[27] One study of college men found that those who indicated a preference for child pornography shared a psychological profile with those who indicated a preference for adult nonconsenting pornography, and that, compared to those who preferred other types of adult pornography, they tended to be higher in dominance and hostility, to have a preference for impersonal sex, and to report aggressive or antisocial tendencies.[2,28]

Most people who are arrested for a child pornography offense do not re-offend subsequently. Studies suggest that 2% to 7% of people arrested for child pornography commit another child pornography offense within 4 to 5 years, while 1% to 3% commit a contact sexual offense.[25,29,30] However, a review of available studies that was published in 2011 assessed 21 separate studies that had information on 4,464 child pornography offenders and found that ap-proximately 13% of offenders had an official criminal record for hands-on sexual crimes, while 55% admitted that they had had hands-on sexual contact with a minor at some point, even if it hadn't resulted in any official criminal case.[31] These results suggest two things. First, not all people who commit the crime of viewing child pornography—in fact, not even most of them—are also perpetrators of hands-on contact sexual crimes. Second, a large percentage of people who view child pornography, as much as slightly over half, may also be contact sex offenders. In other words, the overlap is high, but the correlation is not absolute.

Does Seeing Child Pornography Cause Child Molestation?

It wouldn't be legal or ethical to expose people to child pornography in a labo-ratory setting and then follow up with them to see how many went on to per-petrate child sexual abuse. One research team did get creative and substituted "barely legal" pornography (featuring actresses over 18 years old who looked younger) for child pornography in order to test hypotheses about exposure to child pornography and sexualization of children.[32] But, generally, because experimental research studies that use actual child pornography are out of the question for important reasons, social scientists rely on case-control and co-hort studies to make inferences about the influence of child pornography on the people who view it.

One of the most important questions to answer is whether viewing child pornography increases the odds that the person viewing it will perpetrate child sexual abuse. A review of the literature on child pornography and con-tact sex offending by Malamuth (2018) assessed the findings of nearly 20 re-search studies on child pornography and child molestation and concluded that "at the least, a considerable minority of sexual offenders against chil-dren report that the use of some form of pornography had some salient in-fluence on their criminal behavior" (p. 800).[2] In short, it appears that viewing child pornography may increase the likelihood that some people prone to commit contact sex offenses on children actually do so.[2] Nonconsensual adult pornography may also have an aggravating influence on the people prone to commit hands-on child sexual abuse, as well.[2]

Some people worry that seeing child pornography (accidentally or on purpose) might cause a healthy person to develop pedophilia or to perpetrate child sexual abuse. It's important for public health professionals to know that there is no evidence to suggest that an accidental, one-time, or even multiple-time exposure(s) to child pornography could transform a healthy person into a person with criminal intentions or behaviors. Note, for example, that some civilians and some law enforcement officers classify and analyze seized child pornography to facilitate investigations, and while there is an expectation that they may experience trauma or burnout from this exposure, there is typically little concern that the exposure will turn them into criminal offenders themselves.[33] Some have argued that the fact that child sexual abuse has been steadily decreasing over the same period of time that Internet child pornography has been proliferating suggests that viewing Internet child pornography generally does not lead to hands-on crimes.[33] The catharsis hypothesis, or the idea that would-be hands-on offenders can satisfy their deviant desires with child pornography and that child pornography can therefore *prevent* child sexual abuse, has not been substantiated despite persistent beliefs in it.[34] In short, the consensus from the research experts appears to be that child pornography likely does aggravate sex offending among the users predisposed to contact child sex offense perpetration, which may be between 2% and 55% of those who view it, and that it does not generally inspire hands-on sex offending among otherwise healthy people with no antisocial tendencies and no pedophilic interest.[2,34]

Self-Produced Child Pornography

There are two main types of self-produced child pornography. First, some underage youth voluntarily, or are forced, coerced, or persuaded to, take nude photographs or videos of themselves and share them with others, which is referred to as sexting. Second, a small minority of underage youth may set up a web camera and stream live images of themselves (i.e., "camming") for paying or nonpaying individuals or groups. The results of research surveys with US teenagers suggest that up to approximately 13% to one quarter (28%) have ever engaged in sexting.[35,36] Just as a point of comparison, as many as 62% of emerging adults have engaged in sexting, so it appears that it may be becoming a normative dating or sexual relationship behavior.[37] Accordingly, as adolescents age, the likelihood that they have participated in sexting increases.[38] A recent nationally representative survey of 12- to 17-year-old English-speaking middle and high school students in the United States found that 5% had ever been a victim of "sextortion" (that is, when someone threatened that they would share a nude image of them with other people), and 3% admitted to perpetrating sextortion.[39] A meta-analysis found that 12% of adolescents have ever forwarded a sext without consent.[35]

A problem related to sexting as a subtype of child pornography is that even consensual teen sexting can be prosecuted under state law, or under federal law if the teens involved live in different states.[40] Being prosecuted for a sex crime as a teenager, let alone being convicted of one, can be devastating for a young person and for the families involved.[40] To date, 27 states have passed laws that address sexting.[40] Several of the laws specifically exempt teen sexting from child pornography statutes in certain circumstances, while others have created options for more lenient sentencing of adolescents offenders who sext (rather than subject them to the penalties for child pornography possession or distribution). Many of the state laws take into account the age of the person sending sexts, the age of the person receiving it, and whether the image was made consensually. Public health professionals are urged to incorporate messaging about sexting into safe sex and healthy relationships interventions for adolescents, to encourage parents to discuss healthy and safe digital citizenship at home, to advocate for the decriminalization of consensual sexting between adolescents while working for penalties for adult–child sexting, nonconsensual dissemination of sexually explicit images, and nonconsensual sexting, and to encourage pediatricians to discuss safe and healthy online behavior with patients.[40]

The Link Between Anti-Child-Pornography Activism and Anti-Gay-Rights Activism

Child pornography is in every way abominable, harmful to minors who are victimized, with indirect harms to those who care for them and about them, and with negative effects on the likelihood of child sex offending by people predisposed to offend who view it. Acting in strong, vocal opposition to child sexual abuse imagery is without question the only appropriate public health response. But because public health advocates should not be "single-issue" activists who are so enthusiastic about their one pet issue that they are willing to sacrifice the health of vulnerable populations in other ways as long as their own special topic is getting attention—we have to know, and consider, the full story when we participate in anti-child-pornography activism.

Unfortunately, in recent history, some bad actors have used the issue of child pornography in order to try to find a way to attack GLBTQ+ rights. The problem was that in the 1960s and 1970s, homosexuality was considered deviant. In the 1950s, the American Psychiatric Association (APA) classified homosexuality as a mental disorder.[41] After the Stonewall riots in New York in 1969, which many believe marked the official beginning of the gay rights movement, gay rights activists disrupted an APA convention in San Francisco in 1970 to protest the inclusion of homosexuality in the *Diagnostic and Statistical Manual of Mental Disorders* (DSM).[41] In 1973, the APA finally removed homosexuality from the DSM. But many members of the public still believed that homosexuality was a "sickness" or disorder—a "perversion," just like pedophilia. In fact, some people conflated the issues pedophilia and homosexuality—they erroneously believed that gay people were more likely to be attracted to children than heterosexual people, and that children were more at risk of being sexually abused by a gay adult than by a heterosexual adult.[42] During the 1970s and 1980s, during the same era when gay rights activists were making progress to secure civil rights and liberties, and when the so-called Golden Age of pornography was at its peak, theologically and politically conservative activists lashed out against the changing social norms and often lumped being gay, the availability of adult porn, the availability of child porn, and pedophilia all together as one objectionable issue. As Emily Weissler (2013) wrote in the *Fordham Law Review*:

A ferocious backlash to these more relaxed [child pornography] standards emerged in the late 1970s. This moral backlash was attributable in part to fears that homosexuals would corrupt children by sexually molesting them, and it coincided with a significant conservative campaign launched to reverse the social and political progress made by homosexuals. This moral campaign was justified with statistics that grossly overestimated the number of children being harmed by child pornography. For example, in 1986, an antipornography crusader stated that 'each year, fifty thousand missing children are victims of [child] pornography.' However, these statistics were exaggerated: no major child pornography rings were ever discovered, and all of the figures can be traced back to the rhetoric of well-intentioned activists. This moral panic and outrage were instrumental in elevating child pornography into the national consciousness as a political issue. (p. 1493)

Comments by the celebrity televangelist James Robison, in his 1982 book *Pornography: The Polluting of America*, provide a direct example of how theologically conservative activists attempted to equate pornography use with deviant sexuality and to call out homosexuality as deviant. Robison wrote: "[People who watch pornography] lose their God-given attraction for the opposite sex and begin to lust for persons of the same sex" (p. 31). He also called homosexuality a social ill: "Many studies show empirically that when pornography spreads into a community unchallenged it brings a number of other social ills along with it. Prostitution, drugs, homosexuality, sex-related crimes, such as rape and incest, and all manner of social problems seem to be pornography's fellow travelers" (p. 13). He also wrote that the "anything goes" legal climate of the time, as opposed to strict regulation of pornography, "is far more likely to lead to schoolgate bookstores glutted with picture books of homosexual rape and child torture" (p. 56). In other words, pornography, homosexuality, and "child torture" are essentially described as one and the same.

Conclusions

Child sexual abuse and child pornography, which is also called child sex abuse imagery, are grave problems. It is possible that sexual images of adolescents that they self-produce can also cause legal, social, and psychological problems for the adolescents depicted and for those who disseminate them. Public health professionals should be aware that, historically, outrage about child pornography has been used to galvanize people and to further repressive agendas. For this reason, child pornography prevention strategies need to be carefully devised, in partnership with a wide range of stakeholders, and they need to be studied for effectiveness and unintended consequences.

References

1. Gewirtz-Meydan, A., Y. Lahav, W. Walsh, and D. Finkelhor. 2019. "Psychopathology Among Adult Survivors of Child Pornography." *Child Abuse & Neglect* 98: 11.
2. Malamuth, N. M. 2018. "'Adding Fuel to the Fire?' Does Exposure to Non-consenting Adult or to Child Pornography Increase Risk of Sexual Aggression?" *Aggression and Violent Behavior* 41: 74–89.
3. Seto, M. C., J. M. Cantor, and R. Blanchard. 2006. "Child Pornography Offenses Are a Valid Diagnostic Indicator of Pedophilia." *Journal of Abnormal Psychology* 115, n. 3: 610–615.
4. Tenbergen, G., M. Wittfoth, H. Frieling, et al. 2015. "The Neurobiology and Psychology of Pedophilia: Recent Advances and Challenges." *Frontiers in Human Neuroscience* 9:344.
5. International Centre for Missing & Exploited Children. 2010. *Child Pornography: Model Legislation & Global Review,* 6th ed. Alexandria, VA: International Centre for Missing & Exploited Children.
6. Weissler, E. 2013. "Head Versus Heart: Applying Empirical Evidence About the Connection Between Child Pornography and Child Molestation to Connection Between Child

Pornography and Child Molestation to Probable Cause Analyses." *Fordham Law Review* 82, no. 3: 1–46.

7. Urbina, I. 2007. "Federal Judge Blocks Online Pornography Law." https://www.nytimes.com/2007/03/22/us/22cnd-porn.html

8. US Department of Justice. "Child Pornography." May 28, 2020. https://www.justice.gov/criminal-ceos/child-pornography

9. United States v. Dost. 636 F. Supp. 828 (SD Cal. 1986).

10. Hessick, C. B. 2016. *Refining Child Pornography Law: Crime, Language, and Social Consequences.* Ann Arbor, MI: University of Michigan Press.

11. Seto, M. C., C. A. Hermann, C. Kjellgren, G. Priebe, C. G. Svedin, and N. Langstrom. 2015. "Viewing Child Pornography: Prevalence and Correlates in a Representative Community Sample of Young Swedish Men." *Archives of Sexual Behavior* 44, no. 1: 67–79.

12. Dombert, B., A. F. Schmidt, R. Banse, et al. 2016. "How Common Is Men's Self-Reported Sexual Interest in Prepubescent Children?" *The Journal of Sex Research* 53, no. 2: 214–223.

13. Seigfried-Spellar, K. C., and M. K. Rogers. 2013. "Does Deviant Pornography Use Follow a Guttman-like Progression?" *Computers in Human Behavior* 29, no. 5: 1997–2003.

14. Bissias, G., B. Levine, M. Liberatore, et al. 2016. "Characterization of Contact Offenders and Child Exploitation Material Trafficking on Five Peer-to-Peer Networks." *Child Abuse & Neglect* 52: 185–199.

15. Keller, M. H., and G. J. X. Dance. 2019. "The Internet Is Overrun with Images of Child Sexual Abuse. What Went Wrong?" Accessed January 11, 2020. https://www.nytimes.com/interactive/2019/09/28/us/child-sex-abuse.html

16. Murphy, W. 2009. "Protecting Kids from Scourge of Child Pornography." https://www.patriotledger.com/article/20090330/NEWS/303309996

17. Westlake, B. 2018. "Delineating Victims from Perpetrators: Prosecuting Self-Produced Child Pornography in Youth Criminal Justice Systems." *International Journal of Cyber Criminology* 12, no. 1: 255–268.

18. Westlake, B. 2020. "The Past, Present, and Future of Online Child Sexual Exploitation: Summarizing the Evolution of Production, Distribution, and Detection." In *The Palgrave Handbook of International Cybercrime and Cyberdeviance*, edited by T. Holt and A. Bossler, 1225–1253. London: Palgrave Macmillan.

19. Geary, J. 2011. "Lakeland Woman Gets 60 Years for Making Child Porn." https://www.theledger.com/article/LK/20110408/news/608079395/LL

20. Wolak, J., D. Finkelhor, and K. Mitchell. 2012. "Trends in Arrests for Child Pornography Production: The Third National Juvenile Online Victimization Study (NJOV-3)." http://unh.edu/ccrc/pdf/CV270_Child%20Porn%20Production%20Bulletin_4-13-12.pdf

21. Ward, A. 2009. "Child Pornography." https://www.mtsu.edu/first-amendment/article/993/child-pornography

22. McGraw, C. 1985. "Child Smut Business Going Underground: Grows Uglier as Customers Trade Children, Not Just Pictures, Police Say." https://www.latimes.com/archives/la-xpm-1985-09-16-mn-22002-story.html

23. *Sexual Exploitation of Children: Hearings Before the Subcommittee on Crime of the Committee on the Judiciary*, 95th Congress (1977). https://www.ncjrs.gov/pdffiles1/Digitization/51083NCJRS.pdf

24. Moore, D., and T. Rid. 2016. "Cryptopolitik and the Darknet." *Survival* 58, no. 1: 7–38.

25. Brown, R., and S. Bricknell. 2018. "What Is the Profile of Child Exploitation Material Offenders?" *Trends & Issues in Crime and Criminal Justice* 2018, no. 564: 1–14.

26. Babchishin, K. M., M. C. Seto, S. Fazel, and N. Langstrom. 2019. "Are There Early Risk Markers for Pedophilia? A Nationwide Case-Control Study of Child Sexual Exploitation Material Offenders." *The Journal of Sex Research* 56, no. 2: 203–212.

27. Merdian, H. L., C. Curtis, J. Thakker, N. Wilson, and D. P. Boer. 2014. "The Endorsement of Cognitive Distortions: Comparing Child Pornography Offenders and Contact Sex Offenders." *Psychology, Crime & Law* 20, no. 10: 971–993.

28. Bogaert, A. F. 2001. "Personality, Individual Differences, and Preferences for the Sexual Media." *Archives of Sexual Behavior* 30, no. 1: 29–53.

29. Seto, M. C., J. M. Wood, K. M. Babchishin, and S. Flynn. 2012. "Online Solicitation Offenders Are Different from Child Pornography Offenders and Lower Risk Contact Sexual Offenders." *Law and Human Behavior* 36, no. 4: 320–330.

30. Elliott, I. A., R. Mandeville-Norden, J. Rakestrow-Dickens, and A. R. Beech. 2019. "Reoffending Rates in a UK Community Sample of Individuals With Convictions for Indecent Images of Children." *Law and Human Behavior* 43, no. 4: 369–382.

31. Seto, M. C., R. Karl Hanson, and K. M. Babchishin. 2010. "Contact Sexual Offending by Men with Online Sexual Offenses." *Sexual Abuse* 23, no. 1: 124–145.

32. Paul, B., and D. G. Linz. 2008. "The Effects of Exposure to Virtual Child Pornography on Viewer Cognitions and Attitudes Toward Deviant Sexual Behavior." *Communication Research* 35, no. 1: 3–38.

33. Wortley, R., and S. Smallbone. 2012. *Internet Child Pornography: Causes, Investigation, and Prevention.* Santa Barbara, CA: Praeger.

34. Malamuth, N., and M. Huppin. 2007. "Drawing the Line of Virtual Child Pornography: Bringing the Law in Line with the Research Evidence." *New York University Review of Law and Social Change* 31, no. 4: 773.

35. Madigan, S., A. Ly, C. L. Rash, J. Van Ouytsel, and J. R. Temple. 2018. "Prevalence of Multiple Forms of Sexting Behavior Among Youth: A Systematic Review and Meta-Analysis." *JAMA Pediatrics* 172, no. 4: 327–335.

36. Patchin, J. W., and S. Hinduja. 2019. "The Nature and Extent of Sexting Among a National Sample of Middle and High School Students in the US." *Archives of Sexual Behavior* 48, no. 8: 2333–2343.

37. Drouin, M., M. Coupe, and J. R. Temple. 2017. "Is Sexting Good for Your Relationship? It Depends . . . ." *Computers in Human Behavior* 75: 749–756.

38. Choi, H. J., C. Mori, J. Van Ouytsel, S. Madigan, and J. R. Temple. 2019. "Adolescent Sexting Involvement Over 4 Years and Associations with Sexual Activity." *Journal of Adolescent Health* 65, no. 6: 738–744.

39. Patchin, J. W., and S. Hinduja. 2018. "Sextortion Among Adolescents: Results From a National Survey of U.S. Youth." *Sexual Abuse* 32, no. 1: 30–54.

40. Strasburger, V. C., H. Zimmerman, J. R. Temple, and S. Madigan. 2019. "Teenagers, Sexting, and the Law." *Pediatrics* 143, no. 5: 9.

41. Baughey-Gill, S. 2011. "When Gay Was Not Okay with the APA: A Historical Overview of Homosexuality and its Status as Mental Disorder." *Occam's Razor* 1, no. 2: 5–16.

42. Kort, J. 2016. "Homosexuality and Pedophila: The False Link." https://www.huffpost.com/entry/homosexuality-and-pedophi_b_1932622

11
Pornography and Human Trafficking

Human trafficking is an insidious public health problem that may be worsened by the constant demand for new pornography. However, sex workers' rights—including the rights of pornography performers—are not always served by anti-trafficking efforts. This chapter defines human trafficking, reviews the main arguments that propose how pornography may influence human trafficking, and outlines critiques of the anti-trafficking movement in order to further collective action to address commercial sexual exploitation.

There is indisputable evidence that some people are forced or coerced to appear in pornography.[1,2] For example, several horrific accounts of the brutalization of people who have not consented to appear in pornography—or in some cases, are not even aware that they are being recorded—were relayed by *New York Times* contributor Nicholas Kristof in a widely read expose in 2020.[2] This drew unprecedented public attention to the issue of human trafficking in pornography and forced Pornhub to remove pornographic content from the Internet as well as to implement new procedures to address what has become a possibly widespread problem.

The problem of human trafficking in pornography is not new, but it may be getting worse because the means of pornography production have changed. Until the 2000s, the "pornography industry" generally referred to professional filmmakers and video producers who created sexually explicit media to sell to consumers through production companies. But now, virtually anyone can pick up a phone and record sexually explicit images of themselves or someone else, and they can share that with private buyers or upload it to a pornography website. Some pornography consumers are not content to masturbate to the same material over and over again—they want a continual stream of new material. As a result, there is a thriving market for sexually explicit material and a financial incentive for people who are not employed by pornography production companies (i.e., amateurs) to film and upload pornography. Not every amateur can find willing performers to appear in their sexually explicit content, so some engage in force, fraud, or coercion to make adults do so, or they make pornography involving minors. That's human trafficking, also known as sexual exploitation.

Pornography and Public Health. Emily F. Rothman, Oxford University Press. © Oxford University Press 2021.
DOI: 10.1093/oso/9780190075477.003.0011

One solution to the problem of sexual exploitation is to shut down the pornography marketplace altogether. The thinking goes that if people can't make money from pornography, there would be less incentive for most people to create it and to post it. On the other hand, there are no estimates of the percentage of online sexually explicit material that is made through force, fraud, or coercion versus legitimate methods. To be clear: no amount of sexual exploitation is acceptable, but shutting down entire industries can have unintended consequences, including encouraging illegal markets. By way of comparison, some people might argue for a ban on alcohol sales because even a single death caused by drunk driving is unacceptable. For this reason, public health strategists are needed to join forces with those who are experts in law and public policy, communications—and perhaps particularly those with expertise in Internet communication policy—and business in order to work out the best possible solutions.

What Is Human Trafficking?

There is a common misconception that human trafficking involves transporting people from one place to another and that it tends to involve foreigners or immigrants. That is not correct. Those may be cases of human smuggling or kidnapping, and potentially could be crimes that include trafficking, but human trafficking need not involve any transportation or relocation, and may involve only US citizens. A parent can traffic their child, and a boyfriend can traffic his girlfriend, and the exploitation may take place entirely within the confines of the victims' or perpetrators' residence. People can be trafficked for labor, for organs, or for sex. It is estimated that approximately 4.8 million people around the world are experiencing sex trafficking at any given moment.[3]

According to 22 U.S.C. § 7102(9), the Trafficking Victims Protection Act (TVPA) of 2000, sex trafficking is the recruitment, harboring, transportation, provision, obtaining, patronizing, or soliciting of a person for the purposes of a commercial sex act, "in which a commercial sex act is induced by force, fraud, or coercion, or in which the person induced to perform such act has not attained 18 years of age."[4] To restate a few implications of this law in plain language: If a person is less than 18 years old and they are sexually assaulted, and there is any way in which that assault has a commercial aspect (e.g., it is filmed to be sold or traded for something of value), that qualifies as human trafficking. Also, if a person is less than 18 years old and they are induced to engage in sex because of a gift—like a meal in a restaurant, or a new item of clothing, or a place to stay for the night—that too may qualify as human trafficking. There need not be a third party, such as a pimp, for it to be considered human trafficking under the law. In addition, pertaining to people 18 years old or older, if an adult is forced, tricked, or coerced to engage in sex that has a commercial aspect to it (e.g., it will be sold as pornography, or someone received payment or a gift for the sex), that may also be considered human trafficking. Under the law, while a third party (e.g., a pimp or boy-friend) may broker the commercial sex, *anyone* who engages in a commercial sex act that has been forced or coerced, or arranged through fraud, or involves a victim less than 18 years old, may be guilty of human trafficking.

Human trafficking is a federal crime, which means that cases are heard by federal judges and can result in federal prison sentences. In addition, there are state laws against human trafficking that can stiffen the penalties imposed. At the federal level, for a charge of sex trafficking, there is a mandatory minimum sentence of 15 years and up to life in prison, up to 5 years of supervised release, and a fine of up to $250,000 [see 18 U.S.C. § 1591(b)(1)].[5] By way of comparison, most cases of rape are prosecuted at the state level, by district attorneys, are heard by state court judges, can result in penalties, and typically may result in lesser sentences. The overarching point is that we consider human trafficking to be a very serious crime and attach severe penalties to it, and typically offenders will receive more severe penalties than people convicted of rape and sexual assault.

Ways in Which Pornography May Influence Human Trafficking

There are three main arguments about how the existence of pornography increases human trafficking. These are:

1. The constant demand for new sexually explicit material creates an incentive for individuals to create new pornography and to exploit others to do so.
2. Pornography increases the demand for in-person paid sexual encounters, which supports the sale of sex and therefore human trafficking.
3. All paid sex work is inherently exploitive, therefore all pornography is exploitation.

With regard to the first point, the argument is that people who view pornography become habituated to it and always need novel material in order to achieve the same level of sexual satisfaction. Because this creates a constant demand for new material, there is a financial incentive for human traffickers to exploit people and to generate new pornographic material to meet demand. The evidence in support of habituation is mixed.[6-8] In other words, it's not clear that all people, or even the majority of people who view porn, need a steady stream of novel material in order to experience sexual pleasure. It may be worthwhile for public health researchers to explore whether there are certain subsets of pornography users who are particularly prone to habituation and who are driving the demand for new material, and to determine why there is a high demand for new content. Do most people need novel sexual material on a continual basis? How frequently do they need new material, and why? How might the pornography industry be reshaped if people could go on "pornography diets" where they consume less? This idea represents a harm-reduction approach, or a policy compromise between banning all pornography and the unrestricted approach.

With regard to the second point, the argument is that pornography contributes to a hypersexual culture, and a hypersexual culture is one in which sex trafficking is more likely.[9] In other words, the argument is that pornography increases sexual arousal (i.e., creates a sexualized culture) and normalizes violent sex, which creates a market for sex trafficking. Specifically, some people believe that viewing pornography increases the market for paid sex in order to fulfill sexual fantasies involving violent or atypical sexual behavior.[10] Pornography may be contributing to a cultural environment that normalizes detached sex, casual sex, aggressive sex, and paid sex.[11,12] Given that watching movies and TV shows of people smoking cigarettes and drinking alcohol normalizes those behaviors, and thus there have been public health efforts to ban or reduce cigarette smoking and drinking in entertainment media,[13-15] it is reasonable to believe that our media diet influences what we accept as commonplace and encourages us to imitate it. However, whether seeing pornography translates into people being more likely to pay for sex or to feel motivated to seek out sexual encounters with commercially exploited people is unsubstantiated. Research on this topic is warranted. Public health professionals should also explore whether it is possible for cultural environments that normalize casual sex, or consensual rough sex, or paid sex, to also be ones that promote consent, safety, mutuality, and pleasure. The assumption that a sexed-up society is inherently a worse and more dangerous one can be questioned. Perhaps a society freed from moral strictures that dictate how often we have sex, with whom, how, where, and when would not necessarily be less safe.

With regard to the third point, Catherine MacKinnon and others have made the argument that because people must be paid to be in pornography, it is inherently nonconsensual.[16,17] The suggestion is that paid sex is not given by free choice, it is coerced, and coerced sex is human trafficking. But the idea that people cannot be truly consenting to something if they are being paid is problematic. By that logic, all paid laborers would be labor trafficked individuals. In medical ethics, we offer payments to people for their time and trouble when they participate in research, and we do not view the payment as negating their agency to consent. Ultimately, from a public health perspective, the idea that all pornography is human trafficking because a payment is provided to the performers introduces more problems than it solves by conflating the issue of remuneration with lack of consent.

Criticisms of the Human Trafficking Perspective

The anti-human-trafficking movement has different factions. There are entities within the movement who are as concerned with policing bodies, policing sexuality, promoting religion, and promoting repressive ideology as they are with protecting people from harm.[18,19] While the movement has successfully drawn attention to the issue of human trafficking, anti-trafficking legislation aimed at online advertising of sexual services, such as the controversial bill package including the Fight Online Sex Trafficking Act (FOSTA) and the Senate bill, the Stop Enabling Sex Traffickers Act (SESTA),[20] may have endangered sex workers more than it protected sex trafficking victims.[21–23] As a result, public health professionals should use caution before allying themselves with anti-trafficking entities as they seek to address exploitation in pornography.

The high level of collaboration between anti-trafficking groups and criminal justice entities is viewed by some as reinforcing problems of mass incarceration and neoliberal governance.[24] Panics over sex trafficking, and anti-trafficking efforts, tend to recur in the United States coincident with waves of anti-immigrant sentiment because both reinforce "stranger danger" fears.[25] As such, there are times when anti-trafficking advocacy has provided a vehicle for those who want to promote racist, xenophobic, and extreme right-wing conspiracies or to "put a humanitarian face on their punitive anti-immigration policies."[25,26] Experts studying disinformation subcultures have identified that having legitimate concerns about child abuse and human trafficking can be a risk factor for radicalization into right-wing cults.[19] Even the language of the anti-trafficking movement may be antithetical to public health; the movement has been criticized for refer-ring to commercial sexual exploitation as "modern day slavery," given that this language appropriates Black suffering without regard "for the ongoing Black liberation struggle."[27]

There are, of course, numerous anti-trafficking organizations and efforts that center social justice and operate solidly within an equity-oriented public health framework. Furthermore, it will be tremendously important to the fu-ture of public health to carefully assess the ways in which the present-day por-nography industry exploits individuals and to work actively to stop its harms. A full consideration of structural-level determinants of sexual assault, sexual exploitation, and partner violence should include the possible contributions of sexually explicit media as a societal factor. However, partnering with anti-trafficking agencies, advocacy leaders, and even formerly exploited individ-uals requires an extraordinarily high level of thoughtfulness. There is a serious risk of partnering with entities that simultaneously seek to prevent trafficking while intentionally or unintentionally promoting harmful narratives about sex work and sexuality or engaging in the criminalization of poverty. On the other hand, public health professionals should be aware that the lived expe-rience of trafficking survivors who have had negative experiences in the por-nography industry or because of the market for online pornography cannot be discounted. Deciding how to utilize anecdotal information from both sex workers' rights advocates and human trafficking survivors and how to move toward better science and evidence-informed decision-making will be the key to making progress.

Conclusions

Some pornography is made by human traffickers and depicts sexual abuse. This is an egregious violation of human rights and represents a serious threat to public health. However, the anti-trafficking movement is not uniformly aligned with public health promotion goals, so public health professionals need to use caution before allying themselves with anti-trafficking organiza-tions. It is incumbent upon public health professionals to strategize to ensure the safety of all individuals who perform in pornography, and to advocate for policies that will ensure that those who produce and disseminate sexually ex-plicit material to do so legally and in a manner that safeguards performers from harm and abuse.

References

1. Rivas, M. 2020. "22 Women Just Won $13 Million in Massive Porn Scam Lawsuit." https://www.refinery29.com/en-us/2020/01/9131058/girls-do-porn-lawsuit-judge-ruling-women
2. Kristof, N. December 4, 2020. "The Children of Pornhub." *The New York Times*.
3. International Labor Organization. 2017. "Global Estimates of Modern Slavery: Forced Labour and Forced Marriage." https://www.ilo.org/global/publications/books/WCMS_575479/lang--en/index.htm
4. Trafficking Victims Protection Act (TVPA) of 2000, Pub. L. No. 106–386, Division A, § 103(8), (9), 114 Stat. 1464 (signed into law on October 29, 2000); codified as amended at 22 USC 7102 § 103(8), (9).
5. Doyle, C. 2016. *Sex Trafficking: An Overview of Federal Criminal Law*, 1–40. Washington, DC: Congressional Research Service.
6. Prause, N., V. R. Steele, C. Staley, D. Sabatinelli, and G. Hajcak. 2015. "Modulation of Late Positive Potentials by Sexual Images in Problem Users and Controls Inconsistent with 'Porn Addiction.'" *Biological Psychology* 109: 192–199.
7. Schaefer, H. H., and A. H. Colgan. 1977. "The Effect of Pornography on Penile Tumescence as a Function of Reinforcement and Novelty." *Behavior Therapy* 8, no. 5: 938–946.
8. Voon, V, T. B. Mole, P. Banca, et al. 2014. "Neural Correlates of Sexual Cue Reactivity in Individuals With and Without Compulsive Sexual Behaviours." *PLOS One* 9, no. 7: e102419–e102419.
9. Humphreys, K., B. Le Clair, and J. Hicks. 2019. "Intersections Between Pornography and Human Trafficking: Training Ideas and Implications." *Journal of Counselor Practice* 10, no. 1: 19–39.
10. Beck, J. 2017. "The Link Between Pornography and Human Trafficking." https://everaccountable.com/blog/the-link-between-pornography-and-human-trafficking/ Accessed January 20, 2020.
11. Tokunaga, R. S., P. J. Wright, and J. E. Roskos. 2019. "Pornography and Impersonal Sex." *Human Communication Research* 45, no. 1: 78–118.
12. Cook, M. 2016. "Is Pornography a Public Health Crisis? The Evidence Is Piling up." *Mercatornet*. https://www.lifesitenews.com/opinion/is-pornography-a-public-health-crisis-the-evidence-is-piling-up
13. Sargent, J. D., and R. Hanewinkel. 2015. "Impact of Media, Movies and TV on Tobacco Use in the Youth." In *Tobacco Epidemic*, 2nd ed. Vol. 42, 171–180. Basel: Karger.
14. Koordeman, R., E. Kuntsche, D. J. Anschutz, R. B. van Baaren, and R. Engels. 2011. "Do We Act upon What We See? Direct Effects of Alcohol Cues in Movies on Young Adults' Alcohol Drinking." *Alcohol and Alcoholism* 46, no. 4: 393–398.
15. Strasburger, V. C., G. L. Fuld, D. A. Mulligan, et al. 2010. "Policy Statement—Children, Adolescents, Substance Abuse, and the Media." *Pediatrics* 126, no. 4: 791–799.
16. MacKinnon, C. 2005. "Pornography as Trafficking." In *Pornography: Driving the Demand in International Sex Trafficking*, edited by D. Guinn and J. DiCaro, 31–42. Los Angeles, CA: Captive Daughters Media.
17. Farley, M. 2015. "Pornography, Prostitution, & Trafficking: Making the Connections." http://prostitutionresearch.com/wp-content/uploads/2015/07/Melissa-Farley-Making-the-Connections-7-15-15.pdf
18. Shih, E. 2016. "Not in My 'Backyard Abolitionism': Vigilante Rescue Against American Sex Trafficking." *Sociological Perspectives* 59, no. 1: 66–90.
19. Goldeberg, A., D. Riggleman, J. Baumgartner, et al. 2020. "The QAnon Conspiracy: Destroying Families, Dividing Communities, Undermining Democracy." https://networkcontagion.

us/wp-content/uploads/NCRI-White-Paper-The-QAnon-Conspiracy-%E2%80%93-12-15.pdf

20. Fight Online Sex Trafficking Act (FOSTA) and the Stop Enabling Sex Traffickers Act (SESTA) (FOSTA-SESTA), 115th Congress (2018). https://www.govtrack.us/congress/bills/115/s1693/

21. Souixsie Q. 2018. "Anti-Sex-Trafficking Advocates Say New Law Cripples Efforts to Save Victims." https://www.rollingstone.com/culture/culture-features/anti-sex-trafficking-advocates-say-new-law-cripples-efforts-to-save-victims-629081/

22. Musto, J., A. E. Fehrenbacher, H. Hoefinger, et al. 2021. "Anti-Trafficking in the Time of FOSTA/SESTA: Networked Moral Gentrification and Sexual Humanitarian Creep." *Social Sciences* 10, no. 2: 58.

23. Chapman-Schmidt, B. 2019. "'Sex Trafficking' as Epistemic Violence." *Anti-Trafficking Review* no. 12: 172–187.

24. Baker, C. N. 2019. "Racialized Rescue Narratives in Public Discourses on Youth Prostitution and Sex Trafficking in the United States." *Politics and Gender* 15, no. 4: 773–800.

25. Grant, M. 2021. "QAnon and the Cultification of the American Right." https://newrepublic.com/article/161103/qanon-cultification-american-right Accessed February 19, 2021.

26. Sharma, N. 2020. "Anti-Trafficking Is an Inside Job." https://www.opendemocracy.net/en/beyond-trafficking-and-slavery/anti-trafficking-inside-job/ Accessed February 19, 2021.

27. Beutin, L. P. 2017. "Black Suffering for/from Anti-Trafficking Advocacy." *Anti-Trafficking Review* no. 9: 14–30.

12

The Occupational Safety and Health of Pornography Performers

Concern about workers' health was a primary reason why a US movement to improve public health began in the 1800s.[1] A century later, in 1970, Congress passed the Occupational Safety and Health Act, which established the Occupational Safety and Health Administration (OSHA) in the Labor Department. OSHA sets and enforces workplace safety and health standards in order to reduce work-related injuries, illnesses, and deaths. Today, because of the Occupational Safety and Health Act and OSHA, US employers are obligated to keep workplaces free from recognized hazards, warn employees about possible work-related hazards, keep records of illnesses and injuries, and cooperate with OSHA inspections. Occupational health is a pillar of public health promotion because of the potential to reach diverse subpopulations where they work and to improve health equity by doing so.[2]

When questions about pornography as a public health issue are raised, the focus is almost exclusively on whether and how pornography affects viewers. Typically, relatively little attention is paid to the work-related hazards faced by pornography performers and other laborers in the adult entertainment industry workforce.* A thorough consideration of pornography from a public health perspective, though, should include a review of demographics and characteristics of pornography performers, what health-related and other challenges those in the industry face because of their work, which organized groups support their collective health and safety on the job, and what policies have been drafted that seek to address pornography performers' health and safety.

I begin this chapter with the caveat that I am not a pornography performer. The slogan "Nothing about us without us" is a phrase that has its origins in the disability rights movement of the 1990s,[3] but is one that was adopted by the sex workers' rights movement subsequently.[4] The phrase means that policy should not be crafted or implemented without sufficient participation from the people it will affect. Writing a chapter that describes the working conditions of pornography performers isn't the same thing as crafting policy.

Pornography and Public Health. Emily F. Rothman, Oxford University Press. © Oxford University Press 2021.
DOI: 10.1093/oso/9780190075477.003.0012

However, I want to acknowledge that even the act of writing about performers' and other laborers' experiences without their direct participation is inconsistent with the "Nothing about us without us" philosophy that I seek to uphold in my work as a public health professional. Therefore, I am indebted to my colleagues who have been, and are, part of the pornography industry for their review of this chapter and for having provided invaluable feedback.

Who Are Pornography Performers?

There have been few efforts to investigate empirically the universe of pornography performers. Conducting a census or representative survey is impossible because many performers now operate solo, self-producing content. Even in decades past, when performers were more likely to be affiliated with a pornography production company, it still would have been difficult, time-consuming, and expensive to identify and collect data from a sufficient number of performers to draw valid conclusions about the pornography performers workforce as a whole. For the most part, social scientists have had to settle for what they could learn from small-scale convenience sample studies, interviews with small samples of performers, and case studies.

A psychology researcher, Griffith, has published multiple quantitative studies that characterize pornography performers. In 2006, Griffith and colleagues surveyed 177 female and 105 male pornography performers in California who were patients of the Adult Industry Medical Healthcare Foundation (AIM) located in Los Angeles.[5] AIM was a nonprofit that served the health needs of sex workers and individuals in the adult entertainment industry from 1998 to 2011, and the services it provided included HIV and other STI testing, counseling, information about cosmetic surgery, and educational workshops.[6] It was estimated that in the 2004, there were approximately 1,200 to 1,500 employed pornography performers in Los Angeles who used AIM for HIV and other testing.[6] Griffith and colleagues recruited pornography performers from AIM to complete surveys and created matched comparison groups (matching on age, marital status, and ethnicity) from a university and airport setting. A limitation of the research was that the authors did not report the participation rate for either sample. In other words, it is unclear what percentage of all adult performers who were made aware of the opportunity to participate in the research actually participated, and low participation can be a source of bias that limits the validity of results.

Griffith's team was motivated, in part, to explore the "damaged goods hypothesis," which is the idea that pornography performers choose to perform in pornography because they were sexually abused as children, have mental health problems, have low self-esteem, or have alcohol and drug use disorders. The idea that almost all pornography performers were sexually abused as children was espoused by MacKinnon (1993),[7] and descriptions of pornography actresses as homeless, impoverished, recovering from child sexual abuse, and dependent on illegal substances have been proffered by Dworkin (1989)[8] and anti-pornography activist groups.[9] One mistake that some anti-pornography activists have made when trying to characterize pornography performers is generalizing results from studies of prostitutes/sex workers.[9] (Actually, even generalizing to all sex workers from studies of individuals who sell sex *and* were visible to researchers and willing to volunteer to be in research studies can be a questionable practice.) It is unknown whether pornography performers are a distinct group from sex workers in general, and the degree of overlap between pornography performing and selling sex may be decreasing, given the emergence of websites where individuals can post their own pornographic content, or perform live, without needing to work with a pornography production company, interact with other people, or leave their own house. For that reason, it is not clear that valid inferences about correlates of pornography performance can be made from studies of prostitutes, escorts, or other sex workers.

Griffith and colleagues did not find support for the damaged goods hypothesis. Specifically, the studies found that while pornography actresses on average had an earlier age of first sex, and a higher number of lifetime sexual partners, they had approximately equivalent rates of childhood sexual abuse victimization as the comparison sample (36% vs. 29%).[6] Porn actresses also had higher rates of self-esteem than women in the matched sample, reported higher rates of sexual satisfaction and better social support, and were more spiritual. They were substantially more likely to report alcohol use problems (24% vs. 15%) and marijuana use in the past 6 months, and they were more likely to have tried 10 different illegal drugs in their lifetimes than were women in the matched sample.[6] Focusing on the male performers, Griffith and colleagues found that the rate of childhood sexual abuse victimization was the same for those in their pornography actor and comparison groups (11.4%), that porn actors had higher self-esteem than those in the matched comparison sample, a slightly younger age of first intercourse, a much higher number of lifetime sexual partners, a slightly elevated rate of lifetime alcohol use disorder (31% vs. 23%), lower rates of alcohol use in the past 6 months, and higher rates of marijuana use in the past 6 months.[5] Notably, the majority of men in the study were heterosexual. In short, porn performers, perhaps like other actors and actresses, may be more likely than the general public to use alcohol or illicit drugs, but the results of this analysis did not find support for the idea that they are more "damaged" from childhood abuse or mental health disorders than other people.

Griffith and colleagues also studied why female pornography performers decided to enter the adult entertainment industry. In a sample of 176 performers, they found that the #1 reason was money, but that #2 was enjoying having sex, #3 was attention, #4 was "fun," and #5 was because the women already worked in a related industry (like stripping).[10] Once the women were already part of the industry, reasons that they decided to remain in the industry included money, their fondness for the other people in the industry, the opportunity to have sex, the freedom and independence they were afforded, attention, fun, creative expression, personal fulfillment, and the opportunity to be rebellious.[10] Griffith and colleagues also explored things that the performers did not like about the industry, and they found that 39% reported not liking the other people with whom they had to work, 29% disliked the risk of HIV and other STIs that they faced, 20% felt exploited, 10% did not like their working conditions, and 7% felt social stigma.[10]

A second team also studied the self-reported mental health status and depression in female pornography performers and found markedly different results from Griffith. Grudzen and colleagues (2011) used the Internet Adult Film Database and an adult film jobs website to recruit adult female pornography performers 18 to 40 years old who had performed in pornography in the past 6 months for a self-administered Internet survey in 2008–2009. They compared the porn performers' results to those from respondents to a state women's health survey. The response rate for pornography performers was 16%. The research team analyzed data from 134 adult performers and compared results to those reported by 1,773 California women who served as the comparison group. There were numerous differences between the two samples. Adult film performers were more likely to be non-Hispanic, Black, and US-born, to have attended some college, to be unmarried, to make more than $25,000 per year, to be employed, to have experienced poverty in the past year, to have had a family that received public assistance while they were children, to have been in foster care (21% vs. 4%), to have an earlier age of first sexual intercourse (15 years vs. 18 years), to have had a greater number of sexual partners in the past year, to have experienced forced sex as an adult (27% vs. 9%), and to have experienced forced sex as a child (37% vs. 13%). They were also substantially more likely to have experienced domestic violence in the past 12 months (34% vs. 6%), to have used alcohol in the past month, and to have used tobacco, and they were less likely to have health insurance. Pornography performers had experienced more days of poor mental health in the past month than the general population sample (7 days vs. 5 days), were more likely to meet the criteria for depression (33% vs. 13%), and were more likely to report that they had wanted mental health help in the past year, but they were less likely to have received mental health help in the past year. A multivariable analysis demonstrated that being an adult performer was associated with childhood poverty, forced sex as an adult, domestic violence, and poverty—but it was not associated with having been in foster care or experiencing forced sex as a child.

How do we make sense of the fact that Griffith's team and the Grudzen team found such different results while using similar methods? The surveys were conducted within 2 years of one another and had similar sample sizes of adult performers. There are several strengths of the Grudzen study to note. First, Griffith did not report a participation rate. It could be that only a small percentage of those eligible chose to participate, which is all the more likely because Griffith did not pay all participants for research participation (they put their name in a lottery for two prizes of $300 toward STI testing). Grudzen, on the other hand, paid all participants in the form of a $50 online gift card. Grudzen also recruited participants in a way that likely yielded a wider variety of performers because the team used adult film job boards and databases. The Griffith team recruited from one healthcare setting only (AIM). Performers affiliated with AIM represented a subgroup of performers potentially more likely to be working for larger and more mainstream production companies. Furthermore, Grudzen included only performers who performed in the past 6 months, ensuring that participants were active in the industry, while Griffith did not report that there were eligibility criteria for survey participation other than seeking care at the AIM. Finally, and perhaps most importantly, the comparison sample in the Grudzen study was a general population of California women of the same age as the pornography performers. Griffith recruited 38% of his comparison sample of women from a university setting (i.e., they were college students) and 62% from an airport. College students and travelers are not as likely to be representative of the general population as those who are recruited systematically using random-digit dialing for a health department survey. Taken together, there are more possible limitations of the Griffith team's methodology. The Grudzen study also faced limitations, including a 16% response rate from performers, so if public health and other professionals want to characterize and understand the needs of adult pornography performers, additional rigorous survey research is still needed.

A third study of reasons why people decide to become involved with the pornography industry was conducted by Jill Bakehorn in 2006. Dr. Bakehorn used snowball sampling to identify individuals working for women-run pornography companies in the United States and conducted 72 in-depth interviews with 33 directors and producers, 37 actors, 15 crew members, and 10 with other industry jobs.[11] The study found that reasons why people chose to have a career in women-made pornography could be summarized as falling into one of five main categories: (1) having a background in sex education (50% of the performers), (2) to further sex-positivity, feminist, or identity politics activism, (3) having a background in art, (4) prior involvement in sex work (50% of performers), and (5) being introduced to porn as a career by a friend or sexual partner, although for most this was not their exclusive route into the industry.[11] While the reasons why individuals might choose employment in women-made pornography could be different than the reasons why individuals choose to make pornography in general, one conclusion that can be drawn from the Bakehorn study is that not every person who decides to perform in pornography is coerced or makes the choice for survival-related reasons and in desperation. Some anti-pornography activists argue that it is only a small minority of vocal, relatively privileged, and usually white and college-educated women who choose to perform in pornography, and because of their privilege they are able to command media attention and dominate the public discourse about their labor in pornography. Those activists might argue that the fact that 50% of Bakehorn's performer sample had a background in sex education calls into question the validity and generalizability of her findings. In the end, it's just not possible to know how generalizable Bakehorn's, Grudzen's, or Griffith's findings are because of participation bias that affects all of their studies.

A fourth and fifth study were undertaken by a group of urologists, in collaboration with the industry trade association (the Free Speech Coalition), and were published in 2019.[12] The team sent online surveys to people in a healthcare-related database for pornography performers (PASS, described below). The team sent out one survey, in their words, to people "with biological vaginas," who were at least 20 years old and had experience with pornography performance, and a separate survey for those with "biological penises." The authors estimated that the response rate to the survey was less than 5%, which raises some questions about participation bias.[13] However, of performers who responded to the survey for those with biological vaginas and were eligible, 24% had scores indicative of sexual dysfunction related to sexual desire, arousal, lubrication, or orgasm, which is lower than the percentage of premenopausal women who experience it globally (41%).[12] The researchers also found that 70% of respondents to the survey for men reported that they used erectile aids, and 39% qualified as having erectile dysfunction (ED)—which is higher than the percentage of men in the general population 40 to 50 years old with ED (15%). In the men's study, 29% of the men who performed in pornography reported using erectile aids for their work only.[14]

The main takeaway from these studies of adult pornography performers is that, although performers may have higher self-esteem than people in the general population, in general it appears that they may also be a higher needs population living with numerous stressors, including the lasting effects of childhood poverty and of experiences of interpersonal violence victimization as adults, depression, and lack of access to mental health services. These stressors are undoubtedly compounded if the performers are Black, Latina, transgender, or from another marginalized group.[15,16] Our duty as public health practitioners is to find ways to meet the needs of this population in partnership with them and in ways that do not take away their agency, do not seek to "rescue" them in a way that is disempowering or disrespectful, and do not exacerbate stigma. Also importantly, rates of childhood sexual abuse do not appear to be elevated in this population, and that is an important finding that is consistent across multiple studies. One reason why this finding is important is that the idea that adult women only choose to perform in pornography because they have been "damaged" by experiences of childhood abuse is not borne out. There are logical, rational reasons that some people opt to perform in pornography, although there are cases when others are forced or coerced into it. When performers are characterized as survivors of childhood abuse, it invites pathologizing and condescension that is usually apparent to the performers (who then, no surprise, are not as interested in whatever intervention is being offered) and communicates a fundamental lack of respect for their capacity to steward their own lives toward health. The balancing act that public health professionals need to achieve is to investigate and document the needs of the population and to find ways to communicate about those needs sensitively, without also slipping into paternalistic language and behavior that worsens health inequities. Partnership with present and active pornography performers is one way to try to ensure that the paternalizing does not happen.

Safety and Health Threats Associated with Working in Pornography

The preceding section explores who pornography performers may be and what many may bring to the experience of performing in pornography, based on childhood factors and their circumstances as adults. In this section, I briefly review issues that can affect the safety and health of pornography performers while they are actively engaged in performance work.

Sexually Transmitted Infections

In prior decades, it was somewhat easier to talk about the risk of transmission of HIV and other sexually transmitted infections (STIs) in the pornography industry because the industry, at least in the United States, was centralized in the Los Angeles area of California. Now that virtually everyone, no matter where they live, has access to video-recording and editing tools, and performers do not require production companies to distribute material, the "adult film industry" is less circumscribed and therefore is more difficult to characterize. That said, there have been multiple incidents involving either outbreaks of HIV in the California adult film industry or the positive tests of performers that lead to industrywide production holds, most notably in 2004,[17] 2009,[18] 2014,[19,20] and 2017.[21] HIV is not the only STI that concerns performers, though. Gonorrhea and chlamydia are also more prevalent among pornography performers than among the general population, and according to one study conducted in 2010, performers' risk is elevated compared to brothel workers in Nevada.[22] That study not only found that 28% of pornography performers were positive for gonorrhea and/or chlamydia (which is a high burden), but that 23% of those cases would not have been detected through the type of urogenital testing that is standard in California for the adult industry.[22] To detect a higher percentage of cases, oral and anal swabbing is necessary.

In 2011, the Free Speech Coalition (FSC), which is the trade association for the adult entertainment industry in California, launched an online database called the Performer Availability Screening Services (PASS), which is accessible to some pornography performers, producers, and agents. The database replaced one that formerly had been operated by AIM but was shut down after it was hacked and performers' private medical information was shared online. The PASS system is guided by an advisory council with representation from performers, producers, agents, a workplace safety attorney, and a medical consultant.[23] The way that PASS works is that performers provide evidence of a negative STI test (i.e., HIV, syphilis, gonorrhea, chlamydia, hepatitis B and C, and trichomoniasis) from one of the approved testing facilities every 14 days to remain listed as in good standing in the database. It is a voluntary system. In theory, pornography producers should be making pornography only with performers who are listed in the database, but there are people who produce pornography illicitly and disregard the PASS database. PASS is also US-specific, so performers from other nations may meet up with US-based performers outside the United States for a shoot, and it would be unusual that the PASS system would be used in that case. (NB: In one recent news article, an FSC representative suggested that a parallel database to PASS could be created for European performers in the future.[24]) Students of public health will note that while the PASS system collects results on particular STIs, the system doesn't include results for HPV (genital warts), HSV (herpes), pubic lice, scabies, bacterial vaginosis, or molluscum contagiousum. In addition to checking the PASS database for information about performers' health, on some pornography production sets, a production manager may visually inspect performers' mouths, hands, and genitals to spot visible sores or wounds—although none of the performers with whom I spoke had ever seen this take place on set. In some cases, prior to filming, performers may sign off on attestations that they are comfortable with the STI status check on the other performers.

When people are considering going into pornography, they should consider a few realities about the PASS system. First, unless they receive a subsidy to help offset the cost from the FSC, performers have to purchase their own STI tests every 2 weeks, which cost approximately $150. Use of the PASS system and database is free, but the testing is not. Second, false-negative STI tests occur, so it is possible to acquire an STI on set from another performer even if the production company uses the PASS database—although there may be more risk that performers acquire an STI off set during their personal sexual encounters than on set. In addition, some performers who are HIV-positive take medication that lowers their viral load to the point where they get negative HIV test results and thus are recorded as being HIV-negative in the PASS system.[†] Third, testing every 14 days does not protect someone in the instance where a sexual partner acquired an STI since being tested. Fourth, the STI tests do not include oral and rectal swabs at this time, although there has been some advocacy in support of changing the system to include swabs. In short, the PASS database goes a long way to ensuring performer safety while on set. It would, perhaps, be the best possible system that public health advocates could hope for to mitigate on-set transmission risk if testing modalities were improved to acknowledge the various sex acts that PASS participants engage in, on and off the job. At the same time, it is not a perfect system, particularly without oral and anal testing, so those entering the industry need to be aware that risks remain.

The other infectious disease that has plagued the industry recently is ringworm.[25] Ringworm is a common skin infection that can be easily treated, but it is highly contagious and irritating, and treating it has an associated cost. One performer told me that even though ringworm is easily treated, having to be vigilant about the industry outbreak can be anxiety-provoking.

Violence on Set

The percentage of pornography performers who experience violence and aggression while on set is unknown, and because it is not feasible to conduct a survey of a representative subset of pornography performers, it is hard to know if they are at higher-than-average risk of sexual, physical, and/or emotional abuse at work than other types of laborers. For example, the US Bureau of Labor Statistics estimates that approximately 395 of 10,000 psychiatric technicians were assaulted on the job in 2018, as were 23 of 10,000 elementary school teachers.[26] Sexual harassment and assault are notoriously prevalent among restaurant and hospitality workers. Approximately 30% of European workers in the tourism industry report violence, bullying, and sexual harassment victimization in the past year.[27] Yet, the risk of violence victimization, bullying, and harassment experienced by pornography performers may be worse than for those in other industries, and it may depend very much on the context of the production. Reputable pornography production companies may employ production managers to ensure that performers consent to everything that happens during filming, whereas private individuals who decide to film their friends having sex and upload the content may not even be aware that there are industry standards to which they should adhere. Pornography performers may be at increased risk for experiencing violence and being injured because they are unclothed (i.e., have less personal protection against injury), but more senior performers who are well connected to others in the field may be protected by their ability to do their own informal "background checks" on their fellow performers by communicating with colleagues about their reputations.[28] Performers have told me that while sexual and physical assault can happen on set, it is newcomers to the industry who are typically most vulnerable to experiencing assault because they do not have the means to find out which of their fellow performers, or which directors, to avoid.

There have been multiple pornography performers who have come forward with allegations of sexual assault victimization within the industry, including Stoya (against James Deen), Nikki Benz (against Tony T.), and the nonbinary performer named Rooster.[29] Performers are also at risk when they stay in "model houses," or shared living quarters where performers stay while traveling for pornography-related work, and they may be coerced into having sex with predatory house managers. In one case, an industry veteran who attempted to raise objections to this type of predatory treatment was reportedly doxed and threatened.[28] When performers are assaulted on set, they often have little recourse for injuries sustained on the job.[30] Ineffective policing exacerbates that problem. Like other sex workers, when pornography performers are injured on set and attempt to file police reports, they sometimes face harassment and ridicule by officers that worsens, rather than helps with, their experience.[28]

One factor that puts performers at risk for experiencing coercion on set is that on most pornography production sets performers earn more for engaging in more "extreme" (i.e., hard core) sex acts. For example, a female performer could expect to be paid more for anal sex than vaginal sex. One solution to this is that flat-rate payments, meaning that performers are paid a flat rate for performing in a pornography shoot no matter what they opt to do with the other performers in the scene, reduce pressure to consent to more sex or more extreme sex acts in order to earn more money.[31] A second solution is for pornography producers to use written checklists of sex acts to negotiate consent with performers. A sample checklist is provided by the Adult Performers Actors Guild (APAG), which lists 45 possible sex acts (e.g., hand job, blow job, stomping, facial abuse, nipple clamps, using foot to penetrate) and the statement "I _____ consent to the following sex acts for scene booked today (date)."[32] A third solution is the "On Set Steward Program" (OSS Program), which APAG first proposed in June 2020 in the wake of a number of pornography performers' disclosures that they had experienced abuse on pornography sets. APAG suggests that they will place trained safety stewards on pornography sets to advocate for performers.[33]

Other Challenges of Working in Pornography

In addition to threats to health and safety that pornography performers may experience while on the job, they may also experience additional challenges that subsequently affect their health. A primary issue is that, as of June 2020, most pornography performers in the United States are hired as independent contractors as opposed to salaried workers (i.e., statutory employees). This is true for most pornography production set crew members, as well. As a result, they are not eligible for unemployment benefits or workers' compensation for injuries, and they do not receive sick pay, health insurance from an employer, or a retirement plan. Their working hours are not regulated. Performers do not earn residuals on the pornography videos or films that they make. This could change. On January 1, 2020, a new California state law (called AB5) went into effect that creates more stringent requirements for how workers in any industry are classified. AB5 may mean that more pornography performers are reclassified as employees instead of independent contractors in California—but it is too early to tell if substantial changes in employment practice will result.[34]

There are several problems associated with being employed as a contractor instead of a salaried employee. The financial problems of being paid a cash stipend and receiving no benefits can mount quickly, particularly if work is unsteady or there is a production halt. Many performers may not realize that they are expected to pay tax on their earnings and do not put aside a percentage of their cash stipend for those taxes. Some may decide to underreport earnings or even fail to file, but this can be a costly mistake. There have been cases when pornography performers have been charged with tax evasion and even served short jail sentences because of it (for example, see the case of Janine Lindemulder, who served 6 months for tax evasion in 2008). In other instances, people have harassed pornography performers and other sex workers by attempting to report them to the IRS to be audited.[35]

A second major problem is that sex workers, including pornography performers, are not a protected class and they can be legally excluded from jobs in higher education, politics, teaching, childcare, healthcare, and other fields simply because they work, or previously worked, in pornography. There are numerous cases where people have been terminated because their pornography work came to light and the termination was upheld by judges and commissions even when appealed (see, for example, the cases of Stacie Halas and Kimberly "Houston" Halsey). This discrimination compounds the problem of the lack of job security for those in the industry: anyone who becomes a pornography performer runs the risk that they may be recognized and have difficulty finding other employment. Pornography performers can also face challenges in child custody disputes because of how society views the profession. The stigma of being a sex worker, the experience of being constantly sexualized, and the fear of being "outed" can also cause anxiety and feelings of shame. The intensity of the shame and anxiety about being revealed to be a pornography performer often motivates performers to band together for social and instrumental support, which has undeniable benefits, but it can also make it difficult for individual performers to stand up and speak out against other performers when necessary (i.e., in cases of unfair labor practices or sexual assault).

It's not only employers who can legally discriminate against pornography performers, but also banks and payment-processing companies like PayPal, Square, CashApp, or Google Pay. In 2017, hundreds of current and former porn performers were denied service by Chase Bank and had their accounts terminated—which the bank is within its rights to do if they think that a customer is in a line of work that is high risk for the bank, even if the customer has always been in good standing.[36] Because of the controversy, the Adult Performer

Advocacy Committee (APAC) has formed an alliance with First Entertainment Credit Union to ensure that performers have somewhere to bank their money.[30] But many performers also experience problems with the online payment-processing systems through which customers could pay them for sexually explicit cam performances or other adult content. APAG is reportedly taking legal action against multiple payment-processing companies for discriminating against pornography performers.[37] The American Express company also prohibits customers from using their cards to purchase legal pornography, and some pornography performers have lost Instagram and Twitter accounts without warning and without any violation of terms. The loss of social media accounts can be a major impediment. Performers build massive followings strategically and use their platforms for promotion of their adult websites and to attract sponsorship.[38]

A third problem is that there is little wage transparency in the pornography industry, meaning that without a reputable and trustworthy agent to help negotiate pay, performers are at risk for being paid little. Initially, individuals who are new to the industry can make slightly more money because they are new, although over time their rate will depend on how popular they are and what they are willing to do on screen. More extreme acts are paid more. Women also tend to be paid more than men in the industry. There have been numerous popular press articles written over the past decade about what performers might be paid for various acts.[39,40] The trouble with these articles is that the standard pay rates are changing rapidly now that so many more people have access to producing their own pornography and large production companies are no longer necessary for disseminating the videos. Acts that might have paid $1,000 a decade ago could be paid as little as $50 today, depending upon who is creating the pornography, the experience of the performer, the performer's reputation or following, and the intended distribution channel.[41] Rampant video piracy has contributed to major shifts in the economics of the porn industry in recent years. Performers with whom I have spoken have told me that the lack of wage transparency makes younger and new performers particularly vulnerable to exploitation. Once a performer has close colleagues within the industry, and they begin to share information about what they are paid, they know how to negotiate for fair wages individually.

A History of Some Proposed Legislation that Could Affect Pornography Performers

Until the mid-2000s, most pornography that was legally produced in the United States was made in California. Proximity to the motion picture industry meant that there were experienced directors, crew people, and the other types of related industries and service professionals that one used to need to make a film—hair stylists, makeup artists, and sound and lighting technicians. In addition, in 1998, the California Supreme Court made a decision in the case of *People v. Freeman* that effectively legalized the production of pornography in that state. Today, any individual can get access to video production editing tools, higher quality recorders, and other technologies that make it much easier to produce pornography from wherever they are located. But because Los Angeles County was, for several decades, the center of pornography production in the United States and the world, the Los Angeles County Board of Supervisors and Department of Public Health have been particularly active in implementing measures to regulate the porn industry and porn performers.

In 2012, Los Angeles County passed a mandatory STI testing statute, called Measure B, which officially went into effect on August 1, 2017.[42] Measure B requires pornography performers to wear condoms on set while filming vaginal or anal intercourse scenes with a penis and requires pornography producers to pay an annual fee to the Los Angeles County Department of Public Health. It also requires that app producers and management-level employees take sexual health classes.[42] Producers who produce only girl–girl or solo content for a 2-year period or longer are exempt. Despite constitutional challenges to Measure B raised by the pornography production company Vivid Entertainment, in August 2013 a judge upheld the law as constitutional. The measure was proposed by Michael Weinstein, who is the president of the Los Angeles-based AIDS Healthcare Foundation and who went on to propose that the State of California make the condom mandate statewide. The statewide version was called Proposition 60 and was voted on in 2016, but it did not pass. Proposition 60 included provisions that producers of pornography would need to pay for performer vaccinations, testing, and medical examinations, post the condom requirement at filming sites, get a state health license every 2 years, and notify the state Division of Occupational Safety and Health whenever they shoot a film, with fines up to $70,000 if they were in violation. The cost of enforcing the measure was estimated to be $1 million annually, and other associated costs included the anticipated loss of several million dollars in state and local tax revenue from pornography production leaving the state to be produced in nearby Nevada or elsewhere. Had Proposition 60 passed in 2016, California residents would have been able to sue individual performers for not wearing condoms in pornography scenes.[43]

Students of public health may wonder why pornography performers would object to mandates that the producers pay for their STI testing, require personal protective equipment on set (i.e., condoms), and otherwise reasonable-sounding measures to improve performer health and safety that are in line with standards in the medical industry. Here are a few putative explanations. First, because a porn performer's workday may last between 2 and 12 hours, and they may engage in sexual intercourse for an hour or more on a workday, condom use can cause skin irritations, vaginal dryness, and other problems that make it uncomfortable and potentially riskier for STI transmission. Second, generally speaking, most porn performers tend to have anti-establishment attitudes and are not keen on government mandates related to sexual behavior of any kind. Third, pornography consumers tend to prefer to see pornography without condoms in it, so most pornography producers are opposed to the use of condoms because they fear it will hurt their profits. Some producers are also performers, or are partnered with performers, so a portion of the performer outcry against Measure B and Proposition 60 could relate to what is essentially the producers' concerns about profits. Fourth, Measure B and Proposition 60 were not crafted with input from the performer community. This created a fundamental lack of trust between performers and the proponents of these mandates.

In addition to the measure and proposition related to condom use, in 2020 an additional bill took aim at performers' knowledge of the industry and ways in which they are vulnerable to being exploited. California Assembly Bill 2389 was introduced on February 18, 2020, by Assemblywoman Cristina Garcia (D), who said it was her goal to require training of pornography performers as well as fingerprinting and background check clearance.[44] Although the bill ultimately died in committee, Garciahe explained that, just as the food service industry requires food handlers to take a training course and pass a quiz for health and safety reasons, similar permitting would make working conditions safer for pornography performers in the state as well. The bill was originally proposed by the International Entertainment Adult Union, which is the only US Department of Labor-approved parent union representing the adult industry in the United States. But other pornography performer groups, such as the Free Speech Coalition and Adult Performers Actors Guild, were not consulted by the Union when the bill was being drafted and strongly objected to it. While many performers, particularly those entering the industry, are vulnerable to certain types of exploitation and can benefit from education about sexual health, financial planning, and their legal rights, performers nevertheless object to the proposal that they would benefit by having their personal information entered into a state database, because of the stigma associated with being a sex worker. Many performers see the state's attempt to fingerprint them and to keep other personally identifying information about them as policing them rather than protecting them.[44]

At the national level, students of public health should be aware of the controversial bill package called FOSTA-SESTA, which was passed in 2018.[45] The House version of the bill was known as the Fight Online Sex Trafficking Act (FOSTA), whereas the Senate bill was known as Stop Enabling Sex Traffickers Act (SESTA). FOSTA-SESTA means that third parties, such as websites that host singles advertisements like Craigslist or the now-defunct website that was known as Backpage, can be held liable if their websites post ads for prostitution or consensual sex work. In theory, the goal was to make it more difficult for traffickers to advertise and get new customers, and to make it easier to detect trafficking and to intervene. In reality, many sex workers say that FOSTA-SESTA has made consensual sex work more dangerous for them, as they are unable to connect with potential customers online and are therefore forced to meet in person in the streets or elsewhere. One *Fordham Law Review* paper argues that within a month of its passing, FOSTA-SESTA caused the deaths of two sex workers and 13 additional sex workers to go missing.[46] While FOSTA-SESTA doesn't pertain to pornography specifically, because there is overlap between the pornography performer community and sex worker community, and because legislation aimed at repressing commercial sexual activity may chip away at the rights of those adults who choose to perform in pornography, the reaction to FOSTA-SESTA on the part of pornography performers has generally been unfavorable. Porn performers have also objected to ways in which sexual consent and nonconsent are conflated by anti-trafficking advocates during debates about FOSTA-SESTA. (NB: "Unfavorable" may be putting it too mildly, as many reactions are powerfully emotionally charged and read as something closer to enraged.[47])

A fourth and final piece of legislation that has had a tremendous impact on how pornography performers and producers in the United States operate is 18 U.S.C. § 2257A, on record-keeping requirements for actual or simulated sexual conduct. 2257, as it is commonly called, was approved in November 1988, with amendments approved in 1990, 1994, 2003, and 2006. It mandates that producers of pornography, or any depictions of sexual activity using actual people, are required to verify that the performers are 18 years old or older and to maintain records of the performers' legal names and ages in alphabetical order. Further, pornography producers are obligated to disclose the location of the records and to make the records available to agents of the Attorney General for inspection without advance notice up to once every 4 months or more often if there is a reasonable suspicion that a violation has occurred. Originally, 2257 applied to both the primary producers of pornography and any "secondary producers," such as bloggers who repost pornographic material that they did not create. The goal of 2257 is to prevent the production of child pornography. However, the record-keeping requirements also mean that solo operators and amateurs (for example, individuals who decide to perform as cam-girls from their own home) are obligated to affix their street addresses to their sexually explicit material in at least 12-point font and in a contrasting color to the background of the material, because of the require ment to state where the records are maintained.[48] Violations mean producers can be found guilty of a felony punishable up to 5 years in prison as well as fines for a first offense.[48] In 2018, the constitutionality of 2257 was challenged in the US Third Circuit Court of Appeals, which ruled that most of the record-keeping requirements violated the First and Fourth Amendments. Because it was found unconstitutional, primary producers of pornography are now able to fulfill the requirement using a form, and secondary producers are exempt from record-keeping requirements. In addition, judges must issue a warrant before Attorney General agents can make inspections of records.

Adult Industry Advocacy Organizations

There are several entities in the United States that are organized to protect the rights of adult entertainment industry workers, including pornography performers. While this is by no means a comprehensive list, the entities described here will provide public health advocates with an excellent starting point in the event they want to reach out to performer advocacy groups to collaborate. In addition, the two main trade publications for the pornography industry are *Xbiz* and *AVN*. Public health advocates who want to understand how proposed state or federal legislation is being received by the adult industry, or to keep abreast of the latest developments in the industry, are advised to subscribe.

The Free Speech Coalition (FSC), also known as the North American Trade Association of the Adult Industry, was established in 1991 in the wake of a federal sting operation that targeted 30 adult entertainment companies in 1990.[49] The FSC's mission is to protect the rights and freedoms of the adult industry, which includes the pleasure products (i.e., sex toys) industry. The FSC oversees a network of national testing sites that screen performers for HIV and other STIs.[43] The FSC is the primary political advocacy group for the pornography or "adult entertainment" industry and has focused on issues like censorship, web encryption to reduce hacking of adult websites, zoning laws that limit adult pleasure product stores, regulations related to how lubricants are sold, and condoms in pornographic films. The FSC has had numerous successes blocking anti-pornography film bills at the federal level and was instrumental in helping to defeat the condom-related Proposition 60 in California in 2016. Performers new to the adult industry can become members for anywhere from $5 to $100 per month. To become a member, performers have to provide a tax identification number, but once they are approved as members, performers have access to the INSPIRE "industry new-comer support program," an opportunity to buy personal insurance, and con-sideration for financial support from a performer subsidy fund (available to adult film performers to help subsidize up to three STI tests per month).

The Adult Performer Advocacy Committee (APAC) advocates for worker safety in the adult film industry. APAC recently launched a mentor program that pairs newcomers to the industry or those in need of guid-ance with veteran performers; provides assistance with banking and net-working within the industry; and provides educational videos and written information about performers' rights and responsibilities, navigating on-set experiences, and sexual health; and offers a "model bill of rights" that details what performers have a right to ask when they are hired. These rights include, for example, the right to know the content of the shoot in advance, people that they will be performing with, the expected length of the shoot, and the proposed pay. APAC, like FSC, has a website that provides lists of mental health providers, physicians, accountants, and attorneys who are friendly to porn performers and are knowledgeable about the relevant issues for porn performers' experience. Some performers have criticized APAC for not having any gay men or people involved in creating gay por-nography in leadership positions.[50]

The International Entertainment Adult Union (IEAU) is the only Department of Labor approved parent union representing the adult industry in the United States. There are currently three subordinate chapters of the IEAU, including the Exotic Dancer Guild, the Adult Performers Actors Guild (APAG, easy to confuse with APAC), and the Adult Film Crew.[51] Individuals can apply for membership for $125 per year, with quarterly charges of $50 to remain a member subsequently. Members are then eligible for subsidized health insurance plan participation, discounted accounting programs, mort-gage programs, wholesale prices for dance wear, car rentals, moving services, phone service discounts by AT&T, photo packages, and cosmetic surgery discounts, as well as life insurance, access to a job classified board, and ac-cess to college education programming. IEAU goals include creating retire-ment plans, getting members access to Social Security, and unemployment insurance.[52]

Conclusions

Public health advocates should focus on promoting the safety, health, and well-being of those who work in the pornography industry as performers or crew. This cannot be accomplished without meaningful, long-term, trusting partnership with those presently working in the industry. Those who have exited the industry are not representative of those who choose to remain in it. As a result, anti-human-trafficking and other public health efforts that partner exclusively with former commercial sex and adult industry workers may be out of touch with the needs of those who are presently engaged in pornography-related labor. However, it is also true that some veteran performers, crew members, directors, producers, and allied professionals (e.g., agents, lawyers, and healthcare workers who specialize in service provision to adult entertainment workers) who are no longer active in the industry nevertheless will have important contributions to make. Finding ways of collaborating with both presently active and former industry professionals may strengthen public health advocates' capacity to identify needs, to support stakeholders in developing solutions, and to facilitate their implementation.

Importantly, there may be an excess of financially vulnerable people among pornography performers as compared to the general population, and a higher percentage of performers may be grappling with additional challenges, including depression, intimate partner violence victimization, and alcohol and other drug use disorder. These challenges are made more difficult due to the stigma associated with working in the adult entertainment industry, and for those who are marginalized and oppressed on the basis of their race and ethnicity, they are exponentially more difficult.

A key factor to improving the safety and health of the pornography labor force may be recognition that many of the potential harms faced by workers, including violence or coercion on set, are not always improved through criminal justice system approaches. The largest gains in safety and health may depend upon the capacity of those who work for the legitimate pornography industry to share best practices and set industrywide norms. However, no coalition, association, or union is going to be able to address the harms faced by individuals who work (either voluntarily, or due to force, fraud, or coercion) with nefarious producers who are disconnected from the broader adult entertainment industry community or producers of illegal pornography. Public health professionals can, and should, also prevent people from being harmed in the production of pornography created by unethical autonomous producers and participate in discussions about how to stop them and hold them accountable. Meanwhile, much work needs to be done to characterize and understand the pornography workforce empirically, to quantify their risk of experiencing occupational hazards, and to test workplace interventions to reduce threats to health and safety.

References

1. Davis, L., and K. Souza. 2009. "Integrating Occupational Health with Mainstream Public Health in Massachusetts: An Approach to Intervention." *Public Health Reports* (Washington, DC: 1974). 124 (Suppl. 1): 5–14.

2. Quinn, M. M. 2003. "Occupational Health, Public Health, Worker Health." *American Journal of Public Health* 93, no. 4: 526.

3. Charlton, J. I. 1998. *Nothing About Us Without Us: Disability Oppression and Empowerment*, 1st ed: Berkeley, Los Angeles and London: University of California Press.

4. Vanwesenbeeck, I. 2017. "Sex Work Criminalization Is Barking Up the Wrong Tree." *Archives of Sexual Behavior* 46, no. 6: 1631–1640.

5. Griffith, J. D., S. Mitchell, B. Hammond, L. L. Gu, and C. L. Hart. 2012. "A Comparison of Sexual Behaviors and Attitudes, Self-Esteem, Quality of Life, and Drug Use Among Pornography Actors and a Matched Sample." *International Journal of Sexual Health* 24, no. 4: 254–266.

6. Griffith, J. D., S. Mitchell, C. L. Hart, L. T. Adams, and L. L. Gu. 2013. "Pornography Actresses: An Assessment of the Damaged Goods Hypothesis." *The Journal of Sex Research* 50, no. 7: 621–632.

7. MacKinnon, Catharine A. 1993. *Only Words*. Cambridge: Harvard University Press.

8. Dworkin, A. 1989. *Pornography: Men Possessing Women*, xvii. New York: Penguin.

9. Fight The New Drug. 2020. "What Causes People To Choose To Go into the Porn Industry?" https://fightthenewdrug.org/what-causes-people-to-choose-to-go-into-the-porn-industry/

10. Griffith, J. D., L. T. Adams, C. L. Hart, and S. Mitchell. 2012. "Why Become a Pornography Actress?" *International Journal of Sexual Health* 24, no. 3: 165–180.

11. Bakehorn, J. A. 2010. "Women-Made Pornography." In *Sex for Sale*, 2nd ed., edited by R. Weitzer, 94. New York: Taylor & Francis.

12. Dubin, J. M., A. B. Greer, C. Valentine, et al. 2019. "Evaluation of Indicators of Female Sexual Dysfunction in Adult Entertainers." *The Journal of Sexual Medicine* 16, no. 5: 621–623.

13. Dubin, J. Personal communication.

14. Dubin, J., A. Greer, R. Carrasquillo, I. O'Brien, E. Leue, and R. Ramasamy. 2018. "Erectile Dysfunction Among Male Adult Entertainers: A Survey." *Translational Andrology and Urology* 7: 926–930.

15. Brooks, S. 2010. "Hypersexualization and the Dark Body: Race and Inequality among Black and Latina Women in the Exotic Dance Industry." *Sexuality Research and Social Policy* 7, no. 2: 70–80.

16. Miller-Young, M. 2010. "Putting Hypersexuality to Work: Black Women and Illicit Eroticism in Pornography." *Sexualities* 13: 219–235.

17. Centers for Disease Control and Prevention. 2005. "HIV Transmission in the Adult Film Industry—Los Angeles, California, 2004." *MMWR* 54, no. 37: 923–926.

18. Hennessy-Fiske, M., and R-G. Lin. 2019. "Porn Actor Has Tested Positive for HIV; Industry Clinic Officials Confirm a Quarantine Is in Effect." https://latimesblogs.latimes.com/lanow/2010/10/porn-actor-has-tested-positive-for-hiv-industry-clinic-officials-confirm.html

19. Miles, K. 2014. "Porn Moratorium After HIV-Positive Test From Performer, Cameron Bay." https://www.huffpost.com/entry/porn-moratorium-hiv_n_3792761
20. Wilken, J. A., C. Ried, P. Rickett, et al. 2016. "Occupational HIV Transmission Among Male Adult Film Performers—Multiple States, 2014." *MMWR* 65: 110–114.
21. Free Speech Coalition. 2017. "Preliminary Production Hold Called." https://www.freespeechcoalition.com/blog/2017/04/15/preliminary-production-hold-called/
22. Rodriguez-Hart, C., R. A. Chitale, R. Rigg, B. Y. Goldstein, P. R. Kerndt, and P. Tavrow. 2012. "Sexually Transmitted Infection Testing of Adult Film Performers: Is Disease Being Missed?" *Sexually Transmitted Disease* 39, no. 12: 989–994.
23. Free Speech Coalition. 2020. "PASS." https://fscpass.com/about_us Accessed June 7, 2020.
24. Clark-Flory, T. 2019. "The Porn Industry Is Rethinking How It Works With HIV Positive Performers." https://jezebel.com/the-porn-industry-is-rethinking-how-it-works-with-hiv-p-1833068780
25. Free Speech Coalition. 2018. "Advisory: Warning—Fungal Infection Spreading in the Performer Pool." https://www.freespeechcoalition.com/blog/2018/02/08/advisory-warning-fungal-infection-spreading-performer-pool/
26. US Bureau of Labor Statistics. 2018. "Table R100. Incidence Rates for Nonfatal Occupational Injuries and Illnesses Involving Days Away from Work per 10,000 Full-Time Workers by Occupation and Selected Events or Exposures Leading to Injury or Illness, Private Industry, 2018." https://www.bls.gov/iif/oshwc/osh/case/cd_r100_2018.htm
27. Milczarek, M. 2010. *Workplace Violence and Harassment: A European Picture.* Luxembourg: Publications Office of the European Union.
28. Tiku, N., C. Lewis, and E. Cushing. 2015. "Inside the Porn Industry's Reckoning over Sexual Assault." https://www.buzzfeednews.com/article/nitashatiku/porn-sexual-assault
29. Clark-Flory, T. 2018. "Is 'Feminist' Porn Getting Its #MeToo Moment?" *Jezebel* https://jezebel.com/is-feminist-porn-getting-its-metoo-moment-1828173419
30. Snow, A. 2017. "Porn's Norma Rae Moment." https://www.thedailybeast.com/porns-norma-rae-moment
31. Tarrant, S. 2016. *The Pornography Industry: What Everyone Needs to Know.* New York: Oxford University Press.
32. Adult Performers Actors Guild. n.d. "Model Releases." https://apagunion.com/performer-info/2257-forms-model-releases/
33. Adult Performers Actors Guild. 2020. "APAG Announces On Set Steward Program." https://apagunion.com/2020/06/09/apag-announces-on-set-steward-program/
34. Free Speech Coalition. 2019. "The FSC Guide to AB5." https://www.freespeechcoalition.com/blog/2019/12/20/the-fsc-guide-to-ab5/
35. Alpatrum, L. 2018. "#ThotAduit Is Just the Latest Tactic People Are Using to Harass Sex Workers Online." https://www.theverge.com/2018/11/30/18119688/thotaudit-sex-work-irs-online-harassment
36. Stern, M. 2017. "The Banks' War on Porn." https://www.thedailybeast.com/articles/2014/05/07/the-banks-war-on-porn.html
37. Adult Performers Actors Guild. n.d. "Payment Processor Discrimination." https://apagunion.com/social-media-discrimination/payment-processor-discrimination/
38. Adult Performers Actors Guild. n.d. "Instagram Discrimination." https://apagunion.com/social-media-discrimination/instagram-discrimination/
39. Morris, C. 2016. "Porn's Dirtiest Secret: What Everyone Gets Paid." https://www.cnbc.com/2016/01/20/porns-dirtiest-secret-what-everyone-gets-paid.html
40. Carradori, N. 2020. "This Is How Much Money Porn Stars Really Make." https://www.vice.com/en_uk/article/d3amak/how-much-money-porn-stars-make

41. Dickson, E. J. 2013. "Fired for Doing Porn: The New Employment Discrimination." https://www.salon.com/2013/09/30/fired_for_doing_porn_the_new_employment_discrimination/

42. Free Speech Coalition. 2017. "FSC's Measure B Analysis." https://www.freespeechcoalition.com/blog/2017/09/08/fscs-measure-b-explainer/

43. Comella, L. May 12, 2020. "The Adult Industry Can Survive Without Government Help. Here's Why." *The Washington Post.*

44. Sharp, S. 2020. "'Scarlet Letter Statute': L.A.'s Adult Performers Strike Back Against State Registry Bill. https://www.latimes.com/california/story/2020-02-29/porn-actors-los-angeles-state-registry-bill

45. Fight Online Sex Trafficking Act (FOSTA) and the Stop Enabling Sex Traffickers Act (SESTA) (FOSTA-SESTA), 115th Congress (2018). https://www.govtrack.us/congress/bills/115/s1693/ Accessed August 8, 2020.

46. Chamberlain, L. 2019. "FOSTA: A Hostile Law with a Human Cost." *Fordham University Law Review* 87, no. 5: 2171–2211.

47. Souixsie Q. 2018. "Anti-Sex-Trafficking Advocates Say New Law Cripples Efforts to Save Victims." https://www.rollingstone.com/culture/culture-features/anti-sex-trafficking-advocates-say-new-law-cripples-efforts-to-save-victims-629081/ Accessed August 8, 2020.

48. United States Court of Appeals. 2007. 18 U.S. Code § 2257. Title 18, Part 1, Chapter 110.

49. Free Speech Coalition. 2020. "History." https://www.freespeechcoalition.com/about-fsc/history/

50. Mitchell, T. 2020. "Brokeback Union: The Gay Porn Stars Speaking out About Performer Pay." https://www.dazeddigital.com/life-culture/article/47906/1/gay-porn-stars-speaking-out-about-performer-industry-pay-money

51. International Entertainment Adult Union. 2020. "About I.E.A.U." https://www.entertainmentadultunion.com/?zone=/unionactive/view_page.cfm&page=WHY20THE2020IEAU

52. International Entertainment Adult Union. 2020. "Member Benefits." https://www.entertainmentadultunion.com/index.cfm?zone=/unionactive/view_page.cfm&page=OFFERS

13

The Benefits of Pornography

In 1997, when I started my training in public health, Big Tobacco (as the tobacco industry was called) was a leading foe. Students, faculty, and practitioners were united behind the idea that tobacco and smoking behavior were responsible for needless deaths, illnesses, suffering, and the worsening of numerous health inequities. What's more, tobacco companies like R.J. Reynolds and Philip Morris were being sued (and later found liable) for fraudulently hiding the health risks associated with smoking and for marketing cigarettes to children. There were no two ways about it: tobacco and smoking were reviled. In fact, while I was a graduate student, my school instituted a policy that no faculty or student could accept grant funding from a tobacco company because any collaboration with the tobacco industry was viewed as in direct conflict with the goals of public health. This rule bothered me a bit at the time because Altria group, the parent company of Philip Morris and other tobacco companies, had recently announced that they were willing to fund domestic violence research—which was the topic of my dissertation and was underfunded by government sources. But it also bothered me because as a domestic violence shelter worker, I had seen firsthand the benefits of cigarette smoking. Yes, you read that right. I'm a career public health advocate and I believe that there are circumstances in which cigarette smoking has benefits.

When women came to live in the domestic violence shelter, they were on the run from severely abusive and dangerous partners, and they lived with the fear (as did staff) that at any moment one of the abusive partners might show up with a gun and in a murderous rage. For women who smoked, cigarettes had the benefit of temporary stress reduction. Taking periodic smoke breaks together out on the porch of the shelter also strengthened social bonds between house residents, and sometimes with the staff who joined them, and gave some structure to stretches of time that otherwise felt overwhelming and agonizing. One could argue that healthy alternatives, such as stretch classes or meditation breaks, could have replaced the cigarette smoking. Smoking was increasing the shelter residents' risk of cancer, hypertension, and chronic obstructive pulmonary disease and was polluting the environment. At the same time, it was also a quick, easy-to-obtain, and relatively inexpensive mood

Pornography and Public Health. Emily F. Rothman, Oxford University Press. © Oxford University Press 2021.
DOI: 10.1093/oso/9780190075477.003.0013

booster to many women in acute crisis who had no other opportunity to experience even a moment of pleasure, or calm, or relief from anxiety. In fact, there is evidence that, in low doses, nicotine can have an antidepressant effect.[1] So as a graduate student in public health, I had one of my first chances to experience what it is like to embrace two opposing beliefs at the same time. Smoking is unequivocally bad for human health. There are also times and places when smoking, despite the harm it causes, should be tolerated. I will never take a one-sided view of cigarette smoking—or pornography.

When I began to study the impact of pornography on adolescents, I quickly developed a multidimensional perspective. I could see that a one-sided view on pornography was overly simplistic and inconsistent with both existing literature and my own research findings, and that nuance was needed. I understand that in some academic disciplines scholars are trained to pick one particular side of an issue and to argue vociferously in defense of that viewpoint, even when faced with competing evidence. That is not what we are trained to do in public health. Public health is a scientific field that is concerned with uncovering truth so that people may live healthier, and ideally happier, lives. For example, in the 1980s, the best available data suggested that the saturated fats in butter were harmful to health, so public health advocates promoted margarine as a butter substitute. A decade later, new research revealed that trans fats in margarine were harmful, so nutritional epidemiologists reversed course and provided the public with the updated information about margarine—that it was not a good alternative to butter after all. In public health, we are not embarrassed about "flip flopping" when we have the results of new studies, and we should never be cagey and defensive about the weaknesses in our research studies or limitations of our findings, because what's most important is that we strive to get ever closer to the truth of whatever we are investigating. Generally, public health scientists are OK with saying: "I don't know," "Our conclusions were wrong," and "It's complicated." It comes with the territory of what we do.

I provide this context because I wonder if some readers will be surprised that this book includes a chapter about research that has identified benefits of pornography for human health. Here is why I feel that it is important to include this chapter: Perhaps preceding chapters have persuaded the reader that when it comes to some outcomes (e.g., body acceptance, relationship stability), the research on the influence of pornography is mixed, in that some studies find evidence of an association between pornography and the negative outcome of interest, while others do not. But I would also like to impress upon the reader that when it comes to research about pornography, the evidence is also "mixed" in the sense that there are studies that find that pornography use is associated with positive outcomes of interest as well as with negative ones. I do not argue that the harms of some pornography are canceled out by the fact that there are some people who derive benefits from some of it. These are not equal and opposite propositions! By way of example, that some people feel pleasure or tension reduction from cigarette smoking is not considered a compelling reason to dispense with tobacco use age limits, warning labels, taxes, indoor use prohibitions, and so on. On balance, there may be more reasons for public health professionals to regulate and minimize the role of pornography in people's lives than there are to defend or to celebrate it. But a holistic review of what pornography does, and does not, do to people's health is important—and full consideration of the spectrum of positive and negative impacts that pornography may have on public health is what is often missing from activists' discourse about pornography as a public health issue.

Therefore, in this chapter I review the evidence that pornography can have a positive influence on an individual's sexual wellness, mental health, relationships, body acceptance, self-esteem, and sexual knowledge, that it can increase safer sex behavior, and that it can foster self-acceptance in gay, lesbian, bisexual, and other sexual minority individuals. I do not include a discussion of the benefits of radical and boundary-pushing art to society, or the ways in which materials that are deemed pornographic, sexually explicit, erotic, or obscene may have a helpful role to play in advancing an antiracist and antihomophobic agenda, although these are arguments that can be made and are relevant to public health.

Sexual Wellness

Pornography can cause people to become sexually aroused, increase their sexual excitement, and enable them to have orgasms and experience sexual pleasure. This hardly seems like a controversial statement because sexual arousal and pleasure are, after all, the purpose of pornography. What is controversial about the idea that pornography can cause sexual arousal, though, is the belief that sexual arousal is sometimes bad, that sexual excitement in response to certain materials is wrong, and that orgasms and pleasure are dangerous if they occur in reaction to pornographic material instead of with a human partner.

According to the World Health Organization, sexual health not only is the absence of disease, but also requires "the possibility of having pleasurable and safe sexual experiences."[2] The American Sexual Health Association asserts that is healthy to masturbate, and that sex promotes better sleep, less stress, and more happiness, and that "our bodies thrive on the chemicals released during orgasm, so a healthy sex life is indeed part of a healthy body."[3] At the 2019 World Congress of Sexual Health, it was declared that "sexual pleasure is a fundamental part of sexual rights as a matter of human rights," and governments were urged to promote sexual pleasure because of its importance to global public health.[4] If orgasms are healthful and sexual pleasure is a human right, perhaps the starting assumption of public health advocates should be that sexually explicit material that enables people to experience orgasms and sexual pleasure is beneficial to human health.

There is research to support the contention that pornography can improve sexual well-being. It has been used successfully to treat sexual dysfunction in married women,[5] and more frequent pornography use predicts lower arousal and orgasmic difficulty, greater pleasure, and more masturbation in partnered, adult women.[6] Neurologically, both men and women appear to react similarly to pornography.[7] More frequent pornography use has been found to be associated, cross-sectionally, with the frequency of masturbation, coitus, oral sex, and anal sex in heterosexual men and women,[8] and, in at least in some instances, it encourages some men and women to try new sexual positions and sexual acts, reduces their feelings of sexual guilt, and inspires more direct communication about sexual pleasure with a partner.[8,9] Men have reported moderate positive effects of pornography, including increased sexual functioning, sexual pleasure, relationship enhancement, improved sleep, and other psychosexual health benefits.[10,11] Given the possibility of these direct benefits on sexual well-being, it is not surprising that some therapists recommend the use of pornography to some patients or use sexually explicit material in the therapeutic context.[12]

A study of 151 women Australia who were social media users found that pornography use was generally accepted and normalized within young people's relationships, and that many had positive things to say about pornography. For example, one 27-year-old in the sample said: "[Pornography] can be a great way to engage with my partner, even if just to laugh and wonder how they did what happened in the film. Sometimes it can assist with getting 'in the mood.'"[13] A similar study, which drew upon in-depth interviews with 35 young men from a university in the northeastern United States, also found that pornography had educational benefits for men in the sample. The authors found that pornography use was "an ordinary and unproblematic component of their lives," and that research participants "used pornography to explore their sexual desires [and] emerging sexual identities, and for developing new sexual techniques." One man in the sample reported that his girlfriend had been able to communicate with him about her sexual desires through pornography. He said: "[She's] shown me stuff she likes, and that been fun exploring, too."[14] The idea that pornography may normalize more agentic roles for women, which improves their comfort with sex and arousal and reduces shame and guilt about sexuality, has been proposed by other research teams as well.[15,16]

Relationships

Chapter 7 provides an in-depth review of the evidence that addresses the question of whether pornography viewing by one or both members of a couple harms relationship stability. It concludes that if pornography does influence relationship health, the influence is likely weak, and varies by gender, people's attachment style, overall relationship health, and other factors. But there are a handful of research studies that have found that pornography use by one or both members of a couple can be beneficial for relationship quality. For example, a study of 617 married or cohabiting couples found that female pornography use was positively associated with how satisfied they felt with the physical intimacy in their relationship.[17] Interestingly, the study did not find that the same was true for men in the sample. A study of 217 heterosexual couples found something similar—the more that women used pornography, the more sexually satisfied their male partners were. On the other hand, the more that men used pornography, the less sexually satisfied the men were. Part of the reason for this difference is that women in the sample reported that they primarily used pornography as part of sex with their partners, while men tended to use pornography alone for masturbation. The study also found that shared pornography use was associated with better relationship satisfaction than one person's solitary pornography use.[18]

A third study, which analyzed responses from a convenience sample of 8,376 people who responded to an online survey from *Elle* magazine and MSNBC. com about "online sexual activities," found that both men and women who engaged in online sexual activities were "more open to new things" and found it easier to talk about what they wanted sexually. The study reported negative findings as well, including that men were less aroused by sex with a human partner as a result of their online sexual activities, but the general pattern observed in the findings was that online sexual activities yielded benefits for both men and women, including increased intimacy with their partners and better communication about sex.[19]

In his book about ethical porn viewing for men, author David Ley made the argument that the availability of porn can also protect relationships by offering a sexual outlet to individuals whose partners are not interested in sex (p. 81).[20] In other words, Ley suggested that couples faced with a mismatch in sexual drive or sexual interest could face less relationship strain if the partner with higher sexual interest views porn. Given that disparity in sexual desire is a common and often divisive issue for long-term and married couples, the possibility that sexually explicit and erotic materials could be helpful instead of harmful to the stability of these relationships is a hypothesis to investigate.

Body Acceptance

Chapter 9 provides a review of the evidence that addresses whether pornography viewing causes people to feel less accepting of their own bodies. In that chapter, I conclude that pornography likely harms some people's self-image, has no effect on most people's body acceptance, and for some people improves how they feel about their bodies. In this section, I highlight some of the findings that support the idea that, for some people, there are body acceptance-related benefits of viewing pornography. One small study that involved interviews with 11 adult women recruited through a sexual workshop center in Toronto, Canada, found that pornography helped the women to normalize their own bodies and bolstered their self-esteem and body acceptance. A woman in the sample spoke about the "Big Beautiful Women" (BBW) genre of pornography and reported that seeing it is "a reminder that BBW are sexy and fuckable. So I sort of couch that into boosting my self-esteem."

For those not easily persuaded by an 11-person qualitative study, there are also data from a cross-sectional MTurk study of 393 American young adults that found that, in women, frequency of pornography use was associated with comfort being nude.[21] Women and men who watched more pornography and perceived the pornography as realistic also had better body images than those who didn't perceive pornography as realistic. The study authors explained that they believed that, for men, the reason more pornography viewing was associated with better body image was that those who watched more pornography had higher self-esteem and were more satisfied with their bodies. For women, those who watched more pornography felt more comfortable being nude and had higher self-esteem. The authors explained that while unrealistic pornographic imagery may be associated with negative body image, it is possible that realistic pornography images (i.e., of real people, with realistic bodies, doing real sexual things) may make the performers "good role models for body positivity."[21]

A third quantitative study also found that pornography may have a positive influence on men's acceptance of their bodies. In a sample of 1,274 university students from Norway and Sweden, Kvalem et al. (2014) found that men who perceived pornography as realistic had higher satisfaction with their genital appearance and higher self-esteem than those who did not perceive pornography as realistic.[22] A study of 346 US women similarly found that women who had seen Internet media (pornographic and otherwise) perceived their vulvas as normal-appearing at higher rates that those not exposed to such media (97% vs. 91%, respectively).[23]

Sexual Knowledge

A known public health problem is that too many adolescents and young adults in the United States and elsewhere have inadequate knowledge of sexual anatomy and physiology. Only 71% of US high school districts have adopted a policy that specifies teaching sex education, and two thirds of states and the District of Columbia allow parents to remove their children from sex ed classes that are taught in schools.[24] In the United Kingdom, three quarters of students rate their school-based sex education as "less than fair,"[25] and a recent meta-ethnographic study that covered 25 years of sex education in the United States, United Kingdom, Australia, Canada, Japan, Iran, Brazil, and other nations found that young people report their sex education was generally negative and failed to discuss issues that were truly important, such as sexual pleasure and the details of male and female anatomy.[26,27] A natural consequence of providing inadequate sex education in schools is that adolescents may seek out information about sex elsewhere. Accordingly, the idea that adolescents are learning about sex from pornography, and that that is a problem, has been alleged by various anti-pornography groups since the 1980s—and by me since 2016.[28,29] But there is a possibility that some adolescents and young adults are learning about sex from pornography—and that in some cases it provides them with accurate information about sexual anatomy and physiology.

To test the hypothesis that pornography use may be related to sexual knowledge, Hesse and Pedersen recruited a convenience sample of 337 Canadian university students and social media users and asked them to complete an online survey about pornography and sexual knowledge.[26] They found that pornography use was positively correlated with increased sexual knowledge; more positive attitudes toward sex, sexual behaviors, and the opposite gender; and overall quality of life. The authors were surprised by the finding that the frequency of pornography use predicted more accurate knowledge of anatomy, physiology, and sexual behavior. While they acknowledged that students with better sexual knowledge may have been more likely to seek out pornography, it also is possible that pornography served as a source of sexual information. Interestingly, in this sample, nonheterosexual sexual orientation was associated with greater knowledge and more positive perceptions of pornography, as well.

Because there has been only this single study of pornography and sexual knowledge, and it used a convenience sample, whether pornography can impart accurate anatomical and physiological sexual information to youth or to adults remains unclear. Because pornography is so varied, it may matter very much what kind of pornography is viewed. For example, the casual viewer of mainstream Internet pornography might easily come away with the erroneous idea that women ejaculating or "squirting" during sex is common, or that most women have orgasms quickly and easily from vaginal penetration alone. When the mechanics of sex are staged for the camera, the viewer might not acquire accurate sexual information. However, there remains a possibility that, at least in some basic way, the explicit visual imagery in most pornography provides some accurate information about sex and sexuality to people who are not getting accurate information elsewhere. Importantly, this is not an endorsement of pornography as sex education. As Chapter 8 makes clear, available evidence suggests that pornography is not a good source of information about how to have sex, and if it is viewed as instructional material by adolescents, it likely causes far more harm to their sexual scripts than anything helpful or useful. To my mind, it is an unintended and coincidental side effect that some people may pick up some accurate anatomical information from pornography, rather than a selling point in its favor.

Boredom, Loneliness, and Safer Sex Behavior

Multiple studies have found that one of the reasons that people use pornography is to alleviate boredom.[30,31] When the COVID-19 global pandemic hit in 2020, worldwide traffic to Pornhub increased—and increased even before the website began granting free premium accounts as part of an incentive to attract new users during the pandemic.[32] Pornhub said that they were motivated to offer free premium accounts out of altruism, because it would encourage people to stay indoors and distance themselves socially. While Pornhub may have had other reasons for wanting to offer time-limited free premium accounts, it is also true that during the exceedingly stressful period of 2020, when people had to become accustomed to stay-at-home orders and quarantines, having a sexual outlet may have been helpful to some. Perhaps pornography use encouraged safer sexual behavior because people with access to it were less likely to risk COVID-19 exposure by meeting a hookup partner. Some researchers have conjectured that, in general, increased solo masturbation to pornography could reduce rates of sexually transmitted infections (STIs) or unwanted pregnancies, although designing an observational study to assess this idea would be challenging because pornography use is so common and because it would be difficult to control for the numerous potential confounders.

Self-Acceptance in Sexual Minority Individuals

Just as pornography may help some people accept the appearance of their genitals as normal, it may also help people accept or discover their sexual orientation and sexuality. For example, a study of in-depth interviews with 35 young men from a US university found that porn helped some respondents come to an understanding about, and clarify, their sexual attraction.[14] Similarly, in a mixed-methods study of 526 young men who have sex with men (MSM), Kubicek and co-authors (2010) found that participants reported that pornography was one of their only resources for learning about the mechanics of anal sex and that seeing gay pornography confirmed their sexual attractions— although some participants also expressed disdain for the "nasty" types of sex they saw in porn (e.g., fisting, water sports, bestiality).[33] Similarly, a focus group study involving 10 adult men who had seen gay pornography found that some participants found porn validating. One participant was quoted as saying: "I remember the first time I saw gay porn. I was about nine. I happened to [come across] a magazine in a back alley, and it was so validating. It was like, 'Yeah, that's it. That's what I am. And, look, there's other people doing it; they're having sex; they don't look embarrassed; they don't look grossed out.'"[34] And a recent interview study involving 15- to 19-year-old Black, male, US youths found that participants described using pornography primarily for sexual development, including learning the mechanics of same-gender sex, and to negotiate their sexual identity.[35]

On the one hand, evidence is accruing that suggests some sexual minority individuals (i.e., gay or bisexual individuals) may find pornography helpful because it depicts people with their own sexual orientation and interests engaged in pleasurable sex and normalizes that. On the one hand, given the stigma of being gay or bisexual, and the health-related sequelae of experiencing sexual-orientation-related discrimination, persecution, and shame, material that may have a protective effect could have important, positive value. On the other hand, pornography is diverse, and not all of it depicts realistic sexual positions, sexual acts, or consent, and some of it may shape social norms in ways that ultimately cause harm (see Chapter 5). For this reason, it is hard to celebrate, unqualifiedly, the idea that porn is an important source of self-validation for gay and bisexual men. Materials that boost self-esteem may be essential from a public health perspective, but why should pornography be the only, or best, option? That gay, bisexual, and pansexual people have, in some cases, had to turn to pornography in order to see their sexuality represented positively points to a more fundamental problem with the lack of diversity in mainstream media depictions of people and relationships. From a public health perspective, perhaps pornography does something useful and helpful for some people with same-sex sexual interests and attractions—nevertheless, there may be something problematic about the fact that pornography, which is generally created to make money and not with health education as its goal, is being used to address a health-related need.

Conclusions

Experiencing sexual pleasure is healthful, and pornography offers many people the opportunity to experience sexual pleasure alone or with partners. However, just because something is pleasurable to people does not make it an automatic public health good. Imagine, for example, the argument that the cost to society of the opioid epidemic is offset because opioid users experience pleasure or tension relief from it. This argument is untenable, and similarly, from a public health perspective, the pleasure benefit of pornography only holds up if the health costs to the individual or society are small. But, if we are weighing the possible positives and negatives of pornography use from a public health perspective, we can add to the positive side of the scale that pornography offers viewers the opportunity to see a diversity of body shapes and sexual behaviors celebrated, which some people reportedly find affirming, that some viewers may come away from pornography with more accurate understanding of sexual anatomy and physiology, and that some may be able to communicate better with their partners about their sexuality and sexual interests because of their pornography use. The bottom line is: for some people, there are undoubtedly benefits of having access to pornography, viewing pornography, and using pornography in the context of their relationship or for masturbation. Nevertheless, this should not be misconstrued as conclusive evidence that "porn is good" or that we have no reason for continuing to investigate its potential harms. The research that finds that there are selected benefits of some pornography use by some people highlights the need for public health, public policy, and other professionals to resist the tendency to oversimplify.

References

1. Hughes, J. R. 2008. "Smoking and Suicide: A Brief Overview." *Drug and Alcohol Dependence* 98, no. 3: 169–178.
2. World Health Organization. 2000. "Defining Sexual Health." https://www.who.int/reproductivehealth/topics/sexual_health/sh_definitions/en/
3. American Sexual Health Association. 2020. "Sexual Pleasure." http://www.ashasexualhealth.org/women-and-pleasure/
4. World Association for Sexual Health. 2019. "Declaration on Sexual Pleasure." https://worldsexualhealth.net/declaration-on-sexual-pleasure/
5. Morokoff, P. J., and J. R. Heiman. 1980. "Effects of Erotic Stimuli on Sexually Functional and Dysfunctional Women: Multiple Measures Before and After Sex Therapy." *Behaviour Research and Therapy* 18, no. 2: 127–137.
6. McNabney, S. M., K. Heves, and D. L. Rowland. 2020. "Effects of Pornography Use and Demographic Parameters on Sexual Response During Masturbation and Partnered Sex in Women." *International Journal of Environmental Research and Public Health* 17, no. 9: 16.
7. Stark, R., S. Klein, O. Kruse, et al. 2019. "No Sex Difference Found: Cues of Sexual Stimuli Activate the Reward System in Both Sexes." *Neuroscience* 416: 63–73.
8. Weinberg, M. S., C. J. Williams, S. Kleiner, and Y. Irizarry. 2010. "Pornography, Normalization, and Empowerment." *Archives of Sexual Behavior* 39, no. 6: 1389–1401.
9. Rogala, C., and T. Tydén. 2003. "Does Pornography Influence Young Women's Sexual Behavior?" *Women's Health Issues* 13, no. 1: 39–43.
10. Hald, G. M., and N. M. Malamuth. 2008. "Self-perceived Effects of Pornography Consumption." *Archives of Sexual Behavior* 37, no. 4: 614–625.
11. Hald, G. M. 2006. "Gender Differences in Pornography Consumption Among Young Heterosexual Danish Adults." *Archives of Sexual Behavior* 35, no. 5: 577–585.
12. Darnell, C. 2015. "Using Sexually Explicit Material in a Therapeutic Context." *Sex Education* 15, no. 5: 515–527.
13. Laemmle-Ruff, I. L., M. Raggatt, C. J. C. Wright, et al. 2019. "Personal and Reported Partner Pornography Viewing by Australian Women, and Association with Mental Health and Body Image." *Sexual Health* 16, no. 1: 75–79.
14. McCormack, M., and L. Wignall. 2016. "Enjoyment, Exploration and Education: Understanding the Consumption of Pornography Among Young Men with Non-Exclusive Sexual Orientations." *Sociology* 51, no. 5: 975–991.
15. Vannier, S. A., A. B. Currie, and L. F. O'Sullivan. 2014. "Schoolgirls and Soccer Moms: A Content Analysis of Free 'Teen' and 'MILF' Online Pornography." *The Journal of Sex Research* 51, no. 3: 253–264.
16. McKeown, J., D. Parry, and T. Penny Light. 2017. "'My iPhone Changed My Life': How Digital Technologies Can Enable Women's Consumption of Online Sexually Explicit Materials." *Sexuality & Culture* 22: 340–354.

17. Poulsen, F. O., D. M. Busby, and A. M. Galovan. 2013. "Pornography Use: Who Uses It and How It Is Associated with Couple Outcomes." *The Journal of Sex Research* 50, no. 1: 72–83.

18. Bridges, A. J., and P. J. Morokoff. 2011. "Sexual Media Use and Relational Satisfaction in Heterosexual Couples." *Personal Relationships* 18, no. 4: 562–585.

19. Grov, C., B. J. Gillespie, T. Royce, and J. Lever. 2011. "Perceived Consequences of Casual Online Sexual Activities on Heterosexual Relationships: A U.S. Online Survey." *Archives of Sexual Behavior* 40, no. 2: 429–439.

20. Ley, D. 2016. *Ethical Porn for Dicks: A Man's Guide to Responsible Viewing Pleasure.* Berkeley, CA: ThreeL Media.

21. Vogels, E. A. 2019. "Loving Oneself: The Associations Among Sexually Explicit Media, Body Image, and Perceived Realism." *Journal of Sex Research* 56, no. 6: 778–790.

22. Kvalem, I. L., B. Træen, B. Lewin, and A. Štulhofer. 2014. "Self-Perceived Effects of Internet Pornography Use, Genital Appearance Satisfaction, and Sexual Self-Esteem Among Young Scandinavian Adults." *Cyberpsychology: Journal of Psychosocial Research on Cyberspace* 8, no. 4, Article 4. https://doi.org/10.5817/CP2014-4-4

23. Truong, C., S. Amaya, and T. Yazdany. 2017. "Women's Perception of Their Vulvar Appearance in a Predominantly Low-Income, Minority Population." *Female Pelvic Medicine & Reconstructive Surgery* 23, no. 6: 417–419.

24. Breuner, C. C., and G. Mattson. 2016. "Sexuality Education for Children and Adolescents." *Pediatrics* 138, no. 2: e20161348.

25. National Union of Students. 2014. "Student Opinion Survey: November 2014." United Kindom: National Union of Students.

26. Hesse, C., and C. L. Pedersen. 2017. "Porn Sex Versus Real Sex: How Sexually Explicit Material Shapes Our Understanding of Sexual Anatomy, Physiology, and Behaviour." *Sexuality and Culture* 21, no. 3: 754–775.

27. Pound, P., R. Langford, and R. Campbell. 2016. "What Do Young People Think About Their School-Based Sex and Relationship Education? A Qualitative Synthesis of Young People's Views and Experiences." *BMJ Open* 6, no. 9: e011329.

28. Trostle, L. C. 2003. "Overrating Pornography as a Source of Sex Information for University Students: Additional Consistent Findings." *Psychological Reports* 92, no. 1: 143–150.

29. Rothman, E. F. 2018. "How Porn Changes the Way Teens Think About Sex." https://www.ted.com/talks/emily_f_rothman_how_porn_changes_the_way_teens_think_about_sex Accessed August 12, 2020.

30. Bothe, B., I. Toth-Kiraly, M. N. Potenza, G. Orosz, and Z. Demetrovics. 2020. "High-Frequency Pornography Use May Not Always Be Problematic." *The Journal of Sexual Medicine* 17, no. 4: 793–811.

31. Kraus, S. W., H. Rosenberg, S. Martino, C. Nich, and M. N. Potenza. 2017. "The Development and Initial Evaluation of the Pornography-Use Avoidance Self-Efficacy Scale." *Journal of Behavioral Addictions* 6, no. 3: 354–363.

32. Pornhub Insights. 2020. "Coronavirus Traffic Update." https://www.pornhub.com/insights/coronavirus-update-may-26

33. Kubicek, K., W. J. Beyer, G. Weiss, E. Iverson, and M. D. Kipke. 2010. "In the Dark: Young Men's Stories of Sexual Initiation in the Absence of Relevant Sexual Health Information." *Health Education & Behavior* 37, no. 2: 243–263.

34. Morrison, T. G. 2004. " 'He Was Treating Me Like Trash, and I Was Loving It . . .' Perspectives on Gay Male Pornography." *Journal of Homosexuality* 47, no. 3-4: 167–183.

35. Arrington-Sanders, R., G. W. Harper, A. Morgan, A. Ogunbajo, M. Trent, and J. D. Fortenberry. 2015. "The Role of Sexually Explicit Material in the Sexual Development of Same-Sex-Attracted Black Adolescent Males." *Archives of Sexual Behavior* 44, no. 3: 597–608.

14

Pornography Literacy

In the 1950s, scholars thought that news media had minimal impact on readers' points of view and that most people were able to resist getting sucked into group-think by what they were reading, hearing, or seeing.[1] It wasn't until the 1980s that social scientists understood that media can have profound consequences on public opinion.[1] Today, there are few people who argue that our media diet does not affect our thoughts, beliefs, and opinions. In fact, some people are now worried that media has the power to threaten democracy because it exerts such a powerful influence on what we think.[2]

Decades of media scholarship have demonstrated that media shape how we feel and what we do, and perhaps most worrisomely, ideas that we subsequently generalize.[3] Importantly, not all media are equally influential, and there are factors that make it more or less likely that media will change us. These factors include how much of a particular type of media we consume, whether it elicits positive or negative feelings in us, and whether it is reinforcing a preexisting belief or presenting us with a new one.[4]

The idea that something should be done to mitigate the risk that people are being seduced into a herd mentality by media has been promoted since at least the 1970s. To my knowledge, the earliest written argument in a peer-reviewed journal was made in 1974 by Professor Herb Karl, who wrote in *The English Journal*:

> Just as surely as every person has a right to read, so too has every person a right to know what he is being told and sold through the electronic media. And if—as some claim—electronic media are slowly rendering inoperable the minds of a sizeable portion of the American public by inducing a kind of electronic rapture of the depths, then we have a right to know about that too. . . . What we need, to be sure, is some sort of electronic media education.[5] (p. 7)

What Is Media Literacy?

Karl defined media literacy in two ways, succinctly and in expanded form. His succinct definition is: "Media literacy is the potential result of critical

Pornography and Public Health. Emily F. Rothman, Oxford University Press. © Oxford University Press 2021.
DOI: 10.1093/oso/9780190075477.003.0014

examination of how media mean and how they affect human behavior."[5] His expanded definition suggests that media literacy is the ability to raise questions about what is being communicated through electronic media to the consumer, other than products, services, ideas, news reports, and entertainment. "To put it only slightly differently," he wrote, "what self-concepts, life styles, cultural beliefs, corporate images, socio-political biases, and other hidden assumptions are being transmitted during media presentation?"[5] Media Literacy Now, which in 2020 described themselves as the leading national advocacy organization for media literacy education policy, similarly defined media literacy as teaching the development of critical thinking skills related to all types of media, building an understanding of how media messages shape culture and society, and giving people tools to advocate for changes in media systems.[6]

In lay terms, media literacy can be understood as teaching people to stop taking media like books, movies, shows, videos, etc., at face value, and instead to consider the behind-the-scenes aspects of what went into producing and delivering the media to an audience. A core theoretical principle of media literacy is that if people become aware that media are always coming from a particular viewpoint, and that media are packaged and sold to them in a manner that is designed to make them unquestioningly internalize the values, opinions, and ideas that are embedded in the media, they can make more conscious choices about accepting or rejecting the attitudes that are being foisted upon them.

Theoretically, Why Should Media Literacy Work?

It can be very challenging to change human behavior. Decades of research about the best methods for doing so have produced at least one firm conclusion: even when we are able to educate people and change their knowledge about a subject, we may not be able to change their behavior.[7] For example, we can provide information to people that smoking causes lung cancer, but simply providing that information alone is typically not enough to motivate and enable people to change their smoking behavior.[7] So, why would we expect that educating people about how media are created would change their attitudes about media, alter their media use behavior, or allow them to resist the social norming that takes place through media?

Multiple theories suggest that people learn from what they see other people doing and then behave in ways that they think will earn them others' approval. Bandura's social learning theory (1973) and social cognitive theory (1994) are two such theories.[8,9] Information processing–related theories about how the human mind filters information and makes it personally meaningful and useful also inform our present understanding of why and how media literacy might work.[10] In a nutshell, media literacy education theory proposes that humans can learn to control their media exposures by becoming conscious that they are constantly being exposed to new media and that they have the option of being selective about which media receive their attention. The theory suggests that we often take in media passively and automatically absorb whatever messages are fed to our brain, but that we can train ourselves to notice when we are encoding information from media and through this process become more resistant to some of its possibly pernicious effects.[10] In other words, when we become aware of our own process of acquiring information, and observe ourselves in the act of being influenced by media, we interrupt the direct flow of social norms from the media directly to our unconscious minds, which gives us back some power over ourselves. This theory emerges from what we know about how humans perceive information through their senses (e.g., sight, sound), what grabs our attention (e.g., colors, humor), how we retrieve memories that help us make sense of the images that we are seeing or sounds we are hearing (e.g., the sound of crickets chirping signifies a lack of response from an audience), how we decide to trust information (e.g., did an expert or authority provide it?), and then how we reason with the new piece of information we have just perceived and make the split-second decision to file it away as true, false, useful, useless, or potentially helpful. In summary, media literacy theory proposes that messages get from media into our brains by passing through our senses, getting mixed up with our memories and existing thoughts, and becoming information that has the power to influence us whether we like it or not, but that we are capable of interrupting this chain of events by becoming aware that it is happening.

Does Media Literacy Work?

Adolescents are almost always the targets of media literacy interventions. In part, this is because adolescents are at elevated risk for some so-called risk behaviors like alcohol use, illicit drug use, and non-condom use. It is also because neurodevelopmentally, adolescents are more flexible in their thinking.[11] Media literacy interventions have been designed to address adolescent health issues, including smoking/tobacco, drinking alcohol, use of illicit substances, and unsafe sexual behavior.[12,13] A recent meta-analysis of 35 evaluations of adolescent media literacy interventions on these topics found moderate positive effects of media literacy interventions on media literacy skills, and minor effects on risk-behavior attitudes and attentions.[12] The effectiveness of the media literacy interventions was moderated by several factors, and the interventions that targeted risky sexual behavior were more effective at producing attitude and behavioral intention change than interventions targeting substance use, which is good news for those interested in porn literacy intervention development. Moreover, interventions implemented by peers rather than trained adult facilitators were more effective, but the duration of the intervention (i.e., the number of sessions, over a certain number of weeks) did not seem to influence results.[12] Although not included in the meta-analysis, there have also been evaluations of media literacy interventions that sought to improve adolescents' perspective on a wide range of other topics, including: healthy eating,[13] reactions to stereotypical images of Blacks and Latinos at a predominantly white university,[14] attitudes toward using supplements and performance-enhancing substances,[15] and tanning.[16] There has even been one encouraging study of an intervention to increase skepticism toward advertisements in 4- to 5-year-olds in the United States.[17] In short, there is a lot of enthusiasm for media literacy interventions on a wide range of topics, and the techniques of media literacy education are now being used with youth of all ages.

What Is Porn Literacy?

Porn literacy is media literacy that is designed to teach participants to become aware of, and think critically about, pornography's potential to influence how they think and feel. It is media literacy focused on pornography. Because critical thinking is central to media literacy, authentic porn literacy programs encourage participants to think for themselves and to make their own choices about porn use. There are some anti-pornography education programs that seek to reduce participants' porn use and to build political momentum to ban pornography. Thus far, these programs have not referred to themselves in their marketing materials as "porn literacy" programs—but it is possible that in the future some may co-opt the term and begin to do so. Therefore, an important caveat is that consumers and public health advocates should always investigate porn literacy programs carefully. Unfortunately, some programs may use a judgmental, shaming, sex-negative perspective but nevertheless masquerade as porn literacy programs.

To my knowledge, there are at least five sex-positive porn literacy programs in the world. *PopPorn* is a four-module curriculum for school staff that explores pop culture and pornography, gender differences and teen sex and relationships, online sexual experience, and sexual violence.[18] *In the Picture* is an Australian program that involves a one-session viewing of an educational video about pornography and engaging in a discussion with a trained facilitator.[19] *We Prevent* is a self-paced online educational intervention for US-based sexual minority youth that promotes HIV prevention and porn literacy simultaneously.[20] There is an as-yet unnamed program under development in Ireland that will educate young adults about porn using a sex-positive perspective.[21] Finally, there is *The Truth About Pornography*, which is a nine-session educational program for adolescents that I co-developed and that is the focus of the rest of this chapter.[22] This is by no means an exhaustive list of resources for teaching adolescents about pornography. As mentioned above, several religious and anti-pornography organizations have resources for parents and educators and provide information about pornography from their own perspectives. There are also several sex-positive organizations that have information about pornography literacy on their websites, although they do not train educators or offer workshops directly. For example, the websites Scarlateen and TeenHealthSource provide information for teenagers about pornography.

Our Porn Literacy Intervention in Detail

The Truth About Pornography: A Pornography Literacy Curriculum for High School Students Designed to Reduce Sexual and Dating Violence was created in 2016. The origins of the program are described in my 2018 TEDMED talk.[23] In short, my colleagues Nicole Daley and Jess Alder, who both worked for the Boston Public Health Commission, asked me to make a presentation to high school students about dating violence prevention. When we saw that the students were bored by the violence prevention discussion, but lit up when I started talking about related research I was doing on pornography, we realized that we could harness their energy for talking about pornography in order to raise issues about healthy and respectful dating and sexual relationships. Nicole and Jess had a wealth of experience teaching population activities on media literacy to youth. For example, they used an activity called "sound nutritional label" to educate youth about hidden misogynist or unhealthy relationships messages that are embedded in song lyrics, and an activity called "reel binary" to encourage youth to uncover gender-normative messages in shows and movies.[24] We realized that we could capitalize on their expertise in engaging teenagers in media literacy activities but focus specifically on pornography. Thus, the goal of our porn literacy program was actually *not* to educate youth about pornography! In fact, the goal was to reduce dating and sexual violence, by engaging youth in critical analysis of gender norms, communication norms, and sexual norms that are promoted in some pornography.

One of the defining features of the curriculum is that, much like this book, it attempts to convey the diversity of social science findings about pornography. It is neither anti-pornography nor pro-pornography, although it does take the position that uncritical and indiscriminate viewing of pornography by youth and young adults is antithetical to the goal of promoting healthy relationship behavior. Importantly, youth are not shown pornography during the class and the class does not presume that all youth participants have already seen pornography. That said, approximately 81% of youth ages 15 and older who have taken the class have already seen pornography at least once by the time they enroll.[25] Parents have to give permission for their children to participate in this porn literacy class if their children are minors. Although parents are welcome to review the curriculum before their child participates, we do not permit parents to observe or to sit in on class sessions.

The curriculum was designed to be taught by anyone, including teenagers. One need not be a sex educator, counselor, or public health expert to facilitate it. Training and some practice facilitating the activities before going live with an audience are essential, but our goal was to make the curriculum available for widespread use. Enthusiasm for the nonjudgmental approach is required, though, as is a commitment to uplifting youth without shaming or scolding related to sexuality, gender, and sexual behavior. People who are trained to facilitate the curriculum are invited to make it their own by bringing their own small innovations to the activities and delivery. An important philosophical underpinning is positive youth development, which takes the view that youth should be involved and engaged as equal partners in their own learning. Facilitators do not talk down to youth, and they presume that youth bring many valuable assets into the class, and that they can be trusted to voice opinions, ask questions, joke, laugh, and engage in ways that are optimal for their own learning—even if the classroom environment becomes noisier or less strict than an average school classroom.

The theoretical basis for the curriculum is Ajzen's theory of planned behavior.[26] The theory holds that whether people engage in a new behavior is a function of their attitude toward the behavior, their perceived behavioral control, subjective norms related to the behavior, and their behavioral intentions. In plain language, in order to persuade youth to disregard any unhealthy messages about how to conduct oneself in a dating relationship or in a sexual

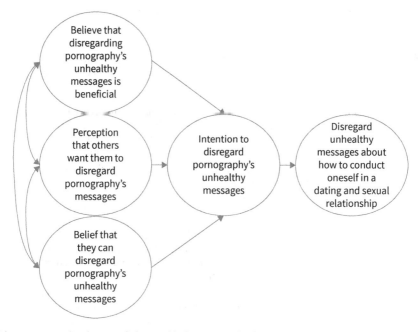

Figure 14.1. The theory of planned behavior applied to the porn literacy curriculum.

encounter that they may receive from pornography, they would first have to be convinced that: (a) they are in control of whether they internalize messages from pornography; (b) peers and other people will think highly of them for disregarding unhealthy messages that are communicated by porn; and (c) they will personally derive benefits from disregarding porn's unhealthy messaging, and in general it is beneficial for society if they do so. In terms of the porn literacy curriculum, we planned session content that addressed each of these factors (see Figure 14.1).

The curriculum presents nine 1-hour sessions (see Table 14.1).

As of May 2020, we had pilot-tested the curriculum with five small groups of adolescents in Boston, Massachusetts, beginning with our first class in July 2016. The primary audience has been youth who were already enrolled in the after-school program of the Boston Public Health Commission called the Start Strong program. We also separately provided the class to a group of lesbian, gay, bisexual, transgender, queer, and pansexual (LGBTQ+) youth at a local nonprofit youth center. We have evaluated the curriculum using a non-experimental, one-group, pretest and posttest design. That means that it has never been tested through a randomized controlled trial (RCT), so changes that we have observed in participants from pretest to posttest cannot be attributed to the curriculum and it would not be correct to say that the

Table 14.1. Content of *The Truth About Pornography* curriculum

Session 1: Why are we talking about pornography?	Session 1 focuses on helping the participants establish their own baseline feelings about pornography, and what they perceive to be the societal values related to pornography where they live. The session also defines terms like hard-core and soft-core pornography (for historical purposes), amateur and mainstream porn, feminist porn, erotica, fetish, BDSM, kink, and obscenity. The idea that pornography is created first and foremost to be entertainment and to make money is emphasized.
Session 2: The history of sexually explicit images in society	Session 2 explores the history of sexually explicit images in society (much like Chapter 1 of this book). Participants consider whether notions of beauty are shaped by media and by sexually explicit media, specifically. Participants also learn about the history of obscenity and pornography in Europe and the United States and about the ways in which claims that art is obscene have been used to persecute politically dissenting and minority groups throughout history.
Session 3: Norms related to violence and double standards about sex	In Session 3, participants learn to recognize that sex acts depicted in some mainstream pornography can reinforce some traditional gender norms. A goal of the session is also to create empathy for porn performers, who work in challenging situations with bright lights awkward camera angles and positions, who must pay taxes, and who may face costly or burdensome STI testing requirements. Understanding that pornography performing is not a quick and easy way to make money is hypothesized to reduce the likelihood that youth will develop unrealistic expectations about a career in pornography. The approach is to have participants learn about performers without denigrating the performers or shaming those who may make that career choice as adults.
Session 4: The adolescent and brain and if pornography use can become compulsive	In Session 4, participants learn about the topic of sexual consent and how it is depicted in some pornography, as well as the likelihood that adolescent brains can be hyperstimulated by media overuse, and they discuss the possibility that pornography use can become compulsive. One activity in this session that is very popular invites participants to touch elbows, fingers, knees, and foreheads in order to learn about boundaries and consent.
Session 5: Healthy intimacy	In Session 5, participants learn about seven types of intimacy (e.g., mutual, affect, cognitive, physical, commitment, self-disclosure, and general closeness) and engage in activities designed to increase positive attitudes about respectful sexual and dating behavior.
Session 6: Healthy flirting, dating, and caring for other people	In Session 6, the learning objective is to increase positive attitudes toward respectful dating and sexual behavior, as well as to impart information about street harassment. Activities include discussion of flirting as it's presented in movies and shows and developing healthy pick-up lines.

Table 14.1. *Continued*

Session 7: Pornography isn't necessarily reality: The link to commercial sexual exploitation	In Session 7, participants receive information about commercial sexual exploitation. An objective is to decrease attitudes that commercial sex is glamorous or an easy way to become rich.
Session 8: So-called revenge pornography and disseminating sexually explicit selfies	In Session 8, participants learn about state laws related to underage sexting and revenge pornography. Norms about sexting and revenge pornography are explored. Understanding how and why some people feel pressured to engage in sexting is explored through activities.
Session 9: Peers and pornography	In Session 9 we increase the perception that others support healthy dating and sexual boundaries.

program is evidence-based. It is a promising program, however, given that pretest and posttest data from those who have participated suggest that many of our knowledge, attitude, and behavior-related objectives changed in the desired direction. For example, the percentage of youth who agree that "being in professional pornography is a good way to make a lot of money" decreased from 52% at baseline to 21% at posttest. At pretest, 26% of youth agreed that pornography is realistic, while 0% agreed at follow-up. Additional evaluation-related findings are available in two peer-reviewed publications.[25,27]

Parental and Other Reactions to the Porn Literacy Curriculum

We have often been asked how parents react to their child's being invited to participate in a pornography literacy class. When we were preparing to offer the class for the first time, our team wondered if some parents would worry that even mentioning pornography to youth would encourage them to seek it out. In fact, comparison of pre- and posttest data from our one-group evaluation study revealed that 81% of our students had seen Internet pornography prior to enrolling in the porn literacy class, and that the percentage who reported the same at posttest was the same.[27] It was comforting to have data that suggest that our class did not cause students who had never seen pornography before to seek it out, and this information might be reassuring for parents as well, although we never did have any parents express to us a fear that our class would encourage pornography use by their children. In fact, and to our surprise, parents have only ever been positive about the class. The typical reaction has been along the lines of: "Thank goodness! I am so glad you are teaching this class and talking to my child about pornography, because someone really should and I definitely don't want to do that."

Have Other Porn Literacy Programs Been Evaluated and Do They Work?

To my knowledge, there have not yet been any RCTs testing the effect of any porn literacy program on youth knowledge, attitudes, or behavior. The *We Prevent* online porn literacy intervention for sexual minority young men is currently being tested through an RCT and results should be available in 2021. It is our hope that the effects of *The Truth About Pornography* may also be tested through an RCT in the future.

The Future of Sex Ed and Porn Literacy

My guess is that pornography is not going to be eliminated and that its availability will not be dramatically reduced anytime soon. Pornography has existed and has been available even during, and sometimes most particularly during, repressive times (see Chapter 1). But the availability of pornography is not the only factor that could change in the near future. The content of pornography may change due to consumer pressures or due to other cultural trends related to what people consider beautiful, sexy, edgy, and so forth. The means of production of pornography have already changed considerably in the past 5 years, and the advent of OnlyFans.com and other websites that permit pornography performers to post their content online and receive payment directly from consumers cuts out the middle-man pornography producer entirely. The change in the business model may also influence what types of pornography are on offer, to whom, and how, and thus has the potential to change what youth see when they seek out sexually explicit material.

Going forward, pornography literacy will need to become, and to remain, extraordinarily nimble in order to stay relevant and useful. I worry about pornography literacy programs that lean heavily on an educational video that was created 2 or more years ago. The popularity of certain genres or subgenres of pornography can change rapidly, the power dynamics within the industry can shift, and laws and policies may influence what is produced, by whom, and how, and where it is used and by whom, too. Because the audience for pornography literacy is generally adolescents, and adolescents can be very sensitive to, and reject, educational programming that seems dated, my first recommendation about porn literacy programs is that they be created in a way that will allow almost continual updates so that they remain both accurate and relevant.

Increasingly, there are calls to incorporate porn literacy into sex ed curricula. For example, the second version of the US National Sex Education Standards, released in 2020, contains recommendations that 6th to 8th graders be educated about "the impact that media, including sexually explicit media, can have on one's body image and self-esteem," that 9th and 10th graders be educated about "the impact media, including sexually explicit media, can have on one's perceptions of, expectations for, a healthy relationship," that 11th and 12th graders be able to "describe the characteristics of unhealthy relationships that media, including sexually explicit media, may perpetuate (e.g., inequality between partners, lack of communication and consent, strict gender stereotypes)," and that 9th to 12th graders understand "the federal and state laws that prohibit the creation, sharing, and viewing of sexually explicit media by minors (e.g., sexting)."[28] None of these recommendations was included in the first version of the US National Sex Education Standards. The updates to the National Sex Education Standards are welcome, although they are in no way binding, because they are not issued by a federal or state government entity. At the very least, the best practices recommended in the standards would require sex educators and health teachers throughout the United States to be knowledgeable about pornography, to be ready to discuss it and to answer questions about it with adolescents, and to be prepared to explain to parents, school administrators, school board members, and others why they educate youth about pornography in whatever way they do. As such, the demand for evidence-based, reliable, easy-to-use, and easily defensible porn literacy curricula can be expected to increase.

Many questions remain about the best ways to provide porn literacy to youth, and what information should be transferred to them through porn literacy classes. Here is a sampling of questions representing what we do not yet know about porn literacy efficacy and effectiveness:

1. Is it more effective to have porn literacy classes delivered as part of a school curriculum, or should they be delivered outside of school through community-based agencies, faith-based groups, or other health educators?
2. Is porn literacy as effective delivered online via asynchronous learning as it is when delivered in person, as part of a usual class session at school?
3. Does it matter who delivers a porn literacy intervention?

    a. Do adolescents learn more from a peer than from an adult?

    b. If a peer is teaching, does it matter if the peer is perceived as a thought leader or sex-positive?

    c. If an adult is teaching, do race, sexual orientation, and gender-matching to student audience influence outcomes?

4. Which topics are essential to produce the desired outcomes?

5. What length of program is required to produce the desired outcomes?

6. What is the most effective way to train an educator to present porn literacy curricula to adolescents?

7. What kind of boosters or follow-up sessions are required over the course of adolescents' secondary school experiences to reinforce particular porn literacy lessons?

8. Do youth who participate in porn literacy interventions disseminate what they learned to friends, sexual partners, and others?

Uncovering the answer to any one of these questions would be useful to the field. I hope that there are sex educators, sexologists, public health students, and others who become interested in investigating them.

References

1. Entman, R. M. 1989. "How the Media Affect What People Think: An Information-Processing Approach." *The Journal of Politics* 51, no. 2: 347–370.
2. Lawson, S. 2019. "Evidence Mounts of Social Media's Negative Impacts for Democracy." *Forbes* https://www.forbes.com/sites/seanlawson/2019/11/07/evidence-mounts-of-social-medias-negative-impacts-for-democracy/#29da63fb14b8
3. Tsfati, Y., and J. Cohen. 2012. "Perceptions of Media and Media Effects." In *The International Encyclopedia of Media Studies*, edited by A. Valdivia. Wiley Online Library.
4. Potter, W. J. 2012. *Media Effects*. Thousand Oaks, CA: SAGE Publications.
5. Karl, H. 1974. "Guest Editorial: Media Literacy—The Right to Know." *The English Journal* 63, no. 7: 7–9.
6. Media Literacy Now. 2020. "What Is Media Literacy?" https://medialiteracynow.org/what-is-media-literacy/
7. Kelly, M. P., and M. Barker. 2016. "Why Is Changing Health-related Behaviour So Difficult?" *Public Health* 136: 109–116.
8. Bandura, A. 1994. "Social Cognitive Theory of Mass Communication." In *Media Effects: Advances in Theory and Research*, edited by J. Bryant and D. Zillman, 61–90. Hillsdale, NJ: Lawrence Erlbaum.
9. Bandura, A. 1973. *Aggression: A Social Learning Analysis*. Englewood Cliffs, NJ: Prentice Hall.
10. Potter, W. J. 2004. *Theory of Media Literacy: A Cognitive Approach*. Thousand Oaks, CA: SAGE Publications.
11. McCormick, E. M., and E. H. Telzer. 2017. "Adaptive Adolescent Flexibility: Neurodevelopment of Decision-making and Learning in a Risky Context." *Journal of Cognitive Neuroscience* 29, no. 3: 413–423.

12. Vahedi, Z., A. Sibalis, and J. E. Sutherland. 2018. "Are Media Literacy Interventions Effective at Changing Attitudes and Intentions Towards Risky Health Behaviors in Adolescents? A Meta-analytic Review." *Journal of Adolescence* 67: 140–152.

13. Austin, E. W., B. Austin, C. K. Kaiser, Z. Edwards, L. Parker, and T. G. Power. "A Media Literacy-Based Nutrition Program Fosters Parent-Child Food Marketing Discussions, Improves Home Food Environment, and Youth Consumption of Fruits and Vegetables." *Childhood Obesity* 16, no. S1: S33–S43.

14. Erba, J., Y. Chen, and H. Kang. 2019. "Using Media Literacy to Counter Stereotypical Images of Blacks and Latinos at a Predominantly White University." *Howard Journal of Communications* 30, no. 1: 1–22.

15. Lucidi, F., L. Mallia, F. Alivernini, et al. 2017. "The Effectiveness of a New School-Based Media Literacy Intervention on Adolescents' Doping Attitudes and Supplements Use." *Frontiers in Psychology* 8: 9.

16. Mingoia, J., A. D. Hutchinson, D. H. Gleaves, and C. Wilson. 2019. "The Impact of a Social Media Literacy Intervention on Positive Attitudes to Tanning: A Pilot Study." *Computers in Human Behavior* 90: 188–195.

17. Stanley, S. L., and C. A. Lawson. 2018. "Developing Discerning Consumers: An Intervention to Increase Skepticism Toward Advertisements in 4- to 5-Year-Olds in the US." *Journal of Children and Media* 12, no. 2: 211–225.

18. Maas, M. K. 2020. "PopPorn: Popular Culture & Pornography Education Program." http://www.meganmaas.com/teaching--training.html

19. Crabee, M. 2020. "It's Time We Talked." www.itstimewetalked.com

20. Nelson, K. M., N. S. Perry, and M. P. Carey. 2020. "The Young Men & Media Project: Developing a Community-Informed, Online HIV Prevention Intervention for 14–17-Year-Old Sexual Minority Males." The 41st Annual Meeting of the Society of Behavioral Medicine, San Francisco, CA.

21. Dawson, K., S. Nic Gabhainn, and P. MacNeela. 2020. "Toward a Model of Porn Literacy: Core Concepts, Rationales, and Approaches." *The Journal of Sex Research* 57, no. 1: 1–15.

22. Alder, J., N. Daley, and E. F. Rothman. 2017. "The Truth About Pornography: A Pornography-Literacy Curriculum for High School Students Designed to Reduce Sexual and Dating Violence." http://sites.bu.edu/rothmanlab/porn-literacy/

23. Rothman, E. F. 2018. "How Porn Changes the Way Teens Think About Sex." https://www.ted.com/talks/emily_f_rothman_how_porn_changes_the_way_teens_think_about_sex Accessed August 12, 2020.

24. Boston Public Health Commission. 2020. "What We Do." https://www.bphc.org/whatwedo/violence-prevention/start-strong/Pages/Resources.aspx

25. Rothman, E. F., A. Adhia, T. T. Christensen, J. Paruk, J. Alder, and N. Daley. 2018. "A Pornography Literacy Class for Youth: Results of a Feasibility and Efficacy Pilot Study." *American Journal of Sexuality Education* 13, no. 1: 1–17.

26. Ajzen, A. 1991. "The Theory of Planned Behavior." *Organizational Behavior and Human Decision Processes* 50: 179–211.

27. Rothman, E. F., N. Daley, and J. Alder. 2019. "A Pornography Literacy Program for Adolescents." *American Journal of Public Health* 110, no. 2: 154–156.

28. Future of Sex Education Initiative. 2020. "National Sex Education Standards, Core Content and Skills, K–12, Second Edition." https://advocatesforyouth.org/wp-content/uploads/2020/03/NSES-2020-web.pdf

Notes

Chapter 3

* In this book, I use the terms "pornography user," "pornography viewer," and "pornography consumer" interchangeably, although one could make the argument that the terms convey different things and that the differences are important. Someone who simply "views" pornography is passive, or their passivity is emphasized. Calling someone a pornography "user" conveys the idea that pornography is used to achieve some ends. We would not refer to a person as a "movie user" because they are a film buff, so the word "user" does attribute to pornography something beyond other forms of entertainment media. A pornography "consumer" is a person who is taking action, and the idea that they have engaged in a commercial transaction (i.e., paid for it) is implied. Each of these words may have different meanings, which I acknowledge, and I employ each of them in various contexts in this chapter.

Chapter 5

* Few embed consent statements throughout a scene, and those that do are not typically found on free, mainstream pornography viewership sites.

Chapter 12

* According to the International Entertainment Adult Union, the adult industry comprises any industry that requires that workers be 18 years old or older, so it also includes cocktail waitresses, bartenders, tattoo artists, boxers, bouncers, security guards, and webcam workers.
† There has been some discussion of creating a separate PASS system for HIV-positive performers whose viral load is so low that they are at exceedingly low risk of infecting other people through sexual contact.

Index

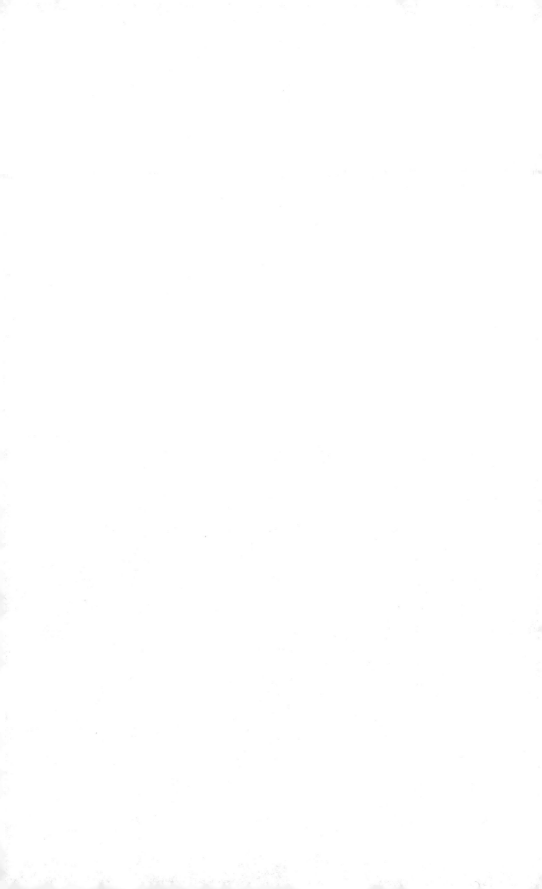